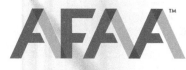

ATHLETICS AND FITNESS ASSOCIATION OF AMERICA

PRINCIPLES OF
GROUP FITNESS
INSTRUCTION

SECOND EDITION

MANAGING EDITOR: ERIN A. MCGILL

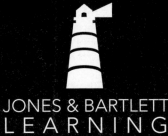

JONES & BARTLETT
LEARNING

World Headquarters
Jones & Bartlett Learning
5 Wall Street
Burlington, MA 01803
978-443-5000
info@jblearning.com
www.jblearning.com

National Academy of Sports Medicine
1750 East Northrop Boulevard
Suite 200
Chandler, AZ 85286
800-460-6276
www.nasm.org

Jones & Bartlett Learning books and products are available through most bookstores and online booksellers. To contact Jones & Bartlett Learning directly, call 800-832-0034, fax 978-443-8000, or visit our website, www.jblearning.com.

Substantial discounts on bulk quantities of Jones & Bartlett Learning publications are available to corporations, professional associations, and other qualified organizations. For details and specific discount information, contact the special sales department at Jones & Bartlett Learning via the above contact information or send an email to specialsales@jblearning.com.

Production Credits
Sr. Director of Product Development, NASM: Erin A. McGill
VP, Executive Publisher: David D. Cella
Publisher: Cathy L. Esperti
Acquisitions Editor: Sean Fabery
Director of Production: Jenny L. Corriveau
Director of Marketing: Andrea DeFronzo
VP, Manufacturing and Inventory Control: Therese Connell

Project Management and Composition: S4Carlisle Publishing Services
Vendor Manager: Molly Hogue
Cover Design: Cynthia Lupoff
Text Design: Jacqueline Werner
Front Cover Image: Getty Images; Back Cover Image: © Athletics and Fitness Association of America
Printing and Binding: LSC Communications
Cover Printing: LSC Communications

ISBN: 978-1-284-40280-3

Library of Congress Cataloging-in-Publication Data unavailable at time of printing

6048

Printed in the United States of America
24 23 22 21 20   10 9 8 7 6 5

Brief Contents

Table of Contents

Contributors

Managing Editors

Erin A. McGill, MA, NASM-CPT, CES, PES,
BCS, AFAA-GFI
Scottsdale, Arizona

Steve Myers, BS, NASM-CPT, CES, PES, FNS,
BCS, GPTS, ACE-GFI
Gilbert, Arizona

Instructional Designers

Jeri Dow, MS, Lead Instructional Designer
Gilbert, Arizona

Casey DeJong, MEd, MBA
Gilbert, Arizona

Contributing Authors

Lawrence Biscontini, MA, Mindful Movement
Specialist
Puerto Rico; Greece

Emily Booth, BM, AFAA-GFI, ACE-GFI, NASM-CPT
Lafayette, Colorado

Melanie Douglass, RD, NASM-CPT, AFAA-GFI,
ACE-GFI
Newton, Utah

Irene Lewis-McCormick, MS, CSCS
Des Moines, Iowa

Angie Miller, MS, LPC, NASM-CPT, AFAA-GFI
and PFT, ACE-GFI
St. Charles, Illinois

Kristen Sokel, BA, NASM-CPT, AFAA-GFI
Chino, California

Foreword

Congratulations on taking the first step on your path to become a Group Fitness Instructor! Fitness instruction is an exciting profession that has continued to evolve since the Athletics and Fitness Association of America (AFAA) published its first edition of *Fitness: Theory & Practice* in 1985 (originally entitled *Aerobics: Theory & Practice*). AFAA has long been recognized as one of the premiere organizations in the group fitness industry. Established in 1983, AFAA released the first nationally standardized guidelines for fitness professionals, guiding instructors to provide new levels of exercise leadership to participants. Today, AFAA has grown into a widely respected international presence in over 73 countries, with licensed, fully operational organizations from China and Japan to Brazil and Turkey. The dream of founder Linda D. Pfeffer, RN and a handful of instructors in 1983 has blossomed into the world's largest fitness educator today through the hard work, selfless contributions, and unbridled enthusiasm of thousands of AFAA Specialists and Presenters.

With over 350,000 worldwide, we are a global leader in movement-based health and fitness. Your decision to start this journey will likely change your life—and the lives of others—in many meaningful ways.

With this new program, we bring to you a culmination of our own history, as well as the experience and knowledge of leading professionals who are shaping the future of the fitness industry.

This text presents recognized leaders and authors in fields that influence fitness instruction: exercise physiology; anatomy; biomechanics; sports medicine; nutrition; weight management; sports psychology; exercise adherence; business management; and instructional technique. Their professional knowledge and hard-earned practical wisdom is passed onto you with the intention that you will use them to develop your own rewarding fitness career or perhaps simply to pursue your personal fitness dreams.

This text works to provide you not only the foundational knowledge you'll need in your early days as a Group Fitness Instructor, but also the context and scientific rationale behind each of the lessons you will be learning. AFAA's mentorship-inspired, learner-centric text shapes a relatable and practical reading experience to help you get what you need to thrive in your new career. Welcome to the AFAA family!

Sincerely,
Erin A. McGill, MA, NASM-CPT, CES, PES, BCS, AFAA-GFI
Senior Director, Product Development

Acknowledgements

Fabio Comana, MA, MS, NASM-CPT, CES, PES, ACE-CPT, HC, NSCA-CSCS, ACSM-EP-C, CISSN
San Diego, California

Marty Miller, DHSc, ATC, NASM-CPT, CES, PES, MMACS
Palm Beach Gardens, Florida

Kyle Stull, DHSc, MS, LMT, NASM-CPT
Austin, Texas

Talent

Isabelle Alexander, Amy Conrad, Luis Guzman, Kayla Hamm, Baylee Hayenga, Autumn Hunt, Jacob McLendon, Madison Murray, Ulyssa Preciado, Annie Souter, Jeffrey Strahan, Eric Thomson, Jo Dee Walker, and Jayme Zylstra.

Gratitude

Additional thanks go to Rebecca Collier, Kristen Radaich, Ian Montel, Marie Roberts, Andrew Payne, Matt Miller, and Shalie Galvin for all the hard work provided in seeing this project to completion.

New Content

Course Overview

AFAA's Group Fitness Instructor certification is built on the foundation of AFAA's reputation of more than 30 years as a leader and innovator of group based fitness. Taking the theory from the exercise library to bring it where it is needed most—the fitness center, the home gym, the street—this new text takes the group fitness industry's successes of the past and realigns them with modern scientific research to effectively help a new instructor navigate a career in fitness.

Not only will AFAA's new course provide for all of the necessary entry-level skills to become an in-demand instructor, it will inform you about format-specific classes and help you navigate various career paths within the fitness industry. The course provides real-life application to specific exercise formats, examples of cueing, communication, and instruction, and comprehensive exercise technique videos.

As you progress through your Group Fitness Instructor program, you will work toward achieving competency in the following areas:

- Demonstrate comprehension of fundamental scientific concepts related to exercise science.
- Design a well-structured and balanced fitness class or workout for a diverse group of participants that is both safe and effective.
- Demonstrate comprehension of key instruction and presentation skills necessary for effective group instruction.
- Demonstrate key traits of professionalism as a Group Fitness Instructor.
- Demonstrate the key skills and knowledge required to be a competent Group Fitness Instructor.

Pedagogical Features

This text employs strategic learning features that not only make the content more digestible but also turn theory into practice. The chapter progression weaves evidence-based research, science, and application throughout the entire text, in order to enhance learning and contextual understanding. The new features are as follows:

- **Caution**—Distinct things instructors should be aware of as they relate to scope of practice and potential pitfalls.
- **Check it Out**—Quick tips and/or facts that have an apparent application and real-world usability. This feature enables the reader a quick insight and application to the concepts read.

- ▾ **Instructor Tips**—Inside-the-industry application tips from experts with years of experience.

- ▾ **Memory Tips**—Tips and tricks for instructors to easily remember complex terms without the extended effort of rote memorization.

- ▾ **Practice This**—On-the-spot activities to help instructors practice and apply the content.

Chapter 1
The Group Fitness Industry

 Learning Objectives

1.1.   **Describe** the history and evolution of fitness.

1.2.   **List** the general benefits of fitness.

1.3.   **Define** the role of Group Fitness Instructor.

1.4.   **Differentiate** between the various methods of group fitness.

1.5.   **Identify** common group fitness formats.

History and Evolution of the Fitness Industry

Fitness has been evolving since the 1950s. It started with male-dominated health clubs and eventually incorporated the first forms of group fitness—coined *aerobics*.

Group fitness became popular in the late 1960s and early 1970s, when dance instructors began combining movement with easy-to-follow, aerobics-based group dance classes. These early fitness instructors organized some of the first group fitness classes and brought intentional exercise to the public. When other forms of group exercise (e.g., aquatic exercise, indoor cycling, Pilates) emerged in the 1990s, many of the new classes did not require any need for dance skills. As a result, the term *group fitness* (or group exercise) replaced the term *aerobic dance*.[1]

Physical activity is recommended for everyone as a part of a healthy lifestyle. However, the United States continues to see rising occurrences of obesity, diabetes, and other chronic diseases. This negative trend has taken its toll on families, the economy, and the healthcare system. As a result, today's fitness industry targets people of all ages, genders, and skill levels through numerous outlets such as fitness facilities, community centers, schools, businesses, universities, and medical centers.

The History of AFAA

In 1983, the Athletics (formerly Aerobics) and Fitness Association of America (AFAA) set out to address the needs of an enthusiastic, emergent profession of fitness instructors. Although new, they were revolutionary for group fitness and started using a growing body of research. AFAA gathered the best among exercise physiologists, cardiologists, physical educators, sports medicine experts, physical therapists, and fitness professionals to compile the first-ever exercise standards and guidelines for Group Fitness Instructors.

On the heels of developing AFAA's Basic Exercise Standards and Guidelines, AFAA published its first textbook in 1985. This gave instructors the information needed to deliver safe and effective classes for both participants and themselves. AFAA offered a definition of fitness that focused on cardiorespiratory endurance, muscular strength, and flexibility. That definition has significantly broadened since those first offerings, keeping pace with research in healthy aging, multicultural interests, and the exponential growth and popularity of the fitness movement worldwide. Today, being fit means having both an active and healthy body, as well as a positive mind and spirit. In addition to the traditional trio (endurance, strength, and flexibility), modern fitness training also encompasses agility, power, speed, balance, and mind-body wholeness.

Throughout its history, AFAA has remained a leader in fitness, issuing over 350,000 certifications in 73 countries around the world. As the industry continues to grow and demand more knowledge and professionalism from practitioners, AFAA continues to elevate its educational standards.

AFAA 5 Questions™

Individuals in a fitness class usually have diverse characteristics and goals. Therefore, more conservative guidelines are recommended. All movement can fall within safe guidelines as long as movements are evaluated from two viewpoints: effectiveness (benefit) and potential injury

---

Obesity

The condition of being considerably overweight; a person with a BMI of 30 or greater or who is at least 30 pounds over the recommended weight for their height.

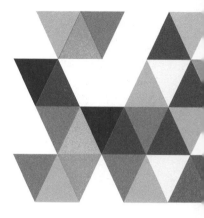

quotient (risk). With this perspective in mind, AFAA presents the historical, and ever-relevant, AFAA 5 Questions™:

1. What is the purpose of this exercise?

    Consider: muscular strength or endurance, cardiorespiratory conditioning, flexibility, skill development, or stress reduction

2. Are you doing the exercise effectively?

    Consider: proper range of motion, speed, body position against gravity, efficient posture, and safe equipment use

3. Does the exercise create any safety concerns?

    Consider: potential stress areas, environmental concerns, or movement control

4. Can you maintain proper alignment and form for the duration of the exercise?

    Consider: form, dynamic posture, stabilization, or balance

5. For whom is the exercise appropriate or inappropriate?

    Consider: risk-to-benefit ratio; whether the participant is a beginner, intermediate, or advanced exerciser; and any limitations noted by the participant

When evaluating the purpose of an exercise, the Group Fitness Instructor should consider the main adaptation of the exercise. Is the exercise for flexibility, movement prep, cardio, endurance, strength, power, etc.? Once the purpose of an exercise is identified, it will dictate how the exercise will be performed and when it will be used within the class.

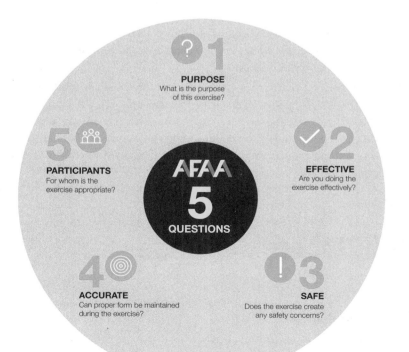

Figure 1.1
AFAA 5 Questions™

Questions #2 and #4 have to do with effective execution of an exercise. Are participants able to perform the exercise with proper range of motion and at the desired speed, all while maintaining correct form? These questions will help the instructor identify if an exercise is appropriate for the participant or if a modification of the exercise would be a better fit. Knowing human movement and how it should look in all forms of exercise is critical in answering these questions.

Recall the two larger objectives of the AFAA 5 Questions™ are *effectiveness* and *assessing risk*. Questions 1, 2, and 4 of the AFAA 5 Questions™ deal with the effectiveness of an exercise, while Questions 3 and 5 are focused on participant safety. Despite how effective an exercise appears to be or how well it fits into a class, if the exercise creates safety concerns for a participant, it is no longer appropriate.

The AFAA 5 Questions™ (Figure 1.1) provide a framework for evaluating a class, allowing the Group Fitness Instructor to examine the appropriateness, effectiveness, and safety of the class objectives and the individual exercises that make up the class.

Changes in Group Fitness

As group fitness has continued to expand, the method of teaching has evolved with it. Key evolutions that enable group fitness to be accessible to anyone who wants to pursue increased physical activity are:

- ▼ **Participant-centered focus:** Design of workouts with the intent of helping participants reach any goal they have; the focus involves encouragement combined with teaching the participants independence.[1]

- ▼ **Emphasis on functional movement:** Use of the growing knowledge of the human body and what is required to improve the communication between nervous and musculoskeletal systems to develop efficient and pain-free movements.

- ▼ **Specific formats:** Incorporation of a variety of formats, including kickboxing, indoor cycling, yoga, dance, resistance training, and boot camp, which provides more ability to explore opportunities long-term.

- ▼ **Movement preparation:** A concept of a comprehensive movement preparation segment that is replacing the traditional warm-up. Instead of generically warming up the body, movement prep takes into account the movements and required range of motion to be included in the main body workout. It also considers common movement impairments and utilizes concepts of corrective flexibility to reduce the risk of injury.

Health Benefits of Fitness

Physical activity can promote myriad of positive benefits, including improved quality of life. Specifically, these benefits include:

- ▼ increased bone density.

- ▼ improved cardiorespiratory efficiency.

- ▼ increased metabolic efficiency (metabolism).

▼ enhanced beneficial endocrine (hormone) and serum lipid (cholesterol) adaptations.

▼ decreased body fat.

▼ increased lean body mass (muscle).

▼ increased tissue tensile strength (tendons, ligaments, muscles).

▼ reduced risk for some chronic diseases.

▼ elevated mood.

▼ improved concentration and cognitive function.

▼ increased energy.

▼ reduced joint pain.

▼ improved sleep habits.

▼ improved self-esteem.

Fitness Concepts

Fitness programs should address all components of health-related physical fitness using scientifically recognized training principles. The strength and stability of a person's musculoskeletal system is directly related to the potential risk of injury, and individuals who are deconditioned are at greater risk of injury.[2] It is important to note that deconditioned is not strictly about weight or cardiorespiratory capacity, but also involves muscle imbalances, decreased flexibility, and a lack of core and joint stability. All of these conditions can inhibit the ability of the human body to produce proper movement and can eventually lead to injury.

Musculoskeletal system

Combined, interworking system of all muscles and bones in the body.

Deconditioned

A state of lost physical fitness, which may include reduced cardiorespiratory capacity, muscle imbalances, decreased flexibility, and a lack of core and joint stability.

Muscle imbalance

Alteration of muscle length surrounding a joint.

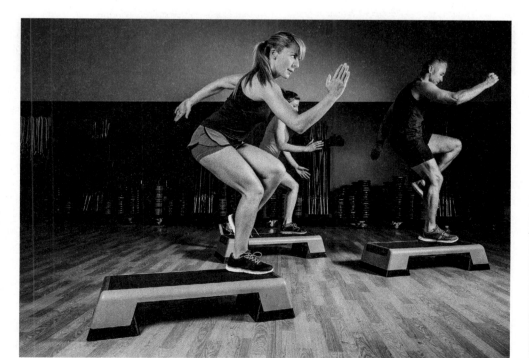

Position Overview

Working as a Group Fitness Instructor requires the ability to create, teach, assess, correct, and modify movement patterns for multiple participants at one time. It is a dynamic position that relies on the ability to coordinate various components, such as movement, speech, music, equipment, temperature, and customer service. It is important to realize that instructors learn and master their teaching skills with time and practice.

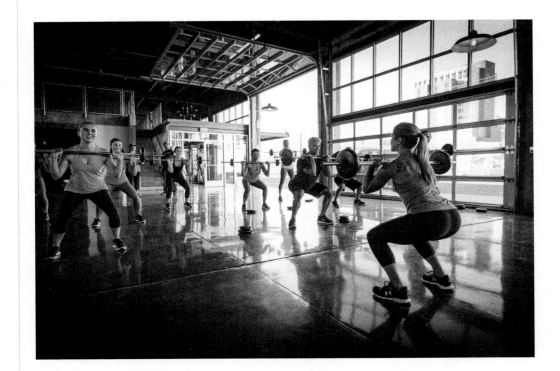

As participation in group fitness increases, more instructors are training to become career instructors. Career instructors may learn and teach multiple class formats. Career instructors may teach anywhere from 5–15 classes per week, often across different formats in order to maintain the energy needed to get through multiple classes each day. Some instructors teach on the side as a hobby instructor. These types of instructors may have a full-time job or family obligations, and typically teach classes 1–5 times per week early in the morning, at night, or on the weekends.

Scope of Practice and Professional Limitations

Health professionals in all settings—from hospitals to rehabilitation centers, to clinics and fitness facilities—focus on one area of practice and work within set guidelines and expectations standardized and legally defined by national and state agencies.

Career Instructor

Instructor who invests the majority of his or her day teaching, researching, and promoting fitness activities.

Hobby Instructor

Instructor who balances teaching with other full-time commitments.

In the group fitness setting, scope of practice refers to what an instructor can legally and ethically do in their professional practice. It includes the knowledge, skills, abilities, processes, and limitations for which an instructor should be held accountable. It helps instructors know where their responsibilities begin and end. For this reason, AFAA has defined the tasks and responsibilities that make up an instructor's scope of practice.

Group Fitness Instructors:

- ▼ Prepare and deliver science-based exercise content for groups of individuals with varying fitness needs and capabilities.

- ▼ Dynamically react to group or individual needs by providing modifications for fitness level, progressions for advancement, and regressions for special populations.

- ▼ Provide adequate energy, enthusiasm, and optimism to create positive associations with exercise.

- ▼ Understand how to use various types of equipment in the group fitness setting, such as hand weights, weighted bars, resistance tubing, stretch bands, stability balls, and other equipment.

- ▼ Work independently and with limited individual interaction.

- ▼ Maintain CPR/AED certification to properly respond to emergencies that may occur before, during, or after class.

- ▼ Answer questions related to the workout, such as: how to do specific moves, why they are beneficial, or how one might modify or progress movements.

- ▼ Avoid one-on-one recommendations regarding health conditions, injuries, nutrition, and remedies for pain. However, pre-class assessments of participants (including observational, postural, and movement assessments) are appropriate for recommending modifications to class movements.

- ▼ Refer personal health questions to appropriate health professionals.

The standard is simple: *all questions outside of the Group Fitness Instructor's scope of practice should be referred to qualified professionals with appropriate training.*

Scope of Practice

Knowledge, skills, abilities, processes, and limitations for which an instructor should be held accountable.

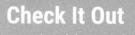

✓ Check It Out

An *instructor* doesn't know each participant's health history or goals. He or she simply knows a participant attends a certain class in order to experience the stated objective of the class (as indicated by class title, description, and content).

A *personal trainer* is trained and qualified to work with individuals or small groups. Personal trainers collect personal health information, understand client goals, and develop personalized programs in order to help individuals achieve their health and wellness objectives.

An instructor who is asked to provide individualized exercise programs in order to achieve specific goals should refer those individuals to a personal trainer.

Diagnosing and Prescribing

Diagnosing involves a comprehensive review and understanding of an individual's health history, current medical conditions, current symptoms, and then—after a complete review—determining a specific condition or disease. *Prescribing* involves providing specific treatment plans in the form of exercise, dietary counseling, nutritional supplementation, meal planning, home remedies, therapeutic aides, or prescription drugs, in order to treat a certain condition or disease.

Group Fitness Instructors should politely refer participants to other appropriate licensed professionals for questions such as (but not limited to):

▼ "I'm experiencing knee pain. Can you tell me what it is?"

▼ "I have high blood pressure and high cholesterol—what's the best workout program for me?"

On the other hand, Group Fitness Instructors should be ready and willing to answer questions about the workout or class being taught. The following types of questions are within the scope of practice of a Group Fitness Instructor:

▼ How to perform movement patterns: "Hey, can you show me again how to do that squat exercise?"

▼ How to modify movement patterns: "Squats hurt my knees. How can I modify them?"

Referring Participants

When participants ask questions or make requests that fall outside the scope of practice for a Group Fitness Instructor, it is important to direct participants to other professionals or organizations that may be able to help. For example:

▼ If participants are asking questions about a personalized training program, they should be referred to a Certified Personal Trainer.

▼ If participants are asking health- or disease-related questions, they should be referred to their medical doctor for clearance and specific recommendations.

▼ If participants are asking questions about pain during movement, they can be referred to a physical therapist or medical doctor.

▼ If participants are asking about other training modalities for which the current instructor is not qualified, they should be referred to certified or trained instructors in that modality, such as kettlebells or yoga.

Group Fitness Methods

Several methods of group fitness can be seen across all kinds of fitness facilities. The method of group fitness found in a certain club typically depends on the interests of the members and the financial and marketing goals of the facility. Most facilities offer a combination of three common group fitness methods:

- ▼ Pre-choreographed
- ▼ Pre-designed
- ▼ Freestyle

These types of group fitness range from providing every detail of how to teach a certain class to providing no detail, allowing absolute creative freedom to the instructor. An understanding of these common types of approaches gives instructors the opportunity to explore various teaching methods and adapt them to the instructor's strengths.

Pre-choreographed

In the fitness industry, *choreography* does not always translate to *dance*. Rather, choreography is used to describe *planned movement patterns*. The main feature of pre-choreographed content is every major component of the class was created by a single person, business, or organization with a connecting theme, brand, and experience in mind (**Table 1.1**).

The instructor is tasked with memorizing and mastering the intended class experience, and presenting that same experience consistently for a set period of time. For this reason, and to ensure brand consistency regardless of who is presenting the class, many pre-choreographed formats now include their own certification processes, often with multiple levels of competency that can be achieved.

Pre-designed

Between the highly detailed pre-choreographed approach and unconstrained freedom of the freestyle approach is the pre-designed approach. Pre-designed content provides a class template that sets overall class direction and standards while allowing instructors to manipulate other

Table 1.1

Benefits of Pre-choreographed Class Method	
For Instructors	**For Participants**
• Gives novice or shy instructors an instant sense of community and confidence • Allows the instructor to focus on the teaching part of the job, leaving the demand for creativity to other sources • Gives those with strong memorization skills the capacity to shine • Has a predictable and consistent timeline for new content delivery • Emphasizes learning from the script or teaching tips provided by the creator, often helping an instructor use new and effective cueing techniques • Demonstrates instant brand recognition and credibility • Provides access to support systems and marketing resources	• Provides a consistent class experience • Allows for practice and mastery of a set routine over a set period of time • Gives advance notice of new choreography • Provides a connected, well-thought-out experience

variables within those standards (**Table 1.2**). Pre-designed classes may have specific standards for one, a few, or *all* of the following class variables:

- Specific exercises
- Order of exercises
- Duration of class components (e.g., warm-up, cardio, strength, cool-down)
- Type of music, specific songs, or playlists
- Length of intervals or sequences
- Modality

Table 1.2

Benefits of Pre-designed Class Method

For Instructors	For Participants
• Provides clear direction and objectives for each class • Requires less time for the pre-class planning stage • Gives ability to experiment with individual variables for career exploration and growth • Gives ability to combine consistency and variety • Provides instant brand recognition and credibility • Marketing tools and resources	• Provides consistency in overall class flow and objectives • Allows for variety in one or more class components to keep things interesting • Provides a branded experience with room to grow • Provides the ability to see, feel, or visualize long-term progress

Table 1.3

Benefits of Freestyle Class Method

For Instructors	For Participants
• Allows instructor to decide every single detail of a class: moves, music, cues, equipment, lighting, etc. • Matches movements to the participants • Slows down or speeds up class flow, movements, cues, or music based on the needs of the class • Changes the workout on the spot if something isn't resonating with participants • Provides an outlet for creative energy • Allows flexibility before, during, or after class • Creates a unique fitness brand, personality, and community • Provides opportunities to learn and try new things	• Provides endless variety that supports both mental and physical growth • Provides cross-training and functional fitness development from a variety of movements • Allows for a tailor-made group fitness experience each and every time • Encourages attending classes that are unique and different • Facilitates feelings of continuous challenge and desire to try and do new things

Freestyle

Freestyle choreography is a method of designing, developing, and delivering movement to participants based on the instructor's personal preferences, skill set, and knowledge of exercise selection. Some freestyle instructors plan out their content the night before, some create a class in their head while commuting to the gym, and some instructors do not plan at all (**Table 1.3**).

Freestyle format options can focus on any type, or combination, of cardiorespiratory, strength, endurance, bodyweight, aquatic, cycling, mind-body, or dance modalities.

Group Fitness Formats

In group fitness, *format* refers to the base organizational structure that connects the components of a class with a particular outcome. A format may differentiate itself by moves, music, teaching style, class size, modality, equipment, and even wardrobe. Six basic formats are prevalent in

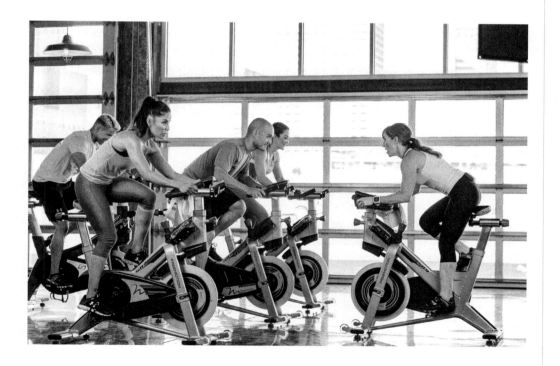

the group fitness arena today, utilizing foundational exercise-science principles and training guidelines for cardiorespiratory, strength, and flexibility improvement:

- ▼ **Strength and Resistance**: Offers participants the opportunity to increase muscular strength and endurance using an opposing force for resistance.

- ▼ **HIIT and Interval**: Involves alternating work periods of higher intensities with recovery periods performed at moderate to low intensities. HIIT workouts are typically shorter in duration, but extremely challenging.

Freestyle choreography

Method of choreography based on the instructor's personal preference, skill set, and knowledge.

Modality

Form or mode of exercise that presents a specific stress to the body.

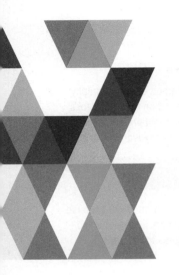

- ▼ **Boot Camp**: Includes a combination of resistance and cardio elements, with a goal of providing a total body workout, with a military-style presentation.
- ▼ **Mind-body**: Includes practices such as yoga, Pilates, T'ai Chi, and more. These formats feature slow, controlled movements that combine strength, stability, flexibility, balance, and breathing techniques. For the purpose of this certification program, and due to its popularity, yoga will be the primary focus when discussing mind-body group fitness formats.
- ▼ **Cycling**: Participants ride stationary bicycles designed to simulate an outdoor cycling experience.
- ▼ **Specialty formats**: Because some formats require additional certification or training, these will be covered only in brief:
    a. *Dance-oriented*: Designed to make cardiorespiratory training more interesting and fun. They rely on exhilarating, energizing moves specifically choreographed to match popular or thematic music.
    b. *Aquatics*: Consists of cardio, strength, and stability movements taught in shallow or deep pools and offer benefits for populations ranging from the overweight and deconditioned to elite athletes.
    c. *Active, aging Adults*: Focus on functional basic movements often through the use of chairs, step decks, water, and lighter resistance.
    d. *Discipline specific*: Relates to a unique form of discipline, such as martial arts or cardio tennis.
    e. *Equipment driven*: Maintains focus on one type of modality, such as suspension training systems or kettlebells.
    f. *Hybrid*: A combination of two or more types of formats to accomplish more than one outcome, such as yogalates.

An instructor is advised to learn and develop skills in one of the eight central formats before specializing further. Specialty formats are created and managed by businesses, education providers, corporate club chains, private studios, and even individual instructors. Common examples of specialty programs include martial arts, cardio kickboxing, barre, Pilates, yoga, athletic performance, injury prevention, and many more that may require experience with specific equipment (e.g., treadmill, rower, balance plate).

Summary

Group Fitness Instructors are active proponents of preventative health care by providing an accessible way to take action against obesity, diabetes, and other chronic health conditions. As a result, Group Fitness Instructors must be qualified with the knowledge and skills to lead participants safely through an effective and challenging workout. Knowledge of the human body, exercise science, communication, and how to connect with participants are just a few of the essential skills required. With these tools and authentic enthusiasm, Group Fitness Instructors can play an important role in helping people achieve a healthier lifestyle.

Chapter in Review

- ▼ History and evolution of group fitness:
  - ▪ 1950s: male-dominated health clubs
  - ▪ 1960s and 1970s: aerobics-based dance classes emerge
  - ▪ 1990s: other forms of group exercise gain popularity; *aerobics* replaced by *group fitness (or group exercise)*
  - ▪ The AFAA 5 Questions™: purpose, effectiveness, safety, alignment and form, appropriateness
  - ▪ Other changes: participant-centered focus, functional movement, specialty formats, movement preparation
- ▼ General benefits of fitness
  - ▪ Increased bone density
  - ▪ Improved body composition
  - ▪ Reduced risk of disease
  - ▪ Reduced pain
  - ▪ Improved cognitive function and mood
- ▼ Scope of Practice
  - ▪ Avoid diagnosing and prescribing
  - ▪ Refer participants to qualified professionals
- ▼ Methods of instruction
  - ▪ Pre-choreographed: components created by third party
  - ▪ Pre-designed: general template provides direction on some class components
  - ▪ Freestyle: components based on instructor preference, skill, & knowledge
- ▼ Formats
  - ▪ Strength and resistance
  - ▪ HIIT and Interval
  - ▪ Boot camp
  - ▪ Yoga
  - ▪ Cycle

References

1. Kennedy CA, Yoke MM. *Methods of Group Exercise Instruction*. Champaign, IL: Human Kinetics Publishers, Inc.; 2005.
2. Barr K, Griggs M, Cadby T. Lumbar stabilization: Core concepts and current literature, Part 1. *Am J Phys Med Rehab*. 2005;84(6):473–480.

Chapter 2
Foundations of Exercise Science

 Learning Objectives

2.1. **Define** biomechanics and its role in the development of a group fitness session.

2.2. **Explain** basic biomechanical principles.

2.3. **Describe** the function of the muscle action spectrum.

2.4. **Identify** joint actions in each of the planes of motions.

The Role of Biomechanics

Group Fitness Instructors must understand biomechanics in the Human Movement System, also known as the kinetic chain. Principles that relate to human movement, such as planes of motion, joint actions, and muscular functions, are critical to designing and delivering effective workouts.

Basics of Biomechanics

Kinesiology and biomechanics are disciplines of the analysis of human movement. Anatomic locations, planes of motion, and joint motions are all key components for learning how the body moves.

Anatomic Locations

Terminology to describe human movement requires the use of a consistent body position, called the anatomic position. Here, the body stands upright with the arms beside the trunk and the palms and head facing forward. The following terms, meanings, and examples of their usage, are highlighted in Figure 2.1.

Anterior: toward or on the front side of the body

Posterior: toward or on the back side of the body

Kinetic chain

The interrelation of the actions of the nervous, muscular, and skeletal systems to create movement.

Kinesiology

Study of human movement.

Biomechanics

Study of how forces affect a living body.

Anatomic position

Standard reference posture where the body stands upright with the arms beside the trunk, and the palms and head both face forward.

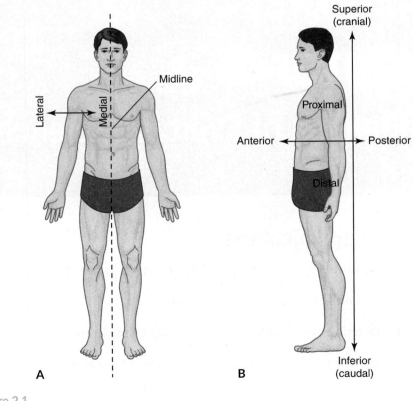

Figure 2.1

(A & B) Anatomic Locations.

Superior: above a landmark or closer to the head
Inferior: toward the bottom part of the body or closer to the feet
Proximal: closer to the center of the body
Distal: farther from the center of the body or a landmark
Medial: toward the midline of the body
Lateral: farther from the midline of the body
Contralateral: on the opposite side of the body
Ipsilateral: on the same side of the body

Planes of Motion

Human movement occurs in three *planes of motion*. They are termed the *sagittal, frontal,* and *transverse* planes, and reflect three basic movement patterns respectively: forward and backward, lateral (i.e., side-to-side), and rotation. Movement of the body is described as running parallel to these planes (Figure 2.2).

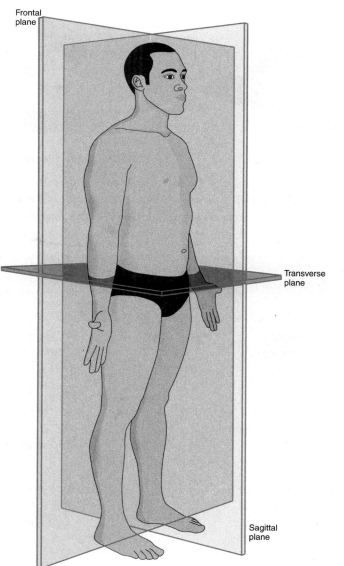

Frontal plane

Transverse plane

Sagittal plane

Midline

Imaginary vertical line that splits the body into equal halves.

Figure 2.2
Planes of Motion

The sagittal plane divides the body into a right half and a left half. Sagittal plane movements move forward and backward, such as walking, cycling, and squatting. In the sagittal plane, one can imagine walls parallel to the left and right side of a person; the only movement that can occur between these imaginary walls is forward and backward.

The frontal plane divides the body into a front half and a back half. In the frontal plane, movements occur from side to side, such as with jumping jacks and side lunges. Here, imaginary parallel walls are in front of the body and behind the body; if a person is restricted by walls in front and behind, movement is limited to side-to-side motions.

The transverse plane divides the body into a top half and a bottom half. Exercises in the transverse plane involve movements parallel to this imaginary line, mostly rotational motions. Lunges with rotation and roundhouse kicks are examples of transverse plane movements.

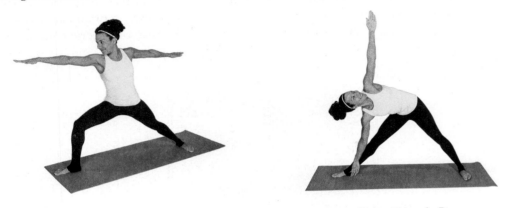

Frontal Plane: Warrior II Pose   Transverse Plane: Triangle Pose

Common exercises primarily occur in one plane of motion; however, the Human Movement System should be conditioned in all three planes of motion to maximize fitness levels and reduce risk of injury. See **Table 2.1** for common exercises and their associated planes of motion and joint actions.

Table 2.1

Sagittal plane

Imaginary plane that divides the body into equal right and left halves.

Frontal plane

Imaginary plane that divides the body into equal front and back halves.

Transverse plane

An imaginary horizontal plane that bisects the body into equal halves, producing a top half and a bottom half.

Planes of Motion and Joint Actions

Plane	Examples of Joint Movements	Examples of Exercises
Sagittal	Flexion Extension	Biceps curl Squat Running
Frontal	Abduction Adduction Lateral flexion Eversion Inversion	Lateral arm raise Side step Side lunge Side shuffle
Transverse	Pronation Supination Internal rotation External rotation Horizontal adduction Horizontal abduction	Trunk rotation Bicycle crunches Lunge with rotation

Joint Movements

The names of joint movements are best learned in terms of the planes of motion.[1]

Sagittal Plane Motions

Joint actions in the sagittal plane (i.e., front to back) include flexion, extension, dorsiflexion, and plantar flexion. Flexion is the bending at a joint where the relative angle between two bones decreases.[1] In the sagittal plane, flexion can occur in both the anterior and posterior directions. Figures 2.3–2.7 include motions occurring in the sagittal plane at the ankle, hip, trunk, arm, and neck (cervical spine).

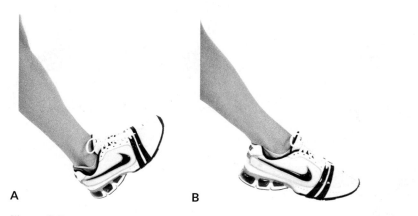

Figure 2.3
(A) Ankle Dorsiflexion. (B) Plantar Flexion.

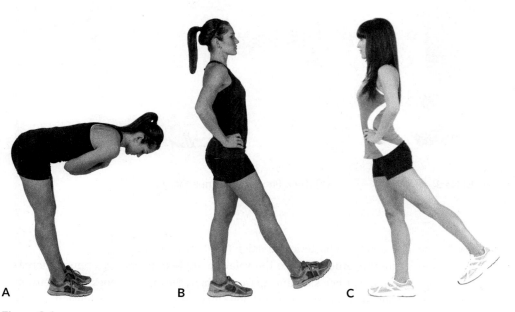

Figure 2.4
Hip Flexion: (A) Femoral-On-Pelvic Rotation. (B) Pelvic-On-Femoral Rotation. (C) Hip Extension.

Flexion

Bending at a joint where the relative angle between two bones decreases.

Extension

Movement at a joint in which the relative angle between two adjoining segments increases.

Dorsiflexion

Anterior flexion of the ankle, where the top of the foot moves up and away from the ground.

Plantar flexion

Posterior extension at the ankle where the top of the foot moves down toward the ground; pointing toes.

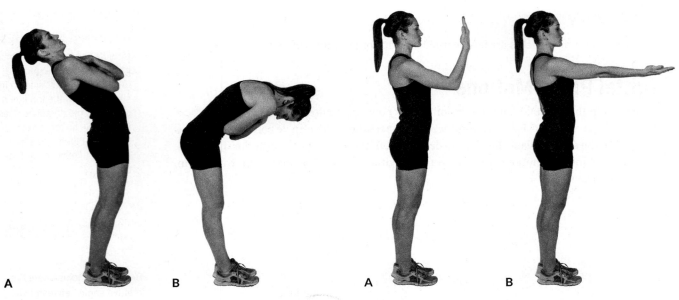

Figure 2.5
(A) Trunk (Spinal) Extension. (B) Trunk (Spinal) Flexion.

Figure 2.6
(A) Elbow Flexion. (B) Elbow Extension.

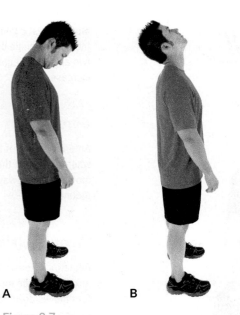

Figure 2.7
(A) Neck (Cervical) Flexion. (B) Neck (Cervical) Extension.

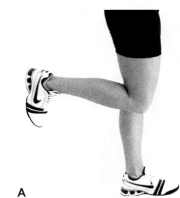
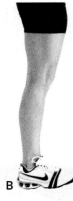

Figure 2.8
(A) Knee Flexion. (B) Knee Extension.

Flexion can also occur in a posterior direction (Figure 2.8A).

Extension is the movement where the relative angle between two bones increases (Figure 2.8B). For example, when standing up from a chair, the hip joint goes into extension as the angle formed by the torso and the upper leg bone increases. In a triceps extension, the lower arm is moving away from the upper arm.

Frontal Plane Motions

Joint actions in the frontal plane (side to side) include abduction and adduction, lateral flexion at the spine, and eversion and inversion of the foot. Abduction means a body segment is moving away from the midline of the body. For example, raising an arm or a leg to the side is abduction of that body part. Conversely, adduction means a body segment is moving toward the midline of the body. Figures 2.9 and 2.10 demonstrate these movements.

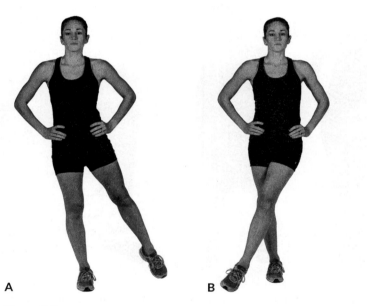

A　　　　　　　　　　B

Figure 2.9
(A) Hip Abduction. (B) Hip Adduction.

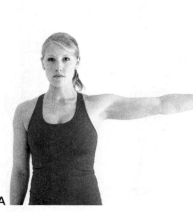
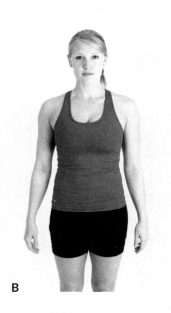

A　　　　　　　　　　B

Figure 2.10
(A) Shoulder Abduction. (B) Shoulder Adduction.

Abduction

Body segment is moving away from the midline of the body.

Adduction

Body segment is moving toward the midline of the body.

Eversion

Bottom of the foot rotates outward (laterally).

Inversion

Bottom of the foot rotates inwards (medially).

Scapular retraction

Movement of the shoulder blades closer to the spine.

Scapular protraction

Movement of the shoulder blade forward and away from the spine.

Internal rotation

Turning of a limb or body segment toward the midline of the body.

Lateral flexion of the spine is also in the frontal plane (Figures 2.11 and 2.12). Lastly, eversion and inversion are related to movements of the foot and ankle complex (Figure 2.13). With eversion, the top of the foot rolls inward, causing the bottom to flatten. During inversion, the foot turns so the top of the foot rolls outward, creating a more visible arch.[2]

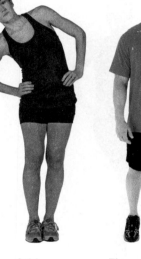

Figure 2.11
Lateral Flexion of the Spine

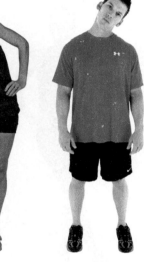

Figure 2.12
Lateral Flexion of the Neck (Cervical Spine)

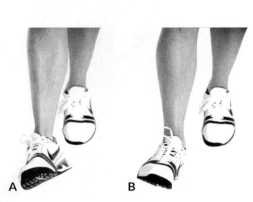

Figure 2.13
(A) Ankle Inversion. (B) Ankle Eversion.

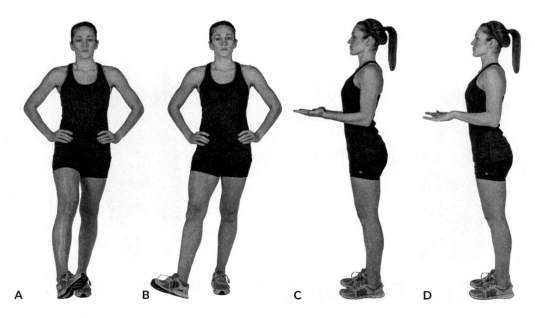

Figure 2.14
(A) Hip Internal Rotation.
(B) Hip External Rotation.
(C) Supination. (D) Pronation.   A   B   C   D

Transverse Plane Motions

Movements in the transverse plane include internal and external rotation, pronation and supination, *horizontal* abduction and adduction, and scapular retraction and protraction.[3,4] Examples of these movements can be seen in Figure 2.14. Internal rotation refers to the inward

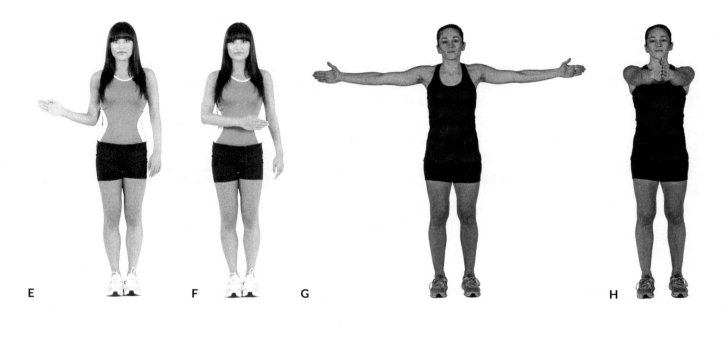

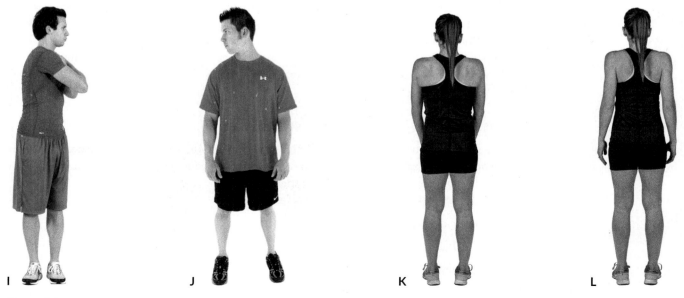

Figure 2.14

(E) Shoulder External Rotation. (F) Shoulder Internal Rotation. (G) Shoulder Horizontal Abduction. (H) Shoulder Horizontal Adduction. (I) Spinal Rotation. (J) Cervical Spine Rotation. (K) Shoulder Protraction. (L) Shoulder Retraction.

External rotation

Turning of a limb or body segment away from the midline of the body.

Pronation

Tri-planar movement (eversion, dorsiflexion, abduction).

Supination

Tri-planar movement (plantar flexion, inversion, adduction).

Horizontal abduction

Lateral-rotational movement *away* from the midline of the body.

Horizontal adduction

Medial-rotational movement *toward* the midline of the body.

Flexors

Muscles that produce flexion of a limb or joint.

Extensors

Muscles that produce extension of a limb or joint.

INSTRUCTOR TIP 👍

Using scientific terminology when teaching may help build credibility with your class, but always explain exercises in a manner that is easily understood and relevant to their fitness needs.

rotation of a limb or body segment. External rotation refers to the outward rotation of a limb or body segment.

Pronation and supination are both tri-planar movements. In relation to the ankle, pronation is the combination of eversion, dorsiflexion, and abduction, while supination is the combination of plantar flexion, inversion, and adduction. The terms are also commonly used when discussing the forearm. In this case, pronation means the forearm is rotating inward toward the body's center with the palm facing down and supination means the forearm is rotating outward from the body's center with the palm turning to face up or toward the body.

Horizontal abduction is a lateral movement away from the midline of the body. This can be seen during the outward motion of a rear deltoid fly. In the opposite direction, horizontal adduction is the same type of movement *toward* the midline of the body. This is demonstrated during the inward motion of a chest fly.

Application of Biomechanics

Muscles can be classified into functional groups based on the actions at joints. Examples of functional muscle groups include:

- ▼ Flexors and extensors
- ▼ Abductors and adductors
- ▼ Pronators and supinators

Muscles are called flexors when they produce flexion of a limb at a joint, whereas extensors are muscles that produce extension of a limb at a joint. Similar naming conventions apply for the rest of the groups: abductors and adductors produce abduction and adduction, while pronation and supination occur through the actions of pronators and supinators. This further reinforces knowing biomechanical terms so the instructor can more instantly recognize what a muscle does when it is activated.

Understanding the structure and function of the human body in a static posture is the basis for studying dynamic postures.[1] Dynamic posture occurs in everyday life and during workouts. It will help instructors quickly assess movement abilities of participants.

Common Exercise Movements

The more an instructor can learn about how the Human Movement System functions, the more he or she can create variations in common gym movements. This empowers instructors to be creative in more functional ways for participants.

Common exercise movements include:

- ▼ Overhead press
- ▼ Pulling
- ▼ Pushing

Table 2.2

Multi-joint vs. Multiplanar	
Multi-joint Exercises (Predominantly Single Plane)	**Multi-joint and Multiplanar Exercises**
Lunge	Lunge with rotation
Squat	Squat to rotational lift
Push-up	Push-up with rotation
Row	Row with trunk rotation

▼ Squatting

▼ Lunging

Although many gym movements incorporate multiplanar joint actions, they tend to occur predominantly in one plane of motion. When creating workouts, the instructor should incorporate exercises that challenge the body through multi-joint and multiplanar training (see **Table 2.2**). The *AFAA 5 Questions* can serve as a guideline for new instructors to evaluate the moves and workouts they are programming.

Exercise Naming Conventions

It is a best practice to describe exercises based on a set of common criteria. In general, the following are widely used criteria when an exercise is named:

▼ Plane of motion

▼ Body position

▼ Type of modality used

▼ Joint action

▼ Primary muscle targeted

It is helpful to break down a name into its separate elements, known as *stems*. The following are examples of stems used to name an exercise and how they are used.

Plane of Motion

Some exercises can be performed in multiple planes. For example, a lunge to balance exercise can be performed in the sagittal, frontal, or transverse planes, so it is to necessary to specify. If all the planes will be used, the word multiplanar applies. See **Table 2.3** for more information.

INSTRUCTOR TIP

It's helpful to tell participants about how and why certain movements are functional, explaining their translation to everyday examples.

Abductors

Muscles that produce abduction of a limb or joint.

Adductors

Muscles that produce adduction of a limb or joint.

Pronators

Muscles that produce pronation of a limb or body segment.

Supinators

Muscles that produce supination of a limb or body segment.

Static posture

The starting point from which an individual moves; a pose in which the body is standing in its natural, relaxed position.

Dynamic posture

Positioning of the body during any movement.

Multiplanar

Occurring in more than one plane of motion.

Table 2.3

Planes of Motion	
Stem	**Example**
Frontal plane	Frontal plane lunge (side)
Sagittal plane	Sagittal plane lunge (forward)
Transverse plane	Transverse plane lunge (rotation then forward lunge)
Multiplanar	Multiplanar lunge (all three)

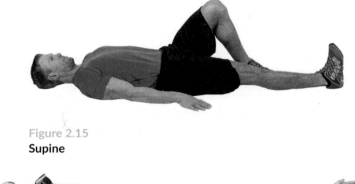

Figure 2.15
Supine

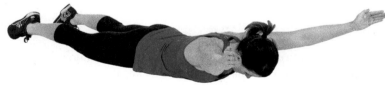

Figure 2.16
Prone

Body Position

Some exercises can be performed in different body positions such as supine (Figure 2.15), prone (Figure 2.16), kneeling, half-kneeling, or standing. Additional variations call for using two legs, a single leg, two arms, or a single arm. Body position stems are listed in **Table 2.4**.

Resistance Modality Used

The type of equipment or modality, such as dumbbells, tubing, stability balls, or kettlebells can be stems. **Table 2.5** provides examples of how exercises may be named based on the modality used to perform the exercise.

Joint Action

Sometimes a joint action is indicated in the name of an exercise. **Table 2.6** shows examples of how exercises may be named based on joint action.

Supine

Body position where one is lying on the back and facing upward.

Prone

Body position where one is lying face downward.

Table 2.4

Body Positions	
Stem	**Example**
Supine	Supine abdominal crunch (floor crunch)
Prone	Prone iso abs (plank)
Kneeling	Half-kneeling hip flexor stretch
Single leg	Single-leg squat
Staggered stance	Staggered-stance band chest press
Alternating arms	Alternating-arm biceps curl

Table 2.5

Resistance Modality Exercises	
Stem	**Example**
Sliding discs	Sliding mountain climbers
Suspension	Suspension push-up
Tubing (TB) or band	Lateral tube walking
Dumbbell (Hand weights) (DB)	Two-arm dumbbell overhead press
Kettlebell (KB)	Two-arm kettlebell swing

Table 2.6

Joint Action Exercises	
Stem	**Example**
Extension	Supine triceps extension
Abduction	Prone iso-abs with hip abduction & extension
Rotation	Walking lunge with rotation

Table 2.7

Primary Muscle Targeted	
Stem	**Example**
Chest	Dumbbell chest press on stability ball
Shoulder	Shoulder press
Triceps	Triceps extension
Legs	Single-leg squat
Calf	Calf raise

Primary Muscle Targeted

Exercises can also be named based on the targeted muscle. See **Table 2.7** for examples.

Muscular Function and Application

Knowing the various functions of muscles allows instructors to create classes aimed to prevent injury, improve flexibility, and increase endurance and strength. This information, and its application, is based on the concepts of the muscle action spectrum, muscle function, and kinetics.

Muscle Action Spectrum

Muscles produce a variety of actions, known as the *muscle action spectrum*. The muscle action spectrum includes three major types of activation:

- ▼ Concentric
- ▼ Isometric
- ▼ Eccentric

Concentric activation means a muscle is producing tension as it shortens to overcome an external resistance.

Isometric activation is when a muscle is producing tension while it maintains the same length. Every movement has a point of isometric activation. It can be seen when the exercise is being held still. The tension produced by a muscle is equal to the force of an external load that is being applied and does not produce joint movement.

Concentric activation

Production of tension while shortening in length.

Isometric activation

Production of tension while maintaining a constant length.

Eccentric activation means a muscle is producing tension while lengthening in order to resist or control an external force. For example, when lowering the arm after a biceps curl, the biceps eccentrically decelerate elbow extension. The biceps become activated in order to resist the downward force of gravity; otherwise, the arm would just fall straight without control.

Muscle Function

Each muscle has a role or function within the body. Memorizing the isolated function of each muscle is helpful when learning functional anatomy. Isolated function refers to a muscle's primary concentric functions (Table 2.8).

Eccentric function refers to the action of a muscle when it is generating an eccentric activation. A muscle that decelerates a movement is reducing the speed in order to maintain control and avoid injury. It is important when landing from plyometric exercises such as a squat or box jump, as the body has to absorb and transfer roughly 15 times the body's weight.[5] Instructors can lead a safer class with increased attention on correctly decelerating a movement.

Eccentric activation

Production of tension while increasing in length.

Isolated function

A muscle's primary functions.

Eccentric function

Action of a muscle when generating an eccentric contraction.

Table 2.8

Isolated Function of Major Muscles

Major Muscle(s)	Isolated Function	Common Exercise
Quadriceps (rectus femoris, vastus lateralis, vastus medialis, vastus intermedius)	Concentrically accelerates knee extension	Squat (the upward phase)
Hamstrings (semitendinosus, semimembranosus, biceps femoris)	Concentrically accelerates knee flexion	Hamstrings curl Ball
Gastrocnemius	Concentrically accelerates plantar flexion	Calf raise
Gluteus maximus	Concentrically accelerates hip extension, and external rotation	Lunge on the upward motion
Rectus abdominis	Concentrically accelerates spinal flexion, lateral flexion, and rotation	Ball crunch
Pectoralis major	Concentrically accelerates shoulder flexion, and horizontal adduction	Push-up
Latissimus dorsi	Concentrically accelerates shoulder extension, adduction, and internal rotation	Band row
Biceps	Concentrically accelerates elbow flexion	Biceps curl
Triceps	Concentrically accelerates elbow extension	Triceps extension

Origin

The relatively stationary attachment site where a muscle begins.

Insertion

The relatively mobile attachment site of a muscle's distal end.

Tendons

Connective tissues that attach muscle to bone and provide an anchor for muscles to produce force.

Location of Muscles: Origin and Insertion

Muscles are attached to body segments and must cross at least one joint in order to create a joint motion. Typically, a muscle attaches to a relatively stationary point on one end of a body segment, such as a bone. This is called the origin. On the other end, the muscle attaches to a relatively mobile attachment called the insertion.[6,7] Muscles attach to the bones via tendons. Tendons are connective soft tissues that provide an anchor for muscles to produce force and are mostly seen at the insertion point of muscles.

Summary

A solid understanding of biomechanics and the Human Movement System will provide the Group Fitness Instructor with information to design, teach, assess, and adapt workout content. By applying the concepts of biomechanics, Group Fitness Instructors can better understand and address common issues such as movement dysfunction and kinetic chain disruption.

Chapter in Review

- Anatomic location terminology
  - Anterior: front
  - Posterior: back
  - Superior: above
  - Inferior: below
  - Proximal: closer
  - Distal: further
  - Medial: to the middle
  - Lateral: to the outside
- Planes of motion: sagittal (forward and back), frontal (side to side), transverse (rotational)
  - Related joint movement (e.g., flexion, extension, abduction, adduction, rotation, supination, pronation, etc.)
- Joint motions
  - Sagittal plane: flexion, extension, dorsiflexion, and plantar flexion
  - Frontal plane: abduction and adduction, lateral flexion at the spine, & eversion and inversion of the foot
  - Transverse plane: internal and external rotation, pronation and supination, horizontal abduction and adduction, & scapular retraction and protraction
- Posture
  - Static: basis for studying posture
  - Dynamic: occurs in everyday life and during workouts
- Common exercise movements
  - Overhead press
  - Pulling
  - Pushing
  - Squatting
  - Lunging

- ▼ Conventions of exercise naming
  - ▪ Plane of motion
  - ▪ Body position
  - ▪ Type of modality
  - ▪ Joint action
  - ▪ Primary muscle targeted
- ▼ Muscle action spectrum
  - ▪ Concentric: shortens muscle length
- ▪ Isometric: maintains muscle length
- ▪ Eccentric: lengthens muscle
- ▼ Muscle function
- ▼ Muscle location
  - ▪ Origin
  - ▪ Insertion

References

1. Hall S. *Basic Biomechanics*. 7th ed. New York, NY: McGraw-Hill Education; 2014.
2. Shier D, Butler J, Lewis R. *Hole's Essentials of Human Anatomy & Physiology*. Boston, MA: McGraw-Hill Higher Education; 2009.
3. Levangie P, Norkin C. *Joint Structure and Function: A Comprehensive Analysis*. 3rd ed. Philadelphia, PA: F.A. Davis; 2001.
4. Neumann D. *Kinesiology of the Musculoskeletal System: Foundations for Rehabilitation*. 2nd ed.
5. Perttunen J, Kyrolainen H, Komi PV, Heinonen A. Biomechanical loading in the triple jump. *J Sports Sci*. 2000;18:363-370.
6. Hamil J, Knutzen K, Derrick T. *Biomechanical Basis of Human Movement*. 4th ed.
7. Saladin K. *Anatomy and Physiology: The Unity of Form and Function*. 4th ed. New York, NY: McGraw-Hill; 2007.

Chapter 3
The Human Movement System

Learning Objectives

3.1.   **Explain** the roles and interactions of the three systems of the kinetic chain.

3.2.   **Identify** common overactive and underactive muscles.

3.3.   **Discuss** other systems related to human movement.

3.4.   **Identify** the different energy systems and their role in exercise.

Introduction to the Human Movement System

The Human Movement System (kinetic chain) is made up of three interconnected components to produce movement in the body: the nervous, muscular, and skeletal systems. In addition to working together these systems use support mechanisms such as the cardiorespiratory, digestive, and endocrine systems to function.

Nervous System

The nervous system tells the musculoskeletal system of the body when and how to move. It collects all sensory information and sends a movement response for a specific outcome. If the nervous system inappropriately fires, it sends misinformation to the muscles and thereby alters movement.

The nervous system is divided into the central nervous system (CNS) and the peripheral nervous system (PNS).[1] The CNS includes the brain and spinal cord, and its primary function is to coordinate activity of all parts of the body. The PNS is the extension of the CNS and includes nerve fibers that branch off from the spinal cord and extend to the body.

Mechanoreceptors

The nervous system is made up of approximately 100 billion specialized nerve cells called neurons (Figure 3.1). The neuron is the functional unit of the nervous system, and it is made of three main parts: the cell body, axon, and dendrites.

Mechanoreceptors are sensory receptors that respond to a change in the position of body tissues. Mechanoreceptors can be stimulated by touch, pressure, stretch, and motion, and they allow the brain to gauge body position. All sensory input to the CNS from the mechanoreceptors in the PNS is called proprioception. Proprioception is the awareness and perception of body position and limb movements. It is what allows a person to close their eyes and still touch the tip of the index finger to the nose. Proprioceptors (body positioning receptors) work constantly throughout the day, especially during exercise.

Muscle spindles are mechanoreceptors found in skeletal muscles that measure the amount and rate of stretch. When the muscle is lengthened too much or too quickly, the muscle spindle sends messages to the CNS, resulting in muscular contraction as a protective response.

Nervous system

A conglomeration of billions of cells to provide a communication network within the human body.

Central nervous system (CNS)

Division of the nervous system comprising the brain and the spinal cord; primary function is to coordinate activity of all parts of the body.

Peripheral nervous system (PNS)

All of the nerve fibers that branch off from the spinal cord and extend to the rest of the body.

Neuron

Functional unit of the nervous system.

Mechanoreceptors

Sensory receptors responsible for sensing change of position in body tissues.

Proprioception

Cumulative sensory input to the central nervous system from all mechanoreceptors.

Muscle spindles

Receptors sensitive to change in length of the muscle, and the rate of that change.

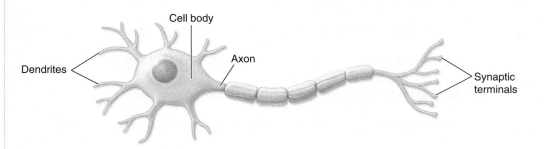

Figure 3.1
The Structure of a Neuron

Golgi tendon organs (GTOs) are located where the muscle and tendon converge. The GTO measures the amount and rate of tension that develops within the muscle. If the tension is too great or develops too fast, the GTO will cause the muscle to relax as a safety response. During static stretching, this happens after the muscle spindle causes the protective muscular contraction. This contraction creates the *tension* the GTO measures, and after 20 to 30 seconds of GTO stimulation, it will signal the brain to have the muscle relax. This is the rationale for holding static stretches for 30 seconds.

Muscular System

The next part of the Human Movement System is the muscular system. It receives messaging from the brain to shorten or lengthen, creating movement to the skeletal system.

Muscles are made up of muscle fibers with smaller tubes held within called myofibrils. Inside the myofibrils are long chains of individual contractile units called sarcomeres. Each sarcomere contains long proteins called filaments that slide past each other to produce muscular contractions (Figure 3.2).

Muscle Fiber Types

There are two major categories muscle fibers: type I and type II. These different muscle fiber types have specific purposes for movement.

Golgi tendon organs (GTOs)

Receptors sensitive to the change in tension of the muscle, and the rate of that change.

Myofibrils

Tubular component of muscle cells containing sarcomeres and protein filaments.

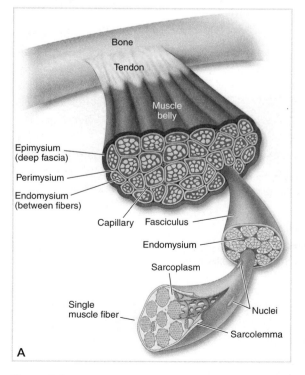

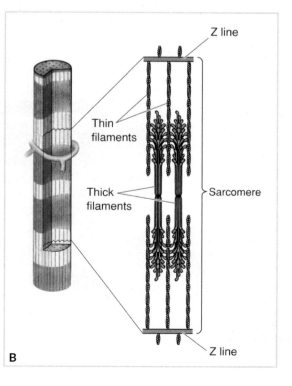

Figure 3.2
(A) Structure of the Skeletal Muscle. (B) Sarcomere.

MEMORY TIP

Use the "S" and the "T" in these terms to help yourself remember their function. A muscle spindle is the "Stretch-O-Meter" and GTO is the "Tension-O-Meter."

Sarcomeres

Individual contractile units made up of actin (thin) and myosin (thick) filaments.

Aerobic

Meaning "with oxygen," the long-term energy production cycle that occurs when sufficient oxygen is present.

Anaerobic

Meaning "without oxygen," the short-term energy production cycle that occurs with insufficient oxygen levels.

Agonist

Muscle that works as the prime mover of a joint exercise.

Synergists

Muscles that assist the prime mover in a joint action.

MEMORY TIP

Mitochondria are nicknamed the "powerhouse of the cell." Mitochondria are organelles that contain genetic material and enzymes necessary for cell metabolism, converting food to energy.

Type I Fibers

A *twitch* is a single contraction of facilitated muscle. Type I fibers are also known as *slow-twitch fibers* because they are slower to reach maximal contraction. The large numbers of capillaries, mitochondria, and myoglobin in these fibers gives them greater ability to obtain and use oxygen; therefore, type I fibers are considered highly aerobic.

Because of their slow twitch speed and high aerobic capacity, type I fibers are more resistant to fatigue. They are also smaller in size, produce less force, and do not respond as well to muscle growth. Distance running, cross-country skiing, and dance-oriented formats are examples of activities that recruit and build type I muscle fibers.

Type II Fibers

Type II muscle fibers are also known as *fast-twitch fibers*. They contain fewer capillaries, mitochondria, and myoglobin than type I fibers. With fewer capillaries, there is less oxygen delivery; type II muscle fibers are considered to be more anaerobic and more susceptible to muscle enlargement. They produce more speed and strength than type I fibers, but the burst of intensity is short-lived. High-intensity interval training (HIIT), sprinting, and plyometric jumping are examples of activities that recruit and build type II muscle fibers. See **Table 3.1** for a summary of the characteristics of type I and type II muscle fibers.

Muscles as Movers

A muscle's function during movement categorizes it as an *agonist*, *antagonist*, or *synergist*. Agonists are the prime movers that produce the most force for a particular joint action. Common agonists are the gluteus maximus at the hip during a squat or the pectoralis major at the shoulder during a push-up.

Synergists are muscles that assist the prime mover in a given joint action. For example, the piriformis, a small deep gluteal muscle, is a synergist at the hip during a squat.

Table 3.1

Muscle Fiber Types	
Type	**Characteristic**
Type I (slow-twitch)	More capillaries, mitochondria, and myoglobin Increased oxygen delivery Smaller in size Less force produced Slow to fatigue Long-term contractions (stabilization)
Type II (fast-twitch)	Fewer capillaries, mitochondria, and myoglobin Decreased oxygen delivery Larger in size More force produced Quick to fatigue Short-term contractions (force and power)

Table 3.2

Muscles as Movers			
Muscle Type	**Muscle Function**	**Exercise**	**Muscle(s) Used**
Agonist	Prime mover	Chest Press Row Squat	Pectoralis major Latissimus dorsi Gluteus maximus, quadriceps
Synergist	Assist prime mover	Chest press Row Squat	Anterior deltoid, triceps Posterior deltoid, biceps Hamstring complex
Antagonist	Oppose prime mover	Chest press Row Squat	Posterior deltoid Pectoralis major Psoas

⊘ Check It Out

Muscle has four behavioral properties that help facilitate movement:
- Extensibility: The ability to be stretched or lengthened.
- Elasticity: The ability to return to normal or resting length after being stretched.
- Irritability: The ability to respond to internal or external stimuli.
- Ability to develop tension: The ability to remain the same length, increase length, or decrease length during tension.

Lastly, the antagonist muscle opposes the prime mover. In a biceps curl, the triceps brachii is the antagonist because it opposes elbow flexion—lengthening to allow elbow flexion.

Table 3.2 provides a summary of the types of muscles based on their role in different types of movement.

Skeletal System

Bones and joints make up the skeletal system. The junction where two or more bones join to create motion is called a *joint*. Ligaments are the connective tissues connecting *bone to bone*. Recall that *tendons* are the connective tissues attaching *muscle to bone* at the insertion point. The skeletal system serves five major roles in the body:

1. *Movement*—Bones are levers, and joints are pivot points where movement occurs.
2. *Support*—Bones provide the framework.
3. *Protection*—Bones encase vital organs and protect them.
4. *Blood production*—Blood cells are formed in the bone marrow.
5. *Mineral storage*—Minerals, such as calcium and phosphorus, are stored in bones.

Antagonists

Muscles that oppose the prime mover.

Ligament

Strong connective tissue that connects bone to bone.

Axial and Appendicular Skeletons

The two divisions of the skeletal system are the axial skeleton and the appendicular skeleton. The axial skeleton includes the skull, rib cage, and spinal column and creates the protective structure. The axial skeleton can be further broken down to its individual segments:

▼   Skull

▼   Hyoid bone

▼   Sternum and ribs

▼   Spinal column

The bones of the spinal column are divided into five major categories (Figure 3.3). From the top down, they are as follows:

Axial skeleton

Portion of the skeletal system consisting of the bones of the skull, rib cage, and vertebral column.

Appendicular skeleton

Portion of the skeleton that includes the bones that support the upper an lower extremities.

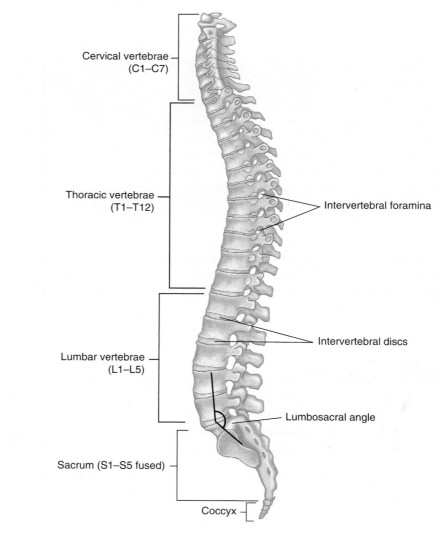

Cervical vertebrae (C1–C7)

Thoracic vertebrae (T1–T12)

Intervertebral foramina

Intervertebral discs

Lumbar vertebrae (L1–L5)

Lumbosacral angle

Sacrum (S1–S5 fused)

Coccyx

Figure 3.3
Bones of the Spinal Column

▼   Cervical vertebrae (C1–C7)

▼   Thoracic vertebrae (T1–T12)

▼   Lumbar vertebrae (L1–L5)

▼   Sacrum

▼   Coccyx

The appendicular skeleton is divided into the upper and lower extremities (see **Table 3.3**).

Joints

Joints are formed where one bone articulates with another bone.[2] They can be categorized by both their structure and their function.[2–4] The three major joint motions are roll, slide, and spin (Figures 3.4–3.6).[3–5]

Table 3.3

The Appendicular Skeleton

Upper Extremity	Lower Extremity
• Clavicle	• Innominate (os coxa, hemi-pelvis)
• Scapula	• Femur
• Humerus	• Patella
• Radius	• Tibia
• Ulna	• Fibula
• Carpals	• Tarsals
• Metacarpals	• Metatarsals
• Phalanges	• Phalanges

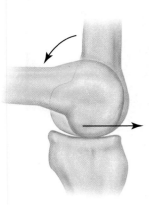

Figure 3.4
Rolling Joint Motion

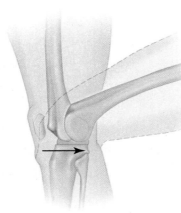

Figure 3.5
Sliding Joint Motion

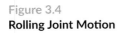

Figure 3.6
Spinning Joint Motion

Classification of Joints

The three main types of joints in the body are *synovial, non-synovial,* and *cartilaginous.* Synovial joints are the most common joints associated with human movement. They comprise approximately 80% of all the joints in the body and have the greatest capacity for motion.[2–4,6] The body has several types of synovial joints, as seen in Figures 3.7–3.12. See **Table 3.4** for examples of each joint type.

Function of Joints

Joints allow for movement while also providing stability. This means joints allow for a functional movement to take place without unwanted movement. All joints in the human body are linked together, which implies movement of one joint directly affects the motion of others.[3,5] This is an essential concept because it creates an awareness of how the body functionally operates and is the premise behind kinetic chain movement.[3,5]

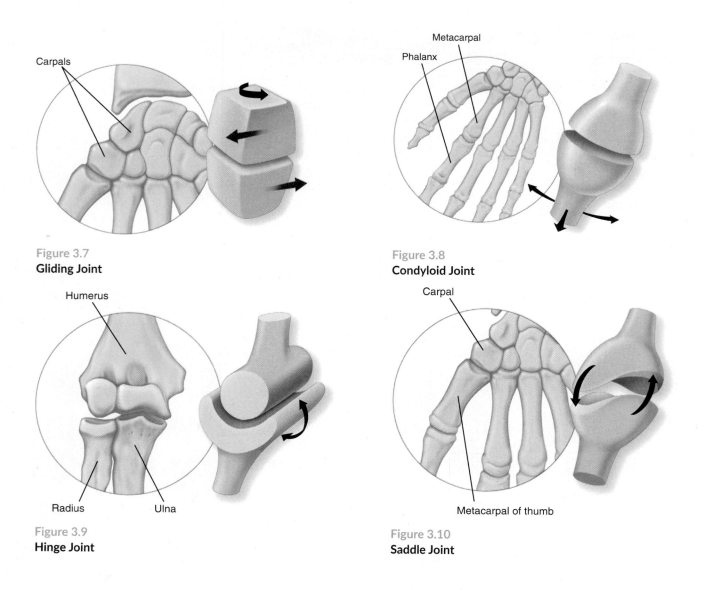

Figure 3.7
Gliding Joint

Figure 3.8
Condyloid Joint

Figure 3.9
Hinge Joint

Figure 3.10
Saddle Joint

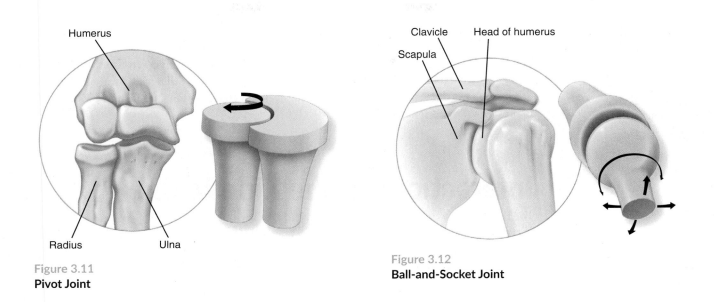

Figure 3.11
Pivot Joint

Figure 3.12
Ball-and-Socket Joint

Table 3.4

Types of Joints

Joint	Characteristic	Example
Non-synovial	No joint cavity and fibrous connective tissue; little or no movement	Sutures of the skull, distal joint of the tibia and fibula, symphysis pubis
Synovial	Produces synovial fluid, has a joint cavity and fibrous connective tissue	Knee*
Gliding	No axis of rotation; moves by sliding side-to-side or back and forth	Carpals of the hand
Condyloid	Formed by the fitting of condyles of one bone into elliptical cavities of another; moves predominantly in one plane	Knee
Hinge	Uniaxial; moves predominantly in one plane of motion (sagittal)	Elbow
Saddle	One bone fits like a saddle on another bone; moves predominantly in two planes (sagittal, joint of thumb frontal)	Only: carpometacarpal
Pivot	Only one axis; moves predominantly in one plane of motion (transverse)	Radioulnar
Ball-and-socket	Most mobile of joints: moves in all three planes of motion	Shoulder

*Note: The knee is only one example of a synovial joint. The vast majority of the joints at each of the kinetic chain checkpoints (as well as the vertebrae of the spine) are synovial.

INSTRUCTOR TIP 👍

Ligaments and tendons have a low blood supply; this is one reason it can take up to 6 weeks for recovery from injuries to these connective tissues.

Exercise and Its Effect on Bone Mass

Like muscle, bone is living tissue that responds to exercise by becoming stronger. Individuals who exercise regularly usually achieve greater bone density and strength than those who do not. Exercise is crucial in maintaining muscle strength, coordination, and balance, which help to prevent falls and related fractures.

Interactions of the Kinetic Chain

The Human Movement System uses the attributes of three systems—the skeletal, muscular, and nervous systems (Figure 3.13). The nervous system acts on the muscular system to contract. The muscular system acts on the skeletal system to create forces for movement. The skeletal system acts as the body's structure and a protective case.

🏃 **Practice This!**

Practice the concept of the kinetic chain. First, start by standing with both feet firmly on the ground and then roll your feet to the right and to the left (i.e., inversion and eversion). Notice what your knees and hips are doing as you perform the movement. Moving one joint will inevitably move the others.

Force-couple relationship

Muscles moving together to produce movement around a joint.

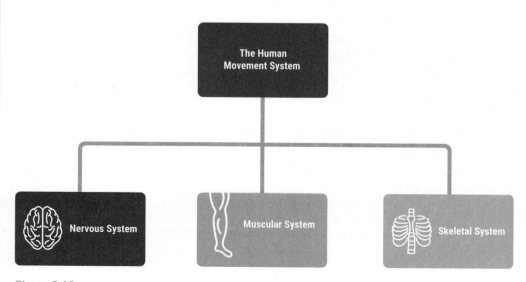

Figure 3.13
The Human Movement System

> ### ✓ Check It Out
>
> Think about a basketball player jumping up to get a ball by going into a deep squat prior to the jump, or a shallow bend of the knees and hips, barely allowing the player to leave the floor in either scenario. For each of these examples, there is an best position from which an athlete can produce the desired result.

Length–tension Relationships

Length–tension relationship refers to the length at which a muscle can create the tension or force.[3,4,6–10] Shortening or lengthening the muscle reduces its ability to produce force. Therefore, there is a strong relationship between the length of a muscle and the tension muscle can produce:

- ▼ If a muscle is too short or too long, it will not be able to produce as much force.
- ▼ A muscle at ideal length can produce the most force.

Force-couple Relationships

The synergistic action of muscles to produce movement around a joint is also known as a force-couple relationship).[3,11,12] When muscles are lengthened or shortened due to an individual's deconditioned state, force-couple relationships can be altered, changing the overall movement and potentially putting too much stress on the synergists.

Reciprocal Inhibition

The word *reciprocal* means *opposite*, and *inhibition* means *restricting*. Reciprocal inhibition occurs when the muscles on one side of a joint relax to allow the muscles on the other side to contract. This process is a normal, functional occurrence during human movement, such as when the triceps relax while the biceps contract. However, altered reciprocal inhibition can also occur, which contributes to muscular imbalances and potential injury. This occurs when a muscle becomes overactive, reducing neural drive from the muscle that should be its functional antagonist in the force-couple relationship.

Kinetic Chain Dysfunction

Because structures of the body are interconnected, if a particular component becomes dysfunctional, it can result in a chain reaction that may cause problems in other parts of the Human Movement System. For example, if a participant walks with externally rotated feet, segments throughout the entire kinetic chain may be affected.

Posture is the alignment of all parts of the kinetic chain with the purpose of countering external forces and maintaining an efficient structure. If any system of the kinetic chain is not functioning properly, movement is affected. To minimize kinetic chain dysfunction, instructors should constantly monitor class participants to ensure they are performing exercises with correct form.

Neutral spine refers to the natural position of the spine when the cervical, thoracic, and lumbar curves are in good alignment. Abnormal curvatures of the spine include scoliosis,

---

Reciprocal inhibition

Simultaneous contraction of one muscle and the relaxation of its antagonist to allow movement to take place.

Altered reciprocal inhibition

Process by which an overactive muscle decreases neural drive to its functional antagonist.

Posture

Alignment of all parts of the kinetic chain with the purpose of countering external forces and maintaining structural efficiency.

Neutral spine

The natural position of the spine when the cervical, thoracic, and lumbar curves are in good alignment.

Scoliosis

Abnormal lateral twisting or rotating of the spine.

> ### INSTRUCTOR TIP 👍
>
> Make sure participants know posture is the constant structure of their body and promotes the ability to move in the most efficient way possible.

Kyphosis

Abnormal rounding of the thoracic portion of the spine, usually accompanied by rounded shoulders.

Lordosis

Sway back; increased or excessive lumbar curve.

MEMORY TIP

When learning dysfunctional muscles, it is helpful to physically perform the movements described by the isolated function. This will allow you to feel what happens when the muscle shortens.

INSTRUCTOR TIP

Just because muscles may be short, tight, or overactive doesn't mean these muscles need to stop being trained. Rather, teach resistance-based classes with an integrated approach that provides balance among all muscle groups, joint actions, and planes of motion.

> **⊘ Check It Out**
>
> Ideal posture and movement relies on flexibility; when flexibility is limited, faulty movement patterns are reinforced while working out. Cueing a participant on correct technique will help increase the participants' awareness of body position in order to create lasting change.

kyphosis, and lordosis. Scoliosis (twisted) is the most common of the three conditionsand is a lateral bending of the spine. Kyphosis (a hump) refers to an exaggerated curve in the thoracic area. Lordosis (swayback) is an increased concave curve in the lumbar portion of the spine. This condition is often accompanied by an increased anterior tilt of the pelvis.

Dysfunctional muscles can disrupt the communication between the nervous system and muscles. This changes the length and tension of muscles and creates patterns of dysfunction. Kinetic chain disruption is typically one part of a chain reaction involving a number of dysfunctional muscles, leading to compensations and adaptations that can lead to pain and injury.[13]

The terms *overactive* and *underactive* will be used when referring to dysfunctional muscles. An overactive muscle is overly tense or tight during movement, and a muscle is considered underactive when it is weak and not being recruited as it should.

Common Overactive and Underactive Muscles of the Foot and Ankle

A number of specific muscles tend to be problematic in the foot and ankle complex, most commonly seen during walking and squatting patterns as feet that externally rotate or flatten. **Table 3.5** lists common overactive and underactive muscles of the foot and ankle. Figure 3.14 displays the muscles of the foot and ankle.

Table 3.5

Common Overactive and Underactive Muscles of the Foot and Ankle	
Common Overactive Muscles	**Common Underactive Muscles**
• Soleus	• Medial gastrocnemius
• Lateral gastrocnemius	• Anterior tibialis
• Peroneus longus and brevis (peroneals)	• Posterior tibialis

Common Overactive and Underactive Muscles of the Knee

Several muscles cross the knee and have attachments at both the thigh and lower leg bones. When there is dysfunction, it can be seen when the knees cave inward or move outward during movement. **Table 3.6** lists common overactive and underactive muscles of the knee. Figure 3.15 displays the muscles of the knee.

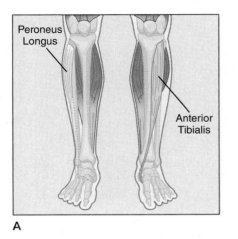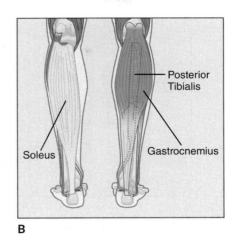

A   B

Figure 3.14
(A) Muscles of the Foot. (B) Muscles of the Ankle.

Table 3.6

Common Overactive and Underactive Muscles of the Knee	
Common Overactive Muscles	**Common Underactive Muscles**
• Biceps femoris (short head) • Tensor fascia latae (TFL)	• Vastus medialis oblique (VMO)

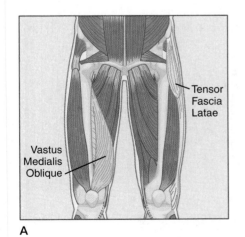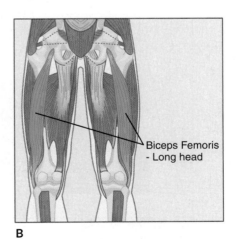

A   B

Figure 3.15
Muscles of the Knee: (A) Anterior. (B) Posterior.

Common Overactive and Underactive Muscles of the LPHC

The lumbo-pelvic-hip complex, or LPHC, is susceptible to imbalance due to the number of muscles that cross the hip (Figure 3.16). Many individuals are in a constant state of hip flexion (from sitting), so stretching these muscles can improve movement for many class participants.

INSTRUCTOR TIP 👍

You can design workouts with exercises, such as hip flexor stretches, that counteract the common dysfunctional patterns many experience from sitting at a desk all day.

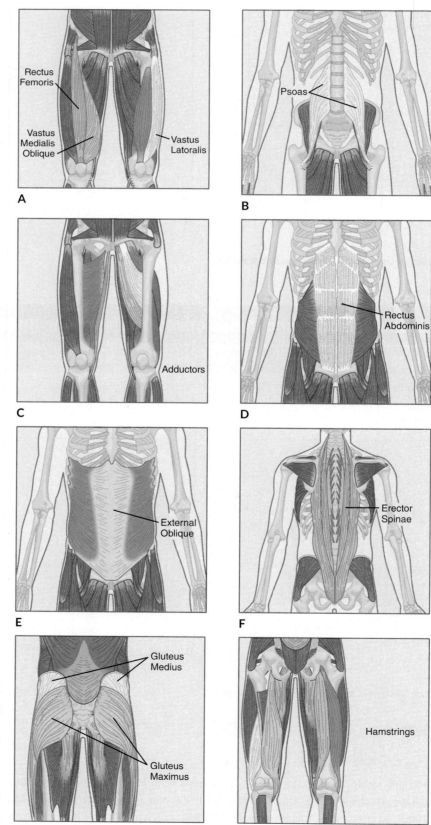

Figure 3.16
Muscles of the LPHC

Muscular LPHC dysfunction can be seen if a participant's low back arches or rounds during exercise. **Table 3.7** lists common overactive and underactive muscles of the LPHC.

Table 3.7

Common Overactive and Underactive Muscles of the LPHC	
Common Overactive Muscles	**Common Underactive Muscles**
• Hip flexors (TFL, quadriceps, psoas) • Adductors • Abdominals (rectus abdominis, external obliques)	• Gluteus maximus • Gluteus medius • Hamstrings • Intrinsic core stabilizers

Common Overactive and Underactive Muscles of the Shoulder

Several muscles have an effect on the stability of the shoulder and provide overall stability during upper body movements (Figure 3.17). When dysfunctional, muscles of the shoulder can contribute

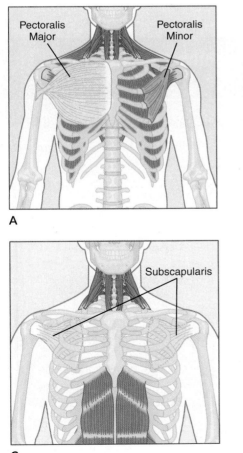

A

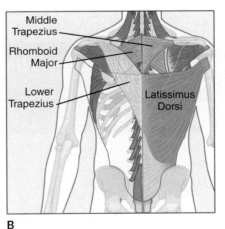

B

C

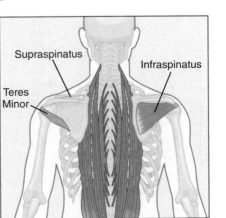

D

Figure 3.17
Muscles of the Shoulder

to shoulders rounding forward, scapulae winging out, or the low back arching during overhead movements (due to the tightness in the latissimus dorsi). **Table 3.8** lists common overactive and underactive muscles of the shoulder.

Table 3.8

Common Overactive and Underactive Muscles of the Shoulder	
Common Overactive Muscles	**Common Underactive Muscles**
• Latissimus dorsi • Pectoralis major/minor	• Middle and lower trapezius • Rhomboids • Rotator cuff

Common Overactive and Underactive Muscles of the Head and Neck

A slouched sitting posture elevates the shoulders and forces the head to protrude forward.[11] **Table 3.9** lists common overactive and underactive muscles of the cervical spine. Figure 3.18 displays the muscles of the cervical spine.

Table 3.9

Common Overactive and Underactive Muscles of the Cervical Spine	
Common Overactive Muscles	**Common Underactive Muscles**
• Upper trapezius • Sternocleidomastoid • Levator scapulae	• Deep cervical flexors

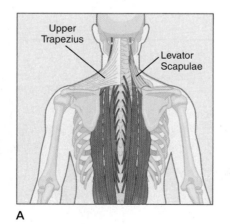

A

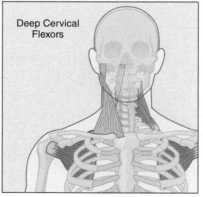

B

Figure 3.18
Muscles of the Cervical Spine

Table 3.10

Common Daily Repetitive Movements

- Talking on the phone and holding it to the same ear each time
- Driving a car with the right foot externally rotated on the gas pedal
- Working on a computer or laptop
- Wearing high-heeled shoes or boots
- Carrying a backpack or purse only on one shoulder

✓ Check It Out

Several studies have shown that sadness and depression have a negative influence on posture, and that movement is an important tool in improving a person's emotional state. The positive effects of exercise on mood are often immediately apparent in a person's posture.[16]

Contributors of Kinetic Chain Dysfunction

The major causes of kinetic chain dysfunction are repetitive movement and frequent lack of movement. Injury and medical issues can also be contributors, but are outside a Group Fitness Instructor's scope of practice to diagnose, assess, or recommend treatment.

Repetitive Movement

Performing the same movement regularly can alter the kinetic chain. For example, repetitive jumping movements in a class can lead to premature fatigue or injury to the muscles of the foot and lower leg, leading to overactive muscles that create imbalances. When fitness sessions are not balanced, individuals' posture will not be either. Overall, the key to avoiding pattern overload is to implement workouts that incorporate a variety of movement patterns and provide equal training time for each muscle group.

Wearing high-heeled shoes, carrying overloaded backpacks, or carrying bags or children on one shoulder or hip are all repetitive movements. Therefore, occupation, recreation, hobbies, and all other activities of daily living play an equally important role in the development of an individual's posture (**Table 3.10**).

Repetitive Lack of Motion

Repetitive lack of motion can also lead to kinetic chain dysfunction. A participant may wake up in the morning and spend the rest of the day sitting — at the breakfast table, in the car, at a desk at work all day, and so on. This repetitive lack of movement increases the risk of injury when engaging in more physical activities.

Cardiorespiratory System

The cardiorespiratory system is a combination of the cardiovascular system (heart, blood vessels, and blood) and the respiratory system (trachea, bronchi, alveoli, etc.). These systems

INSTRUCTOR TIP 👍

Your participants will often overlook daily repetitive movements that contribute to kinetic chain dysfunction. Provide them with examples to aid their self-discovery process.

Repetitive lack of motion

Frequent immobility, which holds the potential for repetitive stress injuries.

Cardiorespiratory system

System of the body composed of the cardiovascular and respiratory systems.

Cardiovascular system

System of the body composed of the heart, blood, and blood vessels.

Respiratory system

System of the body composed of the lungs and respiratory passages that collect oxygen from the external environment and transport it to the bloodstream.

work together to provide the body with adequate oxygen and nutrients and to remove waste products such as carbon dioxide from the cells in the body.[7,9,15–17]

Cardiovascular System

The cardiovascular system is a closed system that circulates blood through a network of blood vessels via the rhythmic pumping action of the heart.

The Heart

The interior of the heart is divided into four chambers: top and bottom, and left and right. The right side of the heart receives blood from the body and sends it to the lungs. The left side of the heart receives blood from the lungs and sends it back out into the body (Figure 3.19).

The top chambers that receive blood from veins are known as atria (right and left atrium). The atria pump blood down into the same-side ventricles, which are larger chambers and are considered the "pumping chambers" of the heart, pumping into arteries.

The chambers of the heart are separated by four major valves (two atrioventricular (AV) valves and two semilunar (SL) valves that prevent blockage, backflow, or spillage of blood back into the other chambers of the heart.

Veins

Vessels that transport blood from the extremities back to the heart.

Atria

Superior chambers of the heart (singular: atrium) that receive blood from outside the heart and deliver it into their corresponding ventricle.

Ventricles

Inferior chambers of the heart that receive blood from their corresponding atrium and, in turn, force blood out of the heart into the arteries.

Arteries

Vessels that transport blood away from the heart.

Atrioventricular (AV) valves

Valves that allow for proper blood flow from the atria to the ventricles.

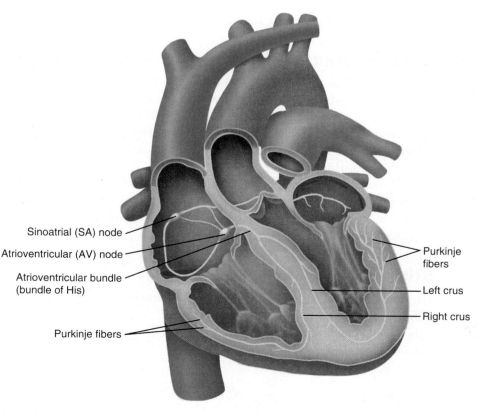

Sinoatrial (SA) node

Atrioventricular (AV) node

Atrioventricular bundle (bundle of His)

Purkinje fibers

Purkinje fibers

Left crus

Right crus

Figure 3.19
Conduction System of the Heart

The following steps outline the path of blood through the heart:

1. The inferior and superior vena cava collect blood from the body and send it to the right atrium.
2. The right atrium pumps blood through the right AV (tricuspid) valve to the right ventricle.
3. The right ventricle pumps out of the heart through the pulmonary valve, into the pulmonary artery, to the lungs.
4. The lungs receive blood from the pulmonary artery and return to the left atrium via the pulmonary vein.
5. The left atrium pumps blood through the left AV (mitral) valve to the left ventricle.
6. The left ventricle pumps blood past the aortic valve into the aorta.
7. The aorta is the artery that transports blood toward the systemic circulation.

Cardiac Muscle Contraction

Cardiac muscle is involuntary, because the heart has its own electrical conduction system. This signal to contract is first received at the sinoatrial (SA) node, also called the "pacemaker of the heart." Then, the SA node sends a delay signal to the atrioventricular (AV) node to offset the contraction timing, thus creating a two-pulse heartbeat.

Cardiac Output

The average number of times the heart beats per minute is known as heart rate (HR), and the average heart rate is 70–80 beats per minute (bpm).[15,17,18] The amount of blood pumped out heart with each contraction is referred to as stroke volume (SV). The SV multiplied by the HR, or the total volume of blood pumped out of the heart per minute, is called the cardiac output ($\dot{Q}$).

$$SV \times HR = \dot{Q}$$

Monitoring heart rate during exercise indicates the amount of work the heart is doing at any given time.[15,19,20] Participants should be taught how to manually check their heart rate. Figure 3.20 illustrates the procedure for manually monitoring heart rate.

Semilunar (SL) valves

Valves that allow for proper blood flow away from the heart to the lungs and body.

Sinoatrial (SA) node

Specialized area of cardiac tissue located in the right atrium of the heart that initiates the electrical impulses that determine the heart rate.

Atrioventricular (AV) node

Small mass of specialized cardiac muscle fibers located on the wall of the right atrium of the heart that receives impulses from the sinoatrial (SA) node and directs them to the walls of the ventricles.

Heart rate (HR)

Rate at which the heart pumps; usually measured in beats per minute (bpm).

Stroke volume (SV)

Amount of blood pumped out of the heart with each contraction.

Cardiac output ($\dot{Q}$)

Heart rate multiplied by stroke volume; a measure of the overall performance of the heart.

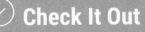 **Check It Out**

The following steps illustrate AFAA's recommended method of pulse taking.
- Locate the radial artery (AFAA preferred site) pulse within 2 to 4 seconds and find the beat of the heart.
- Begin with the count of "1" and continue counting the beats for 10 seconds.
- Multiply by 6 to determine exercise working heart rate.

It is important to continue moving the feet while taking the pulse in order to prevent lightheadedness or blood pooling in the extremities (especially individuals who are less fit or who may be taking anti-hypertension medication).

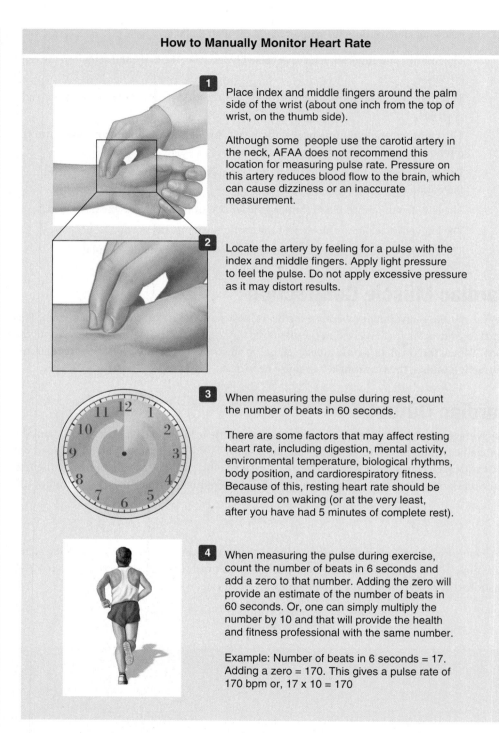

How to Manually Monitor Heart Rate

1. Place index and middle fingers around the palm side of the wrist (about one inch from the top of wrist, on the thumb side).

Although some people use the carotid artery in the neck, AFAA does not recommend this location for measuring pulse rate. Pressure on this artery reduces blood flow to the brain, which can cause dizziness or an inaccurate measurement.

2. Locate the artery by feeling for a pulse with the index and middle fingers. Apply light pressure to feel the pulse. Do not apply excessive pressure as it may distort results.

3. When measuring the pulse during rest, count the number of beats in 60 seconds.

There are some factors that may affect resting heart rate, including digestion, mental activity, environmental temperature, biological rhythms, body position, and cardiorespiratory fitness. Because of this, resting heart rate should be measured on waking (or at the very least, after you have had 5 minutes of complete rest).

4. When measuring the pulse during exercise, count the number of beats in 6 seconds and add a zero to that number. Adding the zero will provide an estimate of the number of beats in 60 seconds. Or, one can simply multiply the number by 10 and that will provide the health and fitness professional with the same number.

Example: Number of beats in 6 seconds = 17. Adding a zero = 170. This gives a pulse rate of 170 bpm or, 17 x 10 = 170

Figure 3.20
How to Manually Monitor Heart Rate

Blood

Oxygen and nutrients are delivered to the body via blood to help regulate body temperature, fight infections, and remove waste products. Thus, blood has three main functions: transportation, regulation, and protection (see **Table 3.11**).

Table 3.11

Support Mechanisms of Blood	
Mechanism	**Function**
Transportation	Transports oxygen and nutrients to tissues Transports waste products from tissues Transports hormones to organs and tissues Carries heat throughout the body
Regulation	Regulates body temperature and acid–base balance in the body
Protection	Protects the body from excessive bleeding by clotting Contains specialized immune cells to help fight disease and sickness

Table 3.12

Structures of the Respiratory Pump	
Bones	Sternum Ribs Vertebrae
Muscles: Inspiration	Diaphragm Exernal intercostals Scalenes Sternocleidomastoid Pectoralis minor
Muscles: Expiration	Internal intercostals Abdominals

⊘ Check It Out

There will be times when participants talk to the instructor and ask questions about specific medical conditions. This is outside of the scope of practice for a Group Fitness Instructor and should be referred to a medical provider.

Respiratory System

The respiratory system moves oxygen *in* and carbon dioxide *out* of the lungs. This is the function of breathing. The lungs pull oxygen into the bloodstream and push carbon dioxide from the bloodstream.

Breathing, or *ventilation*, is the process of moving air in and out of the body using all components of the respiratory pump (**Table 3.12**). Breathing in is called *inspiration* (or *inhalation*). It is an active process involving several muscles, including the following:

▼   Diaphragm

▼   External intercostals

Calorie

A scientific unit of energy.

Metabolism

All of the chemical reactions that occur in the body that are required for life.

▼   Scalenes

▼   Sternocleidomastoid

▼   Pectoralis minor

Respiratory Passages

The purpose of ventilation is to move air in and out of the body. There are two categories of respiratory passages: the conducting airways and the respiratory airways (**Table 3.13**, Figure 3.21).

Table 3.13

Structures of the Respiratory Passages		
Conducting Airways	Nasal cavity Oral cavity Pharynx Larynx	Trachea Right and left pulmonary bronchi Bronchioles
Respiratory airways	Alveoli Alveolar sacs	

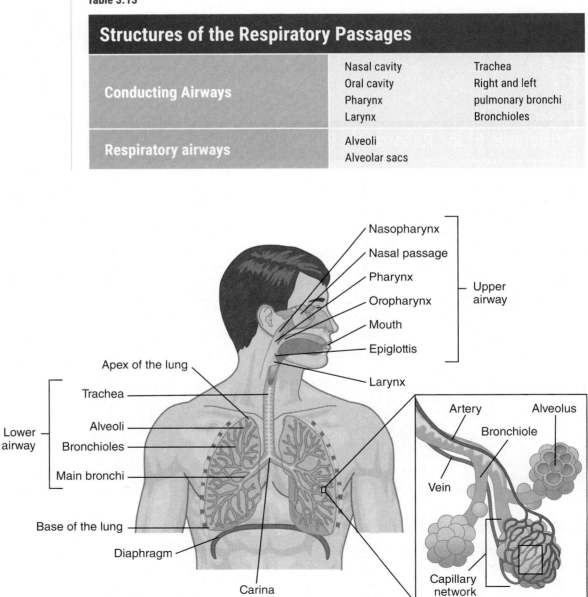

Figure 3.21
The Respiratory Passages

Metabolism and Bioenergetics

The body requires a constant input of energy to maintain basic life activities, such as contraction of the heart and the rise and fall of the lungs, as well as for movement.

Macronutrients (proteins, carbohydrates, and fats) are found in food and contain 4, 4, and 9 calories per gram, respectively. Although carbohydrates, fats, and proteins all provide calories, they do not provide usable energy simply by their ingestion. After food is ingested and the nutrients are absorbed, it must be transformed into usable energy.

Turning chemical energy into a form the body can use requires a series of chemical reactions called metabolism. Metabolism is the sum of biochemical reactions that occur in the cells of the body to obtain usable energy from food in the form of adenosine triphosphate (ATP).

Mitochondria is where most of the energy-producing activity occurs.[21] The associated processes are called metabolic pathways, and refer to a series of steps that work to break down or build up compounds in the body.

Pathways to Energy

There are three pathways by which ATP is produced, depending on the duration of activity and the availability of oxygen in the cells:

1. The ATP-phosphocreatine system
2. The glycolytic system
3. The oxidative system: aerobic glycolysis, Krebs cycle

Processes requiring oxygen are referred to as aerobic metabolism, while those that do not require oxygen are called anaerobic metabolism. The first pathway occurs during the initial 10 to 15 seconds of activity is anaerobic and is called the *ATP-phosphocreatine* (ATP-PC) system. This system is primarily utilized for activities that require high power or strength, such as sprinting.

Glycolysis, after ATP-PC has been used, is the second energy pathway and occurs during the first 2 to 3 minutes of activity. It utilizes glucose without the presence of oxygen (anaerobic) to create ATP. Any activity lasting beyond 2 to 3 minutes will use the third pathway, aerobic processes. Figure 3.22 and **Table 3.14** provide an overview of the different energy systems.

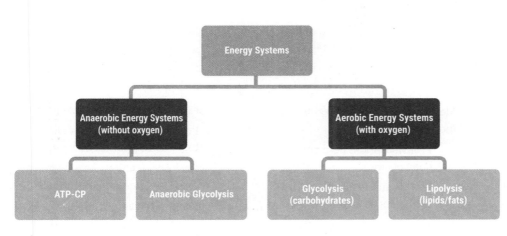

Figure 3.22
Energy Systems

Adenosine triphosphate (ATP)

Energy storage and transfer unit within the cells of the body.

Mitochondria

Organelle found in the cytoplasm of eukaryotic cells that contains genetic material and enzymes necessary for cell metabolism, converting food to energy.

Metabolic pathways

A series of chemical reactions that either break down or build up compounds in the body.

Aerobic metabolism

Chemical reactions in the body that require the presence of oxygen to extract energy from carbohydrates, fatty acids, and amino acids.

Anaerobic metabolism

Chemical reactions in the body that do not require the presence of oxygen to create energy through the combustion of carbohydrates.

Table 3.14

Pathways to Energy	
Pathway	**Description**
ATP-phosphocreatine (ATP-PC) System	• Occurs during the initial 10–15 seconds of activity • Anaerobic • Used for activities that require high power or strength
Glycolysis	• Occurs during the first 2–3 minutes of activity • Glucose without the presence of oxygen (anaerobic) to create ATP
Aerobic Processes	• Used in any activity lasting longer than 2–3 minutes

Summary

It is essential for Group Fitness Instructors to have a robust knowledge of the Human Movement System, the interactions of the kinetic chain, common areas of kinetic chain dysfunction, and other systems that support human movement. Understanding the Human Movement System gives an instructor the insight to create and provide programming that promotes muscular balance, optimal posture, and maximal movement efficiency. In other words, it helps instructors be more knowledgeable, professional, and capable to drive participant results through better planning, teaching, assessing, and motivating large groups of people.

Chapter in Review

- ▽ The Human Movement System: nervous, muscular, skeletal
    - ▪ CNS coordinates activity
    - ▪ PNS extends out through body
- ▽ Mechanoreceptors: GTO = tension; muscle spindle = length
    - ▪ Proprioception: perception of body position
    - ▪ Type I muscle fibers—slow-twitch, more aerobic
    - ▪ Type II muscle fibers—fast-twitch, more anaerobic

- ▽ Muscle movement:
    - ▪ Agonists—prime mover
    - ▪ Antagonists—oppose prime mover
    - ▪ Synergists—assist prime mover
- ▽ Force-couple: muscles working together to produce movement
- ▽ Reciprocal inhibition: antagonist relaxes while agonist contracts
- ▽ Length–tension relationships— muscle too short or long, produces less force.

- ▼ Axial skeleton: skull, spine, and ribs
- ▼ Appendicular skeleton: bones that support upper and lower extremities
- ▼ Joint motions: roll, slide, spin
- ▼ Cardiorespiratory system—cardiovascular (heart, vessels, blood); respiratory (lungs, airways)
  - ▪ Sinoatrial (SA) node—"pacemaker" for the heart
  - ▪ Veins bring blood *to* the heart; arteries move blood *away*
  - ▪ Blood functions: transportation, regulation, protection
  - ▪ "Respiratory pump" muscles for inspiration
  - ▪ Average adult heart rate = 70-80 bpm (to find: take pulse for 6 seconds, multiply by 10
- ▼ Energy systems:
  - ▪ ATP-PC—anaerobic; phosphocreatine; up to 15 seconds
  - ▪ Glycolysis—anaerobic; glucose; up to 3 minutes
  - ▪ Oxidative system—aerobic glycolysis; over 3 minutes

References

1. Tortora GJ, Grabowski SR. *Principles of Anatomy and Physiology*. 8th ed. New York, NY: HarperCollins; 1996.
2. Tortora GJ. *Principles of Human Anatomy*. 9th ed. New York, NY: John Wiley & Sons; 2001.
3. Levangie PK, Norkin CC. *Joint Structure and Function: A Comprehensive Analysis*. 5th ed. Philadelphia: F.A. Davis; 2011.
4. Watkins J. *Structure and Function of the Musculoskeletal System*. Champaign, IL: Human Kinetics; 1999.
5. Clark MA. *Integrated Training for the New Millennium*. Thousand Oaks, CA: National Academy of Sports Medicine; 2001.
6. Hamill J, Knutzen JM. *Biomechanical Basis of Human Movement*. 2nd ed. Baltimore, MD: Lippincott Williams & Wilkins; 2003.
7. Fox SI. *Human Physiology*. 9th ed. New York, NY: McGraw-Hill; 2006.
8. Luttgens K, Hamilton N. *Kinesiology: Scientific Basis of Human Motion*. 11th ed. New York, NY: McGraw-Hill; 2007.
9. Vander A, Sherman J, Luciano D. *Human Physiology: The Mechanisms of Body Function*. 9th ed. New York, NY: McGraw-Hill; 2003.
10. Milner-Brown A. *Neuromuscular Physiology*. Thousand Oaks, CA: National Academy of Sports Medicine; 2001.
11. Neumann D. *Kinesiology of the Musculoskeletal System: Foundations for Rehabilitation*. 2nd ed. St. Louis, MO: Mosby/Elsevier; 2010.
12. Kendall F, McCreary E, Provance P, Rodgers M, Romani W. *Muscles: Testing and Function with Posture and Pain*. 5th ed. Baltimore, MD: Lippincott Williams & Wilkins; 2005.
13. Clark MA. *A Scientific Approach to Understanding Kinetic Chain Dysfunction*. Thousand Oaks, CA: National Academy of Sports Medicine; 2001.
14. Rosário JLP, Diógenes MSB, Mattei R, Leite JR. Can sadness alter posture? *J Bodyw Mov Ther*. 2013;17(3):328–331.
15. Brooks GA, Fahey TD, White TP, Baldwin KM. *Exercise Physiology: Human Bioenergetics and Its Application*. 3rd ed. New York, NY: McGraw-Hill; 2000.
16. Hicks GH. *Cardiopulmonary Anatomy and Physiology*. Philadelphia, PA: W.B. Saunders; 2000.
17. Murray TD, Pulcipher JM. Cardiovascular anatomy. In: Roitman S, ed. *ACSM's Resource Manual for Guidelines for Exercise Testing and Prescription*. 4th ed. Baltimore, MD: Lippincott Williams & Wilkins; 2001:65–72.

18. Tortora GJ, Nielsen M. *Principles of Human Anatomy*. 11th ed. New York, NY: Wiley; 2008.

19. Franklin BA. Cardiovascular responses to exercise and training. In: Garrett WE, Kirkendall DT, eds. *Exercise and Sport Science*. Philadelphia, PA: Lippincott Williams & Wilkins; 2000:104–115.

20. Swain DP. Cardiorespiratory exercise prescription. In: Ehrman JK, ed. *ACSM's Resource Manual for Guidelines for Exercise Testing and Prescription*. 6th ed. Baltimore, MD: Lippincott Williams & Wilkins; 2006:448–462.

21. Hewlings SH, Medeiros DM. *Nutrition: Real people real choices*. Dubuque, IA: Kendall Hunt; 2011.

Chapter 4
Integrated Fitness

 Learning Objectives

4.1. **Describe** the role of integrated fitness in a group class environment.

4.2. **Identify** the various components of integrated fitness.

4.3. **Explain** various principles of applied fitness.

Introduction to Integrated Fitness

Integrated fitness is a comprehensive approach that combines multiple types of exercise to help a participant achieve higher levels of function. Some class formats will focus more heavily on one component than the rest, and some formats balance more than one component of integrated fitness. The components include:

- Flexibility
- Cardiorespiratory
- Core
- Balance
- Plyometric
- Resistance

and, in some instances,

- Speed, Agility, and Quickness

Function is an important component of an individual's everyday performance. It is defined as integrated, multiplanar movement that involves acceleration, stabilization, and deceleration. Integrated fitness addresses function with a well-rounded approach that meets everyday movement needs.

Many causes of movement dysfunction are related to everyday life; the less conditioned the musculoskeletal system is, the higher the risk of injury becomes.[1] Research suggests that musculoskeletal pain is more common now than 40 years ago.[2] An exercise regimen should address as many components of health-related physical fitness as possible. Common incorrect postural and movement patterns suggest the need for multiple components of integrated fitness. It is important to know these components as well as how they relate to someone's overall fitness.

Integrated fitness

Comprehensive approach combining all exercise components to help a participant achieve higher levels of function.

Function

Integrated, multiplanar movement that involves acceleration, stabilization, and deceleration.

Components of Integrated Fitness

Integrated fitness incorporates all forms of exercise as part of a progressive system, and includes flexibility, cardiorespiratory, core, balance, plyometric, speed, agility, and quickness (SAQ); and resistance training components. Its applications should be derived from goals and outcomes of each class.

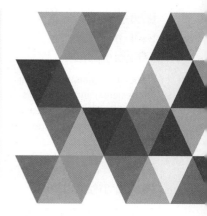

Movement Preparation

Movement preparation is often used interchangeably with *warm-up*, but it has more specific outcomes and purposes for the upcoming workout. A warm-up can be a few minutes of walking or jogging to bring the heart rate up, whereas movement prep takes into account specific exercises to assist in the improvement of movement efficiency, including flexibility, core, balance, plyometric, and, sometimes, SAQ.

Exercises should be chosen that best relate to the format being used. For example, if a resistance training class will be focusing on lower body, it is important to lengthen potentially tight muscles (such as the hip flexors) for full range of motion and glute activation during squatting and lunging. Similarly, in a martial arts-based class, the shoulders need to have full range of motion, and powerful arm and leg movements will require a strong core foundation. Flexibility in this class would focus on the muscles of the shoulder girdle, and a stabilization focus for the core should be incorporated in the movement prep segment.

Flexibility

Flexibility is defined as the normal extensibility of all soft tissue that allows for optimal range of motion (ROM) of a joint. Integrated flexibility incorporates different forms of flexibility (i.e., self-myofascial release [SMR], static, active, and dynamic stretching) based on class format, but SMR and static stretching are commonly used and include the following benefits:

▼ Correct muscle imbalances

▼ Increase joint range of motion

▼ Decrease muscle soreness

▼ Relieve joint stress

▼ Improve muscle extensibility

▼ Maintain the functional length of all muscles

An individual who does not have the proper extensibility and neuromuscular control around a joint will have limited exercise performance. For example, if a person's pectoralis major (chest) is too tight, the shoulder's range of motion is limited, creating internal rotation of the upper arm and lengthening the posterior deltoids. It can be seen during common exercises, such as a push-up. When a participant cannot fully retract his or her shoulder blades at the bottom of the movement and other muscles jump in to assist, it creates errors, such as the shoulders moving up and the head dropping down.

Two important mechanoreceptors involved in flexibility are muscle spindles (Figure 4.1) and the Golgi tendon organs (Figure 4.2).

When stretching a muscle, muscle spindles are stimulated to protect the muscle from stretching too far, causing the muscle to contract. As the stretch is held, more tension is created, stimulating the Golgi tendon organ, which overrides the muscle spindles, causing the muscle to relax. The tightness decreases and there is improved range of motion in proximal joints.

Neuromuscular control

Unconscious trained response of a muscle to a signal regarding dynamic joint stability.

Self-myofascial release (SMR)

Flexibility technique focusing on the neural and fascial systems of the body to decrease receptor excitation and release muscle tension.

Static stretching

A process of passively taking a muscle to the point of tension and holding the stretch for 30 seconds.

Active stretching

Flexibility exercises in which agonists move a limb through a full range of motion, allowing the antagonists to stretch.

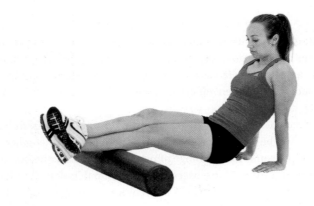

The same concept can be applied to the flexibility technique of self-myofascial release (SMR), commonly accomplished through foam rolling. In this technique, participants use their body weight to apply pressure to tender "knots" (adhesions) for 30 seconds to achieve the relaxation response.

Static stretching should be used in most circumstances because many people have muscle imbalances. Instructors may use active and dynamic stretching in groups of participants with few or no muscle imbalances. Active stretching allows an agonist and its synergists to move a limb

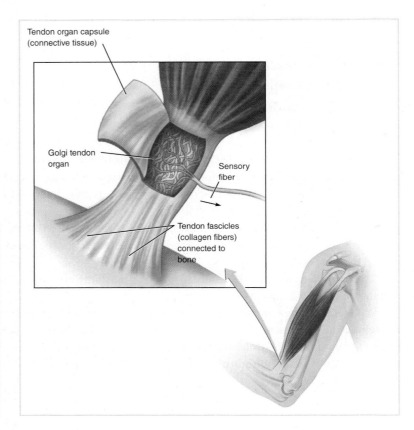

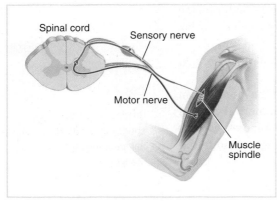

Figure 4.1
Muscle Spindles

Figure 4.2
Golgi Tendon Organs

through a full range of motion while the antagonists are being stretched. The stretch is held for 1 to 2 seconds at the end range of motion and then relaxed for the desired number of repetitions.

Dynamic stretching requires multiplanar extensibility control though a full range of motion at a higher speed. Examples of dynamic stretches include bodyweight squats or walking lunges with medicine ball rotation. Dynamic stretches should be reserved for advanced classes that have progressed to a more conditioned state.

Core Training

All movement begins with the core. Without adequate core activation, participants cannot harness the strength and power of their prime movers. Although core training might occur toward the end of a session as a "cool-down" or transition it is helpful to do core work at the *beginning* in order to send neural drive to the muscles for the more intense period of the class.

Structure and Function of the Core

Anatomically, the core is synonymous to what is termed the *lumbo-pelvic-hip complex* (LPHC). This is the area that lies between the inferior portion of the chest and the inferior portion of the gluteals. The core works to absorb and transfer forces to and from the upper and lower extremities. The core also helps to stabilize the lumbar spine, pelvis, and hips, protecting these regions from excessive stress and injury. Muscles of the core can be classified as either stabilization or movement, as seen in **Table 4.1**.

Activating the Core

Two activation methods often used are the *drawing-in maneuver* and *abdominal bracing*. Although each technique emphasizes the activation of one core system over the other (stabilization vs. movement system), both are crucial in ensuring optimal core stability and strength.

Dynamic stretching

Multiplanar extensibility with optimal neuromuscular control through a full range of motion.

Table 4.1

Stabilization and Movement Muscles	
Stabilization Muscles of the Core	**Movement Muscles of the Core**
• Transverse abdominis	• Latissimus dorsi
• Multifidus	• Hip flexors
• Internal oblique	• Hamstring complex
• Diaphragm	• Quadriceps
• Pelvic floor muscles	• Pectoralis major
• Rotator cuff	• Deltoid
• External obliques	• Gluteus maximus
• Quadratus lumborum	• Triceps
• Psoas major	• Biceps
• Rectus abdominis	• Erector spinae
• Gluteus medius	
• Adductor complex	

CAUTION ⚠

Take care with abdominal bracing, which can increase intra-abdominal pressure if participants hold their breath while bracing (Valsalva maneuver). This pressure can increase blood pressure and may cause fainting.

Practice This!

In order to experience the drawing-in maneuver, stand up and pull your navel toward your spine. Make sure you are looking in the mirror and there is no other external movement. You should have felt your stomach move away from the waist line of your clothing. This is the drawing-in movement.

The drawing-in maneuver is performed by drawing the navel back toward the spine without spinal flexion, like pulling the stomach in to button a pair of tight jeans. The premise behind the maneuver is that it contracts the transverse abdominis to form a corset to increase the segmental stability of the lumbar spine.[3] The maneuver also helps to activate the inner unit of the core, creating stability.[4,5]

The second technique to activate the core for optimal stability is abdominal bracing. Bracing is a co-contraction, commonly described as a "tightening," of the outer unit muscles. The premise behind this technique is that contraction of the more superficial core muscles (movement system) will improve lumbo-pelvic stiffness, which, in turn, will lead to spinal stability.

Balance Training

Proprioceptively enriched environments

Unstable, yet controllable environments.

Balance

Ability to maintain the body's center of gravity within its base of support.

Balance training simulates proprioceptively enriched environments (i.e., unstable, yet controlled), teaching the body how to recruit the right muscle, at the right time, with the right amount of force. A balance component can be added to any workout by making the base of support less stable—by standing on a balance plate or simply standing on one foot instead of two while performing upper body resistance exercises.

Importance of Balance Training

Static balance

Ability to maintain equilibrium in place with no external forces.

Regardless of the type of activity, balance is required to execute the task. Balance can be divided into two forms: static and dynamic. Static balance refers to the ability to maintain a static equilibrium through a perturbation while remaining still. Dynamic balance refers to the ability to maintain the intended path of motion following an external perturbation, or force placed on the moving body.

Balance is influenced by age, inactivity, and injury. As age increases, the ability to maintain postural control decreases. The task of maneuvering stairs can create a significant risk of injury for older adults, who may lack the ability to control their center of gravity, leading to a fall. The more inactive an individual is, the less efficient their nervous system will be at responding to unstable surfaces and maintaining center of gravity.

Perturbation

A disturbance of equilibrium; shaking.

Inefficient balance can create a pattern of overload and stress throughout the kinetic chain due to faulty movement patterns and compensations. Research supports the use of balance to increase postural stability and reduce the risk of injury.[6,7,8]

Science of Balance Training

Dynamic balance

Ability to maintain equilibrium through the intended path of motion when external forces are present.

The human body goes through a dynamic process of controlling its center of mass upon a continually changing base of support. Balance is a necessity because the body's base of support shifts with

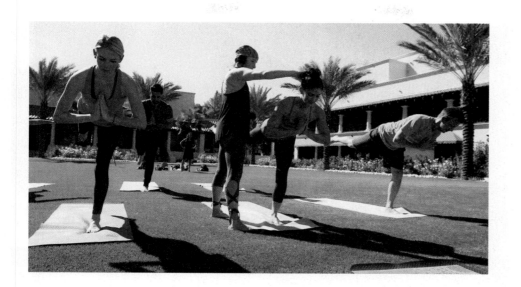

every step. To obtain postural control, the body uses a complex interaction among the muscular system, peripheral nervous system (PNS), and central nervous system (CNS).

The body controls posture through a series of complex processes that involve visual, vestibular, and proprioceptive inputs from the Human Movement System.[9,10] Maintaining postural equilibrium requires sensory detection of motion, sensorimotor integration, and the execution of appropriate musculoskeletal responses, all of which can be challenged during balance training to improve dynamic postural stability.[9,11]

Plyometric Training

Plyometric training enhances the rate of force production (i.e., the speed at which motor units are activated). Integrated plyometric training teaches the body how to respond at realistic speeds to changes in the environment encountered during functional activities. Most high-intensity formats, such as high-intensity interval training (HIIT) or kickboxing, have a robust reactive component due to the frequent jumping and landing movements used. Plyometric training can be used as part of movement prep in order to prepare the body for its application at greater intensities or can be used as the body of the workout in advanced classes.

Importance of Plyometric Training

Plyometric training is important because it develops a rapid, powerful neuromuscular response to allow safe movement at functionally applicable speeds. Plyometric training has been shown to provide benefits such as increased jumping ability, and rate of force development, as well as injury prevention.

Science of Plyometric Training

The neuromuscular system must react quickly and efficiently following deceleration in order to produce a contraction and impart the necessary force and acceleration in the appropriate direction.

Sensorimotor integration

Ability of the nervous system to gather and interpret information to anticipate and execute the proper motor response.

Plyometric training

Uses quick, powerful movements involving an eccentric contraction, followed immediately by an explosive concentric contraction.

Rate of force production

Ability of muscles to exert maximal force output in a minimal amount of time.

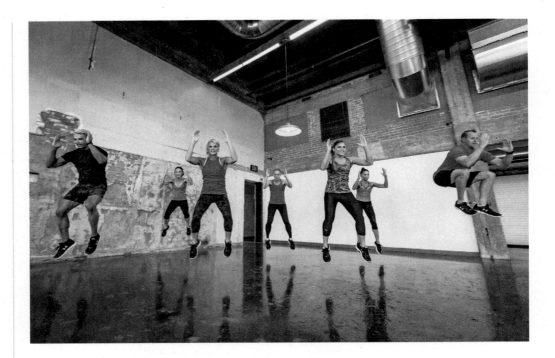

Integrated performance paradigm

A forceful cycle of muscle contraction that involves eccentric loading of the muscle, isometric muscle contraction, and concentric muscle contraction.

Speed

The straight-ahead velocity of an individual.

Agility

Ability to maintain center of gravity over a changing base of support while changing direction at various speeds.

Quickness

Ability to react to a stimulus with an appropriate muscular response without hesitation.

The goal of plyometric training is to improve this reaction time by improving neuromuscular efficiency and the range of speed set by the nervous system. The focus is on developing quick, powerful movements involving an eccentric contraction, followed immediately by an explosive concentric contraction. This is accomplished through the stretch–shortening cycle, also known as the integrated performance paradigm (Figure 4.3).

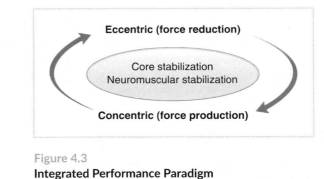

Figure 4.3
Integrated Performance Paradigm

SAQ Training

Integrated fitness includes Speed, Agility, and Quickness (SAQ) training has been used to prepare athletes for the demands of their sport. While in some instances a typical participant can benefit from SAQ training to improve their daily functioning and overall conditioning, most Group Fitness Instructors will use SAQ sparingly based on class format.

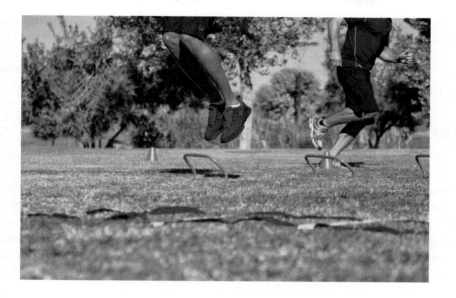

Cardiorespiratory Training

The following are the most common goals of cardiorespiratory training:

▼ To reduce cardiovascular risk factors (e.g., unhealthy body composition, poor blood lipid profile, high blood pressure)

▼ To assist in weight management

▼ To improve performance in work, life, and sports

▼ To reduce mental anxiety

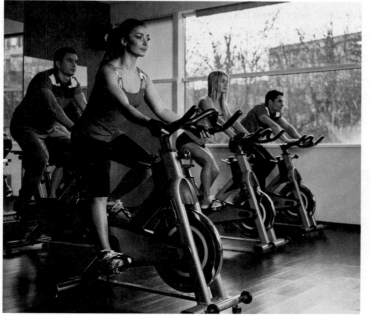

© Stasique/Shutterstock

Anaerobic threshold

The point during high-intensity activity when the body can no longer meet its demand for oxygen and anaerobic metabolism predominates; also called the *lactate threshold*.

Interval training

Training that alternates between intense exertion and periods of rest or lighter exertion.

Resting heart rate (RHR)

Number of contractions of the heart occurring in 1 minute while the body is at rest.

Stabilization

Body's ability to remain stable and balanced over the center of gravity in a changing environment.

To meet the goals outlined above, cardiorespiratory training must train *both* the aerobic energy system *and* the anaerobic energy system, especially for participants who constantly switch between their aerobic and anaerobic energy systems, maximizing performance and minimizing fatigue. This type of conditioning is referred to as *interval training* and is the foundation for group formats such as HIIT.

Interval and Zone Training

To achieve the desired physical and physiological adaptations of cardiorespiratory overload, zone training may be employed (**Table 4.2**). Zone 1 consists of an individual maintaining a training heart rate of approximately 65–75% of his or her maximum heart rate (HR_{max}). This zone is referred to as the recovery, or cardio base, zone. Participants who stay in this zone without variation will initially improve, but will plateau.

Zone 2 is close to a person's anaerobic threshold at 76–85% of HR_{max}. In this zone, the body can no longer produce enough energy for the working muscles with just the aerobic energy system. Thus, one of the main goals of cardiorespiratory training is to increase the anaerobic threshold. However, as with Zone 1, if a participant continues to only train in this zone, plateaus will occur. To improve fitness level or increase metabolism, the participant must overload the body and transition to Zone 3 training.

Zone 3 approaches peak exertion levels; a true high-intensity workout reaches 90% of HR_{max}, which may require several short sprints. Participants should exercise in Zone 3 for 30–60 seconds and then recover in Zones 1 or 2 before repeating (i.e., interval training). For most individuals, exercising in Zone 3 once per week is enough to obtain the benefits without overtraining.

Preventing Overtraining

A participant's resting heart rate (RHR) can be used to determine if the participant is being over-trained. Participants and instructors can use the following steps to determine the onset of overtraining:

1. For five days, record true RHR (i.e., heart rate upon waking in the morning)
2. Calculate the average RHR for that time period
3. Record resting pulse in a fitness setting
4. Fitness resting pulse should be no more than 8 bpm higher than that of the time recorded

Table 4.2

Cardio Training Zones	
Zone	**Training Heart Rate**
One	65–75% of HR_{max}
Two	76–85% of HR_{max}
Three	86–90% of HR_{max}

Resistance Training

Resistance training is an integral part of disease and injury prevention. Resistance training programming comes with four major adaptations: stabilization endurance, strength, hypertrophy, and power.

Stabilization Endurance

Stabilization endurance adaptations require the recruitment of tissues in the body responsible for postural stability (primarily type I muscle fibers). Type I muscle fibers are slow to fatigue and are important for long-term contractions required for postural control and stabilization. These muscle fibers are emphasized in training for stabilization endurance. Research has shown that resistance training protocols with higher repetition ranges and lower loads demonstrate a greater propensity for improving measures of local muscular endurance.[12]

Creating muscular endurance is critical to increasing core and joint stabilization because these muscles need to have the ability to fire over prolonged periods of time. Without this, one cannot effectively build muscle size, strength, and power.

Strength

The ability of the neuromuscular system to provide internal tension and exert force against external resistance is strength. Strength gains can occur rapidly in beginning participants and can increase with a structured, progressive resistance training program.

Skeletal muscle fiber enlargement (hypertrophy) occurs as a response to increased volumes of tension created by resistance training. Resistance training protocols use low to intermediate repetition ranges with progressive overload to create changes in measures of hypertrophy. Structured, progressive resistance training programs, using multiple sets, will help to increase hypertrophy.[12]

Power

The ability to react, explode, and jump all rely on the body's ability to generate the greatest possible force in the shortest amount of time. Power is defined as the neuromuscular system's ability to increase the rate of force production (i.e., the speed at which the motor units are activated). Power depends on stabilization and strength because it requires neuromuscular efficiency (as gained through stabilization adaptations) and increased motor unit activation (as gained through strength adaptations). Power can be enhanced through an increase in force or an increase in speed: The higher the force (heavier load), the slower the movement, and vice versa. To maximize this type of training, both heavy and light loads must be moved as fast as possible to create the adaptation of power.[13,14]

Principles of Applied Fitness

The General Adaptation Syndrome (GAS), the principle of specificity, the overload principle, and concept of periodization are scientific principles of fitness. When understood and correctly applied, physical and physiological adaptations occur.

Strength

Ability of the neuromuscular system to provide internal tension and exert force against external resistance.

Power

Ability to produce a large amount of force in a short amount of time.

General adaptation syndrome

Kinetic chain response and adaptation to imposed demands and stress.

Principle of specificity

States that the type of exercise stimulus placed on the body will determine the expected physiological outcome.

Principle of overload

To create physiological changes, an exercise stimulus must be applied at an intensity greater than the body is accustomed to receiving.

Periodization

Division of a training program into smaller, progressive stages.

Alarm phase

First stage of the GAS; the initial phase of response to a new stimuli within the Human Movement System.

Adaptation phase

Second stage of the GAS in which physiological changes take place in order to meet the demands of the newly imposed stress.

Exhaustion phase

Third stage of the GAS in which stress continues beyond the body's ability to adapt, leading to potential physiological and structural breakdown.

Overtraining syndrome (OTS)

Excessive frequency, volume, or intensity of training, resulting in fatigue.

MEMORY TIP

Think of the alarm phase as an alarm clock. The alarm phase wakes your body up and alerts the kinetic chain to a new stimulus, much as an alarm clock wakes you up and alerts you to a new day.

General Adaptation Syndrome

The Human Movement System adapts to the demands imposed by physical activity through the General Adaptation Syndrome. Exercise places physical stress on the body involving three phases:[15]

1. Alarm phase: The alarm phase, also referred to as the *shock phase*, is the initial response to the imposed demands of exercise, lasting approximately 2–3 weeks.

2. Adaptation phase: In the adaptation, or resistance, phase, the body adapts to the applied stimuli by changing structures within the human body and their physiological function. This phase is characterized by progressive improvements in strength and can last approximately 4–12 weeks after the introduction of the training stress.

3. Exhaustion phase: In this phase, the body can no longer tolerate the physiological stresses and imposed demands of the applied training stimulus. Once an individual has reached the exhaustion phase, further adaptations may halt, and the risk of overtraining increases. Overtraining syndrome (OTS), sometimes described as being "under-recovered," can affect various parts of the kinetic chain. OTS can lead to a host of physiological problems, including recurring illness, loss of sleep, moodiness, decreased physical performance, and overuse injuries.

The GAS establishes the rationale for changing acute variables on a regular basis.

Principle of Specificity

The Human Movement System will adapt and change in response to the specific types of movement, and applications of those movements is known as the *principle of specificity* (also referred to as the Specific Adaptation to Imposed Demands (SAID) principle). This principle states the type of exercise stimulus placed on the body will determine the expected physiological outcome. Each system of the body (e.g., neural, endocrine, muscular, skeletal, etc.) will respond and adapt to the specific physical demands applied.

Types of Specificity

The three types of specificity the body will adapt and respond to are mechanical, neuromuscular, and metabolic. Achieving specific results may require adjustment of any or all three.

1. **Mechanical specificity** refers to the weight and movements placed on the body. For example, to develop endurance in the legs, lighter weights would be used with a higher number of repetitions.

2. **Neuromuscular specificity** refers to specific exercises using different speeds and movement patterns performed. For example, to increase power, high-speed exercises are used to develop the ability to contract muscle fibers as fast as possible.

3. **Metabolic specificity** refers to the energy demand placed on the body. In endurance events, it is important for the body to efficiently utilize the aerobic energy system.

Overload Principle

To create physiological changes, an exercise stimulus must be applied at an intensity greater than the system is accustomed to receiving—thus the overload principle. This increased stimulus results in the system adapting to the increased demands, and providing a desired change. When the body is not overloaded, it does not change.

Adjusting the acute variables will provide the added stimulus needed to overload the system and push it out of homeostasis. Group Fitness Instructors should therefore change a workout routine after a certain number of sessions.[16-18]

Periodization

Periodization refers to the planned changes in the acute variables of the exercise program over a designated period of time. The planned changes are designed to result in physical changes that align with participants' goals. One of the most important aspects of periodization is to prevent injuries due to overtraining.

A Group Fitness Instructor teaching a strength class could apply periodization on a weekly, monthly, or even bi-monthly basis, changing up the exercises and movements so regular participants do not end up doing the same routine over and over. Or, in the case of a weight-loss boot camp, the class could be periodized over three separate 9-week cycles, each becoming progressively more advanced than the last.

Acute Variables

Each element of an integrated fitness program is based on training areas of the body essential for daily function (e.g., the stabilizing muscles of the hips, trunk, and neck) and proper progression of acute variables (e.g., sets, repetitions, and rest periods).

The acute variables determine the amount and kind of stress placed on the body, and what changes the body will experience. The most commonly addressed acute variables are: exercise selection, load (weight/resistance) and intensity, volume (repetitions × sets), rest periods, and tempo.[19]

Volume

Training volume is the total amount of work performed within a specified time. Training volume is typically the number of repetitions multiplied by the number of sets in a group class. More training volume leads to better strength adaptations.

Acute variables

Components that specify how each exercise is to be performed.

Set

A group of consecutive repetitions.

Repetition

One complete movement of a single exercise.

Rest period

The time taken between sets or exercises to rest or recover.

Training volume

The total amount of work performed within a specified time; number of repetitions multiplied by the number of sets in a training session.

⊘ Check It Out

Load vs. Volume:
As the load increases, the number of repetitions decreases.

Load vs. Rest Period:
As load or intensity increases, the rest period must also increase. This is due to the amount of adenosine triphosphate (ATP) accessible to the muscles during activity.

INSTRUCTOR TIP 👍

A benefit of using slow tempo is helping the participant be aware of and correct their form. Slowing down helps reinforce good movement patterns to allow the use of faster tempo later on.

Load

Amount of weight lifted or resistance used during training.

Training intensity

An individual's level of effort, compared with his or her maximal effort; usually expressed as a percentage.

Exercise Tempo

Repetition tempo refers to the speed with which each repetition is performed (**Table 4.3**). This is an important variable for achieving specific training goals such as endurance, muscle growth, strength, and power. The movement occurs at different speeds in order to get the appropriate results from the training.

Slower training tempos are better for increasing endurance and initially developing motor control. A slower tempo, especially during eccentric contractions, is recommended for stabilization endurance training and with untrained individuals.

Tempo is listed with three numbers representing the eccentric/isometric/concentric (E/I/C) phases of an exercises (for example: 2/1/1, 2/0/2, and so on). The first number represents the seconds for the eccentric portion (**E**/I/C) of the exercise. The middle number represents an isometric hold at the transition point of the exercise (E/**I**/C). The last number represents the number of seconds spent on the concentric portion of the exercise (E/I/**C**). The tempo x/x/x indicates the exercise should be performed as fast as can be controlled.

Load and Intensity

Load is the amount of weight lifted, or resistance used, during an exercise. Training intensity is an individual's level of effort compared to his or her maximal effort, usually represented as a percentage of the estimated one-repetition maximum (1RM) for a strength class or the estimated maximal heart rate for a cardio class. The load or training intensity used is dependent on several other acute variables (**Table 4.4**).

Table 4.3

Assigned Tempos for Adaptations of Integrated Fitness			
Speed	**Exercise Tempo (E/I/C)**	**Exercise Tempo with Music (E/C)**	**Adaptation**
Slow	4/2/1	3/1	Endurance
Moderate	2/0/2	2/2	Strength
Fast	x/x/x	1/1 or ½/½	Maximal strength, Power

Table 4.4

Load vs. Intensity	
As Load Increases	**As Load Decreases**
Volume decreases	Volume increases
Rest period increases	Rest period decreases

Table 4.5

Rest Period and Percent Recovery	
Amount of Rest	**Percent Recovery**
20–30 seconds	50%
40 seconds	75%
60 seconds	85–90%
3–5 minutes	100%

Rest Periods

A rest period is the time taken between sets or exercises to rest or recover. The amount of time taken for rest can influence the adaptations and response to exercise. Rest periods are directly related to bioenergetic pathways and energy production, and are indirectly related to load and training intensity. Exercises at lower intensity can be performed for longer periods of time because the body is able to use oxygen, and therefore does not require much rest to recover. When exercises are performed at much higher intensity for shorter periods of time, the body is not able to use oxygen and energy stores are quickly depleted; thus, the body requires longer rest periods. **Table 4.5** provides estimated recovery times following depletion of ATP.[20]

Exercise Selection

Exercise selection is the process of choosing exercises that allow for achievement of the desired change, or adaptation. Exercises should be specific to the desired outcome of the class. Choice of exercise determines the muscle groups to be worked, the position in which they will be worked, and the component of integrated fitness being developed.

Summary

Robust understanding of the components of integrated fitness enables Group Fitness Instructors to design and implement effective class formats. Regardless of format, all components of integrated fitness can be incorporated into each workout to ensure good results and reduce the risk of injury. By manipulating the acute variables of each exercise selected, group fitness classes can be tailored to meet participants' goals.

Chapter in Review

▼ Integrated Fitness: combines components of exercise for optimum performance

▼ Components of Integrated Fitness:
  ▪ Flexibility: increases ROM, relieves joint stress, improves extensibility

Exercise selection

Process of choosing exercises that allow for achievement of the desired adaptation.

INSTRUCTOR TIP 👍

Think about the *why* behind building a class, and select exercises that best support the class objective. Share that objective with the class, and then connect the purpose of each exercise to it.

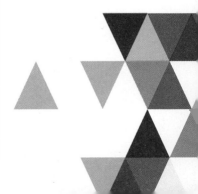

- Cardiorespiratory: reduces cardiovascular risk, improves performance
- Core: stabilization, protects body from stress and injury
- Balance: improves postural stability, reduces risk of injury
- Plyometric (reactive): improves response to changes in environment
- Resistance: postural stability, improves strength, reaction time, and ability to produce force
- Speed, Agility, and Quickness (SAQ): improves daily functioning and overall conditioning

▼ Movement preparation (warm-up): improves movement efficiency

▼ Principles of Applied Fitness
- GAS: response to stimuli(alarm, adaptation, exhaustion, overtraining syndrome)
- Principle of Specificity (SAID): type of stimulus will determine physiological outcome
- Overload: to create change, stimulus must be greater in intensity

▼ Acute variables
- Volume
- Tempo
- Load/Intensity
- Rest
- Exercise selection

References

1. Barr KP, Griggs M, Cadby T. Lumbar stabilization: Core concepts and current literature, part 1. *Am J Phys Med Rehabil.* 2005;84(6):473–480.
2. Harkness EF, Macfarlane GJ, Silman AJ, McBeth J. Is musculoskeletal pain more common now than 40 years ago? Two population-based cross-sectional studies. *Rheumatology (Oxford).* 2005;44(7):890–895.
3. Hodges PW, Richardson CA. Feedforward contraction of transverse abdominis is not influenced by the direction of arm movement. *Exp. Brain Res.* 1997;114:362–370.
4. Aroski JP, Valta T, Airaksinen O, Kankaanpää M. Back and abdominal muscle function during stabilization exercises. *Arch Phys Med Rehab.* 2001;82(8):1089–1098.
5. Hodges PW, Richardson CA. Contraction of the abdominal muscles associated with movement of the lower limb. *Phys. Ther.* 1997;77:132–142.
6. Hewett TE, Lindenfeld TN, Riccobene JV, Noyes FR. The effect of neuromuscular training on the incidence of knee injury in female athletes: a prospective study. *Am J Sports Med.* 1999;27(6):699–706.
7. Olsen OE, Myklebust G, Engebretsen L, Holme I, Bahr R. Exercises to prevent lower limb injuries in youth sports: Cluster randomised controlled trial. *BMJ.* 2005:330(7489):449.
8. Wedderkopp N, Kaltoft M, Holm R, Froberg K. Comparison of two intervention programmes in young female players in European handball—with and without ankle disc. *Scand J Med Sci Sports.* 2003;13(6):371–375.
9. Lephart SM, Riemann BL, Fu FH. Introduction to the sensorimotor system. In: Lephart SM, Fu FH, eds. *Proprioception and Neuromuscular Control in Joint Stability.* Champaign, IL: Human Kinetics; 2000.
10. Riemann BL, Lephart SM. The sensorimotor system, part I: The physiologic basis of functional joint stability. *J Athl Train.* 2002;37(1):71–79.
11. Peterka RJ. Sensorimotor integration in human postural control. *J Neurophysiol.* 2002;88(3):1097–1118.
12. Campos GE, Luecke TJ, Wendeln HK, et al. Muscular adaptations to three different resistance training regimens: Specificity of repetition maximum training zones. *Eur J Appl Physiol.* 2002;88(1–2):50–60.

13. Ebben WP, Watts PB. A review of combined weight training and plyometric training modes: Complex training. *Strength Cond J*. 1998;20(5):18–27.

14. Hoffman JR, Ratamess NA, Cooper JJ, Kang J, Chilakos A, Faigenbaum AD. Comparison of loaded and unloaded jump squat training on strength/power performance in college football players. *J. Strength Cond. Res*. 2005;19(4):810–815.

15. Selye H. *The Stress of Life*. New York, NY: McGraw-Hill; 1976.

16. de Hoyo M, Pozzo M, Sañudo B, et al. Effects of a 10-week in-season eccentric-overload training program on muscle-injury prevention and performance in junior elite soccer players. *Int J Sports Physiol. Perform*. 2015;10(1):46–52.

17. Ramírez-Campillo R, Henríquez-Olguín C, Burgos C, et al. Effect of progressive volume-based overload during plyometric training on explosive and endurance performance in young soccer players. *J Strength Cond Res*. 2015;29(7):1884–1893.

18. Tous-Fajardo J, Gonzalo-Skok O, Arjol-Serrano JL, Tesch P. Change of direction speed in soccer players is enhanced by functional inertial eccentric overload and vibration training. *Int J Sports Physiol. Perform*. 2015;11(1):66–73.

19. Hayes LD, Bickerstaff GF, Baker, JS. Acute response exercise program variables and subsequent hormonal response. *J Sports Med. Doping Stud*. 2013;3(2):1–10.

20. Harris RC, Edwards RH, Hultman E, Nordesjö LO, Nylind B, Sahlin K. The time course of phosphorylcreatine resynthesis during recovery of the quadriceps muscle in man. *Pflugers Arch*. 1976;28(367):137–142.

Chapter 5
Teaching Basics

Learning Objectives

5.1. **Identify** the five components of a workout.

5.2. **Describe** general considerations for various group fitness formats.

5.3. **Explain** the components of a workout in relation to various formats.

Introduction

Instructor engagement with participants and explanation of the workout and class expectations.

Movement prep

Activities to increase body temperature and prime the body for workout demands.

Body of workout

Majority of the fitness class; activities with a singular or integrated focus on cardio-respiratory fitness, muscular strength, muscular endurance, flexibility, or mindfulness.

Transition

Safely takes participants through the gradual physiological change from exertion to rest.

Outro

Final class segment to conclude the workout, praise participants' effort, and invite participants back for the next session.

Workout Design Considerations

Today's Group Fitness Instructors need to be prepared to teach movement, demonstrate proper form, and deliver appealing classes to a variety of fitness levels and formats. Approaches to help an instructor achieve goals can vary widely based on class format. Popular class designs help promote education, workout success, and long-term exercise adherence. The implementation of a safe and effective group fitness class follows an established organizational format.

AFAA recommends incorporation of five components that work together to create a connected, holistic workout experience. The five components vary in time and complexity, though each is important for the implementation of a safe and effective group workout. The five components of class design are:

1. Introduction
2. Movement prep
3. Body of workout
4. Transition
5. Outro

The Introduction

The introduction should be succinct, yet informative, to capture the attention of the participant. A good introduction should be no more than 60 seconds and include:

▾ a warm welcome.

▾ the instructor's name and class title.

▾ an overview of the workout and equipment.

▾ a motivating segue into movement prep.

⊘ **Check It Out**

A smooth introduction should flow something like this:

"Hi everyone, welcome! My name is ____, and I'll be your instructor for 'Strength 101.' We're going to start with some movement prep and core work; do 45 minutes of strength training with dumbbells and kettlebells, and then finish with some flexibility. The goal is to increase your strength and burn calories. It's going to challenge you, but I'll coach you every step of the way. Let's get started!"

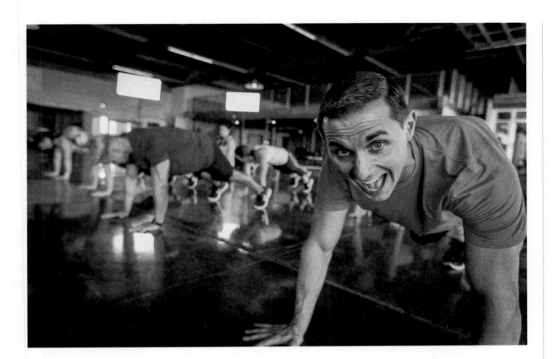

**General
movement prep**

Consists of simple, move-
ments of integrated fitness
(such as flexibility, core,
and balance) to gradually
increase intensity.

**Format-specific
movement prep**

Activities that initiate
body-of-the-workout
movements at a lower
intensity and/or complexity.

Movement Prep

To reduce the risk of injury, preview upcoming movements, and move participants from resting to steady state, movement prep should be applied after the class introduction. This also might be called *warm-up*. Efficient movement prep should:

▼   Increase the core body temperature

▼   Increase blood flow and breathing rate

▼   Prime the body for the class movements

Typically, movement prep will include elements of integrated fitness such as flexibility, core, balance, and (if appropriate) plyometric. Depending on class format, these can be used as long as the intended outcome is aligned with the goals of movement prep. If possible, movement prep should incorporate all three planes of motion to ensure the body is prepared for dynamic, multi-planar movements.

General movement prep consists of simple, movements of integrated fitness (such as flexibility, core, and balance) to gradually increase intensity. Formats such as strength, dance, and HIIT benefit from a combined movement prep approach that progresses from general movement prep to *format-specific movement prep*. Other formats (such as cycling, yoga, and aqua) use only format-specific movement prep.

Format-specific movement prep introduces base movements and establishes coordination requirements unique to a specific format, such as a down stroke in cycling or a punch combo breakdown in kickboxing. These movements should be introduced at a slower pace and smaller range of motion. Format-specific movement prep, like general movement prep, also reduces the risk of injury and promotes movement efficiency but has the added benefit of providing participants with increased skill and confidence needed to master more complex movements.

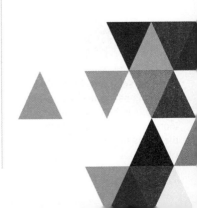

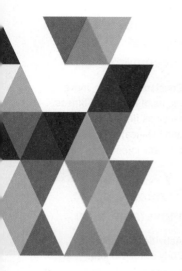

Check It Out

General-to-format specific movement prep in a kickboxing class begins with an instructor incorporating general movement prep activities such as stretching the hip flexors and lats and performing planks and roundhouse kick chambers (for balance). Then the instructor can introduce format-specific movements and combinations such as punches, jabs, upper cuts, and hooks.

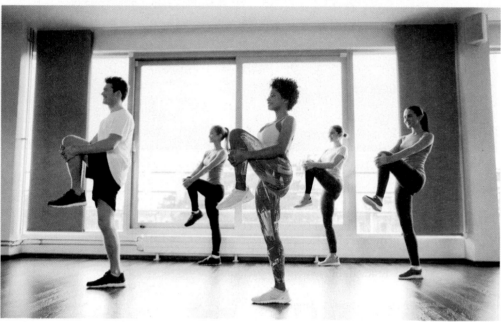

© Syda Productions/Shutterstock

Rating of perceived exertion (RPE)

A technique used to express or validate how hard a participant feels he or she is working during exercise.

INSTRUCTOR TIP 👍

Allow time to transition between supine and standing positions as it can cause a decrease in blood pressure, increase heart rate, and cause dizziness in participants (Tse, et al., 2005).

Body of the Workout

The focus of the class format occurs during the body of the workout. At this point, exercises and combinations can be executed at full intensity. The workout body should be designed with a specific population or goal in mind but must also be adjusted to meet the needs of the actual participants. Because the body of the workout takes up the majority of time, it takes the most effort in planning.

The body of the workout may be focused on a single outcome or a combination of outcomes, such as:

- ▼ Achieving or maintaining a certain heart rate or rating of perceived exertion (RPE) level
- ▼ Completing a specific choreography pattern
- ▼ Performing a certain number or sets, reps, or intervals
- ▼ Burning an approximate number of calories
- ▼ Dissipating stress or anxiety
- ▼ Practicing athletic skills

Monitoring Intensity

Instructors need to monitor the work intensity of participants, specifically in the body of the workout. Participants of various fitness levels need benchmarks of how hard they should be working at different points in the class so they can pace themselves and complete the experience. Instructors can choose from several ways to educate the group on how to self-monitor intensity.

RPE

The rating of perceived exertion (RPE) is a subjective technique for participants to evaluate how hard they are working based on the overall physical sensations a during physical activity, including increased heart rate, respiration rate, sweating, and muscle fatigue.

There are two versions of the RPE scale. The first is the Borg Scale (Figure 5.1), based on a 6–20 rating scale associated with heart rates. Based on the rating, participants add a 0 to the end of their number. This creates a subjective estimate of their heart beats per minute. The average adult has a resting heart rate of 70–80 bpm, making this a representation of where a participant's heart rate might be before the workout begins. If the 6–20 Borg scale is difficult for participants to understand, it may be easier for a participant to use a modified Borg scale using the numbers 0–10 (**Table 5.1**). In this case, 5–6 would equate to "hard," 7–9 to "very hard," and 10 to "extremely hard" and "maximal exertion."

6	No exertion at all
7	Extremely light
8	
9	Very light
10	
11	Light
12	
13	Somewhat hard
14	
15	Hard (heavy)
16	
17	Very hard
18	
19	Extremely hard
20	Maximal exertion

Figure 5.1

Rating of Perceived Exertion (Borg Scale)

Table 5.1

The 0–10 RPE Scale

Rating	Description
0	Nothing at all
1	Very light
2	Fairly light
3	Moderate
4	Somewhat hard
5	Hard
6	
7	
8	Very hard
9	
10	Very, very hard (Maximal)

Table 5.2

Methods for Recommending Exercise Intensity	
Method	**Formula**
Peak $\dot{V}O_2$	Target $\dot{V}O_2 = \dot{V}O_{2max} \times$ intensity desired
Peak heart rate (HR)	Target HR (THR) = $HR_{max} \times$ % intensity desired
Heart rate reserve (HRR)	Target heart rate (THR) = $[(HR_{max} - HR_{rest}) \times$ % intensity desired] $+ HR_{rest}$
Ratings of perceived exertion (RPE)	6- to 20-point scale
Talk test	The ability to speak during activity can identify exercise intensity and ventilatory threshold

If an exercise feels too easy, it likely is. Therefore, if the perceived intensity is low, a participant will realize they can increase their effort level. Participants can use either of the perceived exertion scales to establish exercise intensity at the start of the class, and continue to monitor throughout the workout.

Talk Test

The talk test is another way to estimate intensity of effort and is helpful in classes that reach near-maximal exertion. The foundation of this scale implies if a participant is working so hard they can't speak, the intensity is too high.

A number of studies have reported a correlation among the talk test, oxygen consumption ($\dot{V}O_2$), the ventilatory threshold (T_{vent}), and heart rate during exercise.[1,2] A summary of the methods for recommending exercise intensity is provided in **Table 5.2**.

Dyspnea Scale

This method uses a subjective scale to represent how participants perceive their relative difficulty in terms of breathing (dyspnea refers to difficulty breathing).

- ▼ +1 Mild and noticeable to participant, but not to an observer
- ▼ +2 Mild, with some difficulty noticeable to an observer
- ▼ +3 Moderate difficulty, but participant can continue to exercise
- ▼ +4 Severe difficulty, and the participant must stop exercising at that level

This scale is helpful for participants who have pulmonary conditions (such as asthma or emphysema) or who feel limited because of breathing difficulties. The scale should be used in

INSTRUCTOR TIP 👍

Try this cue to determine if participants are training at the correct intensity using the talk test: "For this effort I am looking for all-out intensity. You could not sustain this intensity for longer than 30 seconds, and if you had to talk, you would be breathless. This rate of intensity should be a 9 or a 10 on a 0-to-10 scale."

Perceived intensity

Perceived exertion is used by participants to guide participants in subjectively defining their training intensity.

Talk test

A self-evaluation of intensity associated with the ability to talk while exercising.

conjunction with RPE and HR, and participants should reduce intensity when their breathing becomes more labored (+3). Participants with breathing difficulties should consult with their primary care physician regarding their exercise goals and methods.

Dyspnea

Difficulty or troubled breathing

Observation

Observing participants in a class is another way to monitor intensity levels. Normal physical reactions to exercise include increased breathing rate, sweating, and a red face from increased blood flow to the surface of the skin. Signs a participant might be overexerting themselves include rapid breathing; becoming disoriented, dizzy, or lightheaded; losing color in his or her face; and lack of sweating. These physical signs could indicate a medical issue and should be addressed immediately.

Transition

The transition component of the class offers a steady, gradual change in intensity. The transition is focused on a downward trajectory, and it is sometimes referred to as cool-down. The overall objectives of the transition are:

- ▼ Reduce workout intensity to pre-workout levels
- ▼ Complete the experience (start-to-finish connectivity).

Flexibility is a common component in the transition section of class. Group Fitness Instructors should include static or SMR-based movements to improve joint range of motion, increase muscle length, and promote relaxation and recovery.[3]

Transitions should be paced to allow adequate time for the body to safely move out of an exercising state and into a resting state. The transition should be about the same length as the movement prep segment. Transitioning too quickly from intense movement can cause dizziness, lightheadedness, and even fainting.

Outro

The outro only takes moments and should leave an impression on participants. Exercise is not easy for most people and time is valuable, so participants in a class deserve praise. A few words at the end can shape a positive view of exercise and fitness. The outro should be brief (about the same time as the intro) and cover the following points:

- ▼ Confirmation the workout is complete
- ▼ Compliments or positive statements on effort in class
- ▼ Invitation to come back
- ▼ Request for participants to provide feedback and ask questions

INSTRUCTOR TIP 👍

A positive outro might flow something like this:
"We're done! You did great today, especially hitting your target heart rate zones when you needed to. Please come see me with questions or feedback. Have a great day, and see you next week!"

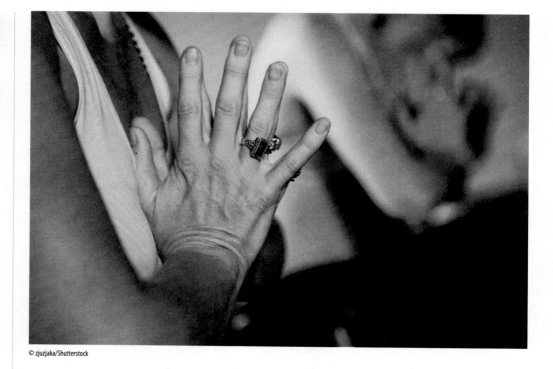

© zjuzjaka/Shutterstock

Maintaining Class Flow

Cohesive group fitness experiences have a plan that provides a safe and efficient route. To do this, the Group Fitness Instructor should work backward, starting with the class vision and then determining *how* the vision will be accomplished, as discussed in other chapters.

Group Fitness Instructors follow a roadmap that covers the *journey* and the *destination* for each class. The *destination* involves the overall purpose of the class (cardio, flexibility, strength, etc.). The *journey* is the experience that flows, motivates, and makes sense to the participant. Leading successful group fitness experiences involves creating a structured plan and implementing it in a smooth, connected manner, called flow. Flow refers to the Group Fitness Instructor's ability to connect all five components of workout design to accomplish a goal.

Efficient flow allows participants to be focused on following directions and enjoying the workout. Instructors can master class flow with the following techniques:

- ▽ Planning
- ▽ Practice
- ▽ Preparation
- ▽ Modifications
- ▽ Presentation personality

Flow

Instructor's ability to create a seamless experience from start to finish.

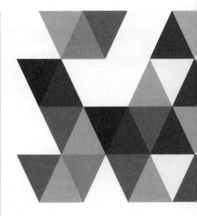

Workout Components for General Class Formats

Although the five components of a group fitness class will remain the same, the delivery method will change depending on the type of format and design. Freestyle and pre-designed classes have common considerations and applications for general formats which are listed in this section.

The Strength and Resistance Workout

Strength-based classes can have the goals of endurance and stabilization, general strength, power, or a combination of these. Additionally, these classes will incorporate a variety of equipment and music.

General Considerations for Strength

Strength classes attract a wide variety of participants due to the general health benefits and simplicity of exercise movements. Participants will have varying conditioning levels, so modifications should be planned in advance. General considerations for a strength class include:

- ▼ Kinetic chain alignment (e.g., foot and ankle, knee, LPHC, shoulders, head)
- ▼ Core engagement
- ▼ Proper foot positioning (e.g., wide, staggered, single leg)
- ▼ Controlled speed and tempo
- ▼ Adequate time under tension in the muscle
- ▼ Movement coaching from start to finish

Training Intensities for Strength

Intensities in strength-based classes will vary depending on the goal. Intensity in strength classes can be thought of in terms of percentage of an individual's one-rep maximum (1RM). Most participants will not know their 1RM, so the following guidelines should be used: A strength class with a focus on endurance or stabilization should have a low intensity, with lighter resistance and increased repetitions; increased overall strength or muscular development classes will have a higher intensity, using more resistance and fewer repetitions.

See **Tables 5.3** and **5.4** for more detail.

Components of Strength Workouts

When the instructor conducts the intro, the general goal of the class should be stated and equipment needs identified. Guidance should be given on the general amount of weight appropriate for a beginner, intermediate, and advanced exerciser.

One-rep maximum (1RM)

The maximum force that can be generated in a single repetition.

Table 5.3

Endurance Training in Strength-based Classes

		Reps	Sets	Tempo	% Intensity	Rest Interval
Movement Prep	Flexibility	1	1–3	30 sec hold	N/A	N/A
	Core	12–20	1–4	Slow	N/A	0–90 sec
	Balance	12–20 6–10 (SL)	1–3	Slow	N/A	0–90 sec
Resistance		12–20	1–3	Slow	50–70% 1RM	0–90 sec

Table 5.4

Overall Strength or Muscular Development in Strength-based Classes

		Reps	Sets	Tempo	% Intensity	Rest Interval
Movement Prep	Flexibility	5–10	1–2	1–2 sec hold	N/A	N/A
	Core	8–12	2–3	Medium	N/A	0–60 sec
	Balance	8–12	2–3	Medium	N/A	0–60 sec
Resistance		6–12	3–5	Medium	75–85% 1RM	0–60 sec

During the movement prep segment of the workout, attention should be given to improving muscle imbalances, activating the core, and incorporating balance (as needed). This will accomplish the benefits of preparing for greater intensity. Common movement prep exercises for strength-based classes can include:

▼ Kneeling hip flexor stretch

▼ Lat stretch

▼ Floor planks

▼ Floor bridges

▼ Single-leg squats

As the instructor segues into the body of the workout, there are general ways to program resistance training classes:

▼ Alternate upper and lower body exercises (peripheral heart action training)

▼ Total body movements

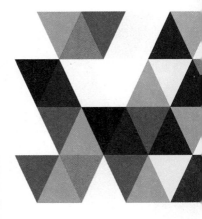

▼ Alternate opposing muscle groups, such as a push exercise followed by a pull exercise.

▼ Use industry-standard methods, such as circuit training

Common exercises to be used in the body of a strength-oriented class include:

▼ Squat to overhead press

▼ Push-ups

▼ Bent-over rows

▼ Biceps curls

▼ Lunge variations

The transition and outro of a strength-based workout will mirror general workout considerations.

The HIIT and Interval Workout

Many formats offer cardiorespiratory training (dance, aqua, cycle, kickboxing), and HIIT is a common one even if it is applied differently (cycle, boot camp, etc.). HIIT can enhance performance, change body composition, and support overall improvements in health and fitness.

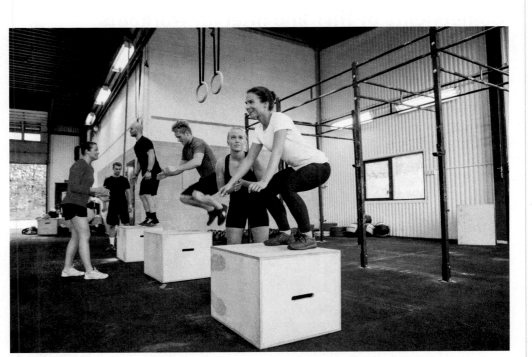

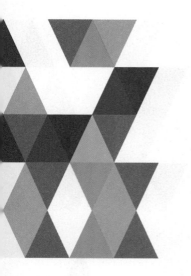

General Considerations for HIIT and Interval

A variety of people will attend HIIT classes because of general cardio improvements and the ability to provide self-modifications as needed. One consideration in a HIIT workout is joint impact, as many movements require high-impact, repetitive actions. General considerations for a HIIT or interval class include:

▼ Kinetic chain alignment

▼ Control based on intended intensity and

▼ Systematically challenging heart rate zones

Training Intensities for HIIT and Interval

HIIT classes imply a high-intensity interval that is short in duration and preceded and followed by a moderate-intensity time period to allow the body to actively recover. Based on the advancement of the group, participants will spend 3 minutes training at 65–75% of their maximum heart rate (HR_{max}) and immediately transition into a 1-minute interval of 76–85% of their HR_{max}. When teaching a more advanced HIIT class, an interval of 86–95% can incorporated (lasting no longer than 1 minute) so long as the active recovery periods allow 1–3 minutes of work (at 65–85%, depending on fitness levels). See Figure 5.2.

Components of HIIT and Interval Workouts

Because HIIT and intervals are short, timed segments, the intro should include specific descriptions of what is going to be done and for how long. Then general movement prep activities should be included, such as:

▼ Static stretch calves and adductors

▼ Abdominal crunches

▼ Push-ups

Figure 5.2
HIIT Training Parameters

Zone 1	Zone 2	Zone 3
HR_{max} (65%–75%) RPE = 12–13	HR_{max} (76%–85%) RPE = 14–16	HR_{max} (86%–95%) RPE = 17–19

Warm-up/Cool-down   Zone 1: Recovery   Zone 2: Lactate Threshold   Zone 3: Peak/Interval

Warm-up 5–10 min
1 min
1 min
1 min
1 min
1 min
Cool down 5–10 min

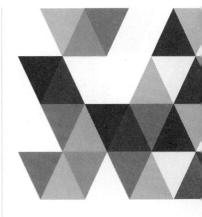

- Walking lunges
- Squat jump to stabilization

The body can alternate low- and high-intensity intervals, gradually increase difficulty with each interval, or change the demands with each interval. Some general ways to program HIIT or interval classes include various work-to-rest ratios. The first number in the sequence represents the amount of time spent working and the second represents resting time. Examples include:

- 20:10 seconds
- 60:30 seconds
- 60:60 seconds
- 120:60 seconds

Common exercises to be used in the body of a strength oriented class include:

- Jogging (stationary or in place)
- Burpees
- Shuffles
- Repetitive squat jumps

Because of the high-intensity nature, extra time may be required during the transition.

The Boot Camp Workout

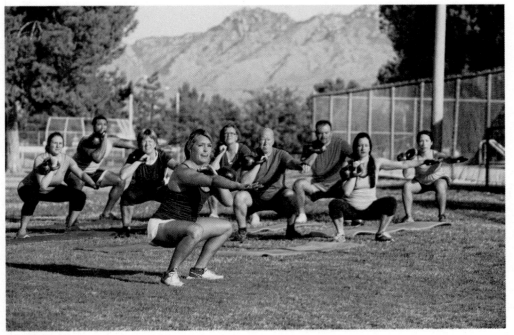

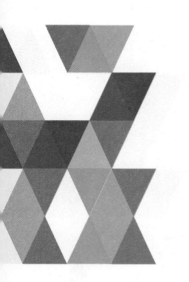

Boot camp workouts offer instructors an opportunity to be creative in exercise selection, equipment use, circuit flow, and location. They often incorporate HIIT and other interval techniques with an aggressive but team-oriented approach. These classes typically use music for background rather than timing repetitions and incorporate a variety of equipment.

General Considerations for Boot Camp

Participants usually attend boot camps because they want to be pushed to new levels or feel competitive. They will arrive with varying levels of conditioning, so modifications should be planned in advance. General considerations include:

▾ Kinetic chain alignment

▾ Core engagement

▾ Strong motivational focus

Training Intensities for Boot Camp

Training intensities can follow recommendations similar to strength- and HIIT-based classes. The intensity level is usually determined by the vision and goal of the class rather than the format, with a focus on completions (x minute mile, 150 push-ups, etc.)

Components of Boot Camp Workouts

Participants should be informed about how hard the workout *should* feel and the level of effort expected. Movement prep should preview unique moves without equipment or with a reduced load, in order to learn the movement pattern before the body of the workout begins. Instructors should emphasize core endurance and strength for safe and effective movement execution. Movement prep in a boot camp class might consist of:

▾ Abdominal crunches

▾ Push-ups

▾ Walking lunges

▾ Prisoner squats

The body of a boot camp workout varies by location and equipment available. The workout should have a clear direction and flow to avoid confusion or frustration. Examples of boot camp activities include:

▾ *High-Rep Goals*—The instructor motivates the class to complete 100, 200, etc. reps with structured rest.

▾ *Poker Cards*—The number on the card designates the number of reps or type of exercise.

▾ *Group Tasks*—The group has to stay at a specific station until every participant has completed the task before moving on.

▾ *Pyramid Circuits*—The circuits gradually get harder, then peak, then gradually get easier.

INSTRUCTOR TIP 👍

It's helpful for boot camp instructors to bring whistles, visible timers, or other props to keep the momentum and fun going in a boot camp class.

Transitional moves in a boot camp class should consist of stretches that increase joint mobility at the hip and shoulder to ensure participants can continue to improve movement efficiency. The outro should recap the goals accomplished in class, as they are usually significant or dramatic.

The Yoga Workout

Yoga workouts can vary in type, duration, level, and ambience. Considerations will vary based on these factors, but some common factors are seen.

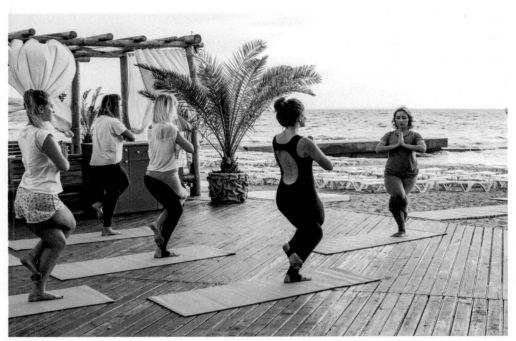

© Osadchaya Olga/Shutterstock

General Considerations for Yoga

Yoga primarily works muscles isometrically. Concentric and eccentric movements exist when moving into and out of postures, but the most traditional forms of yoga emphasize holding stability within posture, to train balance and improve range of motion. General considerations for a yoga class include:

- ▼ Kinetic chain alignment
- ▼ Postures begin at the pelvic floor to increase core stability and balance
- ▼ Intra-abdominal pressure and core bracing
- ▼ Grouping postures according to spinal movement
- ▼ Differing training intensity based on outcomes

Components of Yoga Workouts

A yoga intro should include what the participant should *feel* coming out of class. Movement prep will often begin with the instructor asking participants to focus on their current state and to bring awareness to the integration of one's mind, body, and breath. Then preparatory motions that rehearse the body for up-coming positions and patterns are used. Common poses and flows that work well for movement prep in yoga include:

- ▼ Child's Pose
- ▼ Cat/Cow Flow
- ▼ Spinal Balance
- ▼ Chair Pose

The class body should consist of movements appropriate to the goals of the yoga class being taught. Additional training and certification may be required; however, for the purpose of familiarization, the following are common examples of sequences, patterns, or experiences that work well in the body of a yoga workout:

- ▼ Sun Salutation A
- ▼ Warrior 1, 2, and 3 (Warrior Series)
- ▼ Mountain Pose to Goddess Pose
- ▼ Plank Flow

The transition in a yoga workout often consists of meditation, breathing, or other methods that reduce stress and improve clarity of thought. The outro should be a gentle shift for those in a relaxed state, be spoken lightly, and include validation of the work performed.

The Cycle Workout

Cycling workouts are typically 45–60 minutes in duration and include various drills, work sets, and intervals to drive intensity and proper recovery. Instructors manipulate leg speed (RPM), bike resistance, and body position to meet class objectives. Cycling will generally focus on one movement pattern at various intensities in seated or standing positions.

General Considerations for Cycle

Participants will be attracted to cycling for health benefits and simplicity of movements. The physiological objectives of the workout will determine the types of sets, drills, or intervals performed.

General considerations for a cycle class include:

- ▼ Kinetic chain alignment
- ▼ Potential overactivity in the hip flexor complex

▼ Proper bike fit

■ Seat at hip height

■ Handlebar should support proper upper body alignment

▼ Core engagement

▼ Proper foot position

Training Intensities for Cycle

When determining intensity, the instructor must decide if the workout will focus primarily on the aerobic or anaerobic energy systems. If the goal is aerobic, then intervals and work sets will be longer in duration. If the instructor chooses to include work for the anaerobic system, then shorter, high-intensity intervals with proper recovery ratios will be the focus. This is similar to the heart rate zones discussed with HIIT.

Components of Cycle Workouts

The introduction of a cycle class should include a brief overview of proper bike fit, and how to increase or decrease resistance. It should also include information about the goal of the workout so riders can best manage their energy.

The movement prep segment should avoid undue fatigue in the legs or prematurely spiking the heart rate. It will also give them time to get comfortable on the bike and resistance changes.

Depending on the objective, the body of the workout may include steady-state efforts, aerobic intervals, lactate threshold intervals, and various drills that focus on speed, strength, or power, and utilize both seated and standing postures. Intensity is created by manipulating

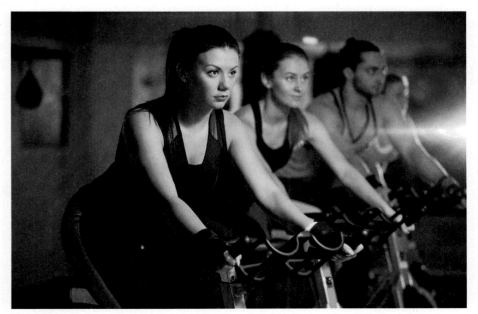

© RomanSo/Shutterstock

resistance, speed (RPM), and body position. Common exercises to be used in the body of a cycle-oriented class include:

- ▼ Seated or standing flats
- ▼ Seated or standing climbs
- ▼ Sprints
- ▼ Attacks
- ▼ Jumps

After heart rates have recovered and the pre-class physical state is achieved, flexibility techniques like SMR and static stretching can be performed off the bike. In general, attention should be paid to the primary muscles used during class, as well as the lower back and neck.

The outro should congratulate the class on a job well done, tell the class how to clean and care for the equipment, and invite participants to come chat while everyone packs up.

Summary

The five components (intro, movement prep, body, transition, and outro) of a workout are the foundation from which an instructor should teach common formats. The intro and outro are the soft skills instructors should apply, like bookends. The movement prep and transition components of the workout aim to bring the body to an ideal state where it can complete the workout and then safely exit from the higher-intensity body. The body is where the majority of teaching occurs and should accomplish the ultimate goal of the class. The understanding of format specific considerations will help an instructor establish safe, effective practices while allowing for creativity in approach.

Chapter in Review

- ▼ Components of a workout & common elements of each
  - ▪ Intro
  - ▪ Movement prep (warm-up)
  - ▪ Body of the workout
  - ▪ Transition (cool-down)
  - ▪ Outro
- ▼ Monitoring intensity
  - ▪ Rating of perceived exertion (RPE)—scale of perceived work intensity

- ▪ Talk test—helps estimate maximal exertion
- ▪ Dyspnea—scale related to difficulty of breathing
- ▼ Class flow: connecting workout components
  - ▪ Planning
  - ▪ Practice
  - ▪ Preparation
  - ▪ Modifications
  - ▪ Presentation personality

▼ General considerations by format

  ■ Kinetic chain alignment (foot and ankle, knee, LPHC, shoulders, head)

  ■ Posture & core engagement

▼ Considerations and exercise selection for a workout

  ■ By component (intro, movement, prep, body, transition, outro)

  ■ By format

    ❖ Strength and resistance

    ❖ HIIT and cardio

    ❖ Boot camp

    ❖ Yoga

    ❖ Cycle

▼ Training intensities by format

  ■ Strength: percentage of 1RM

    ❖ Stabilization: low intensity, lighter resistance, increased repetitions

    ❖ Strength/Muscular development: higher intensity, more resistance, fewer repetitions

  ■ HIIT and interval

    ❖ High intensities in short durations followed by moderate intensities to recover

  ■ Boot Camp, Yoga, and Cycle

    ❖ Vary depending on outcomes

References

1. Foster C, Porcari JP, Anderson J, et al. The talk test as a marker of exercise training intensity. *J Cardiopulm Rehabil Prev.* 2008;28(1):24–30.

2. Persinger R, Foster C, Gibson M, Fater DC, Porcari JP. Consistency of the talk test for exercise prescription. *Med Sci Sports Exerc.* 2004;36(9):1632–1636.

3. Clark M, Sutton BG, Lucett S. *NASM Essentials of Personal Fitness Training.* 4th ed. Burlington, MA: Jones & Bartlett Learning; 2014.

Chapter 6
Teaching Multi-training and Exercise Technique

 Learning Objectives

6.1. **Identify** proper techniques to improve strength, cardiorespiratory fitness, flexibility, and overall well-being.

6.2. **Identify** appropriate exercises aligned to outcomes and format.

6.3. **Explain** proper exercise technique.

6.4. **Identify** appropriate exercise modifications, including regressions and progressions.

Introduction to Multi-training

The Group Fitness Instructor should know common exercises associated with each format, perform them correctly, effectively cue, and provide modifications (progressions and regressions) for all exercises. With a solid knowledge of these, Group Fitness Instructors are equipped to teach safe, effective classes and build credibility with participants. This chapter focuses on the body of the workout and exercises for common formats (strength, cardio, yoga, and cycle).

Cueing will always follow correct alignment of the five kinetic chain checkpoints: starting with the feet straight ahead (knee in line with the second and third toe), knees straight, LPHC, shoulder girdle, and head aligned with the upper arm.

Flexibility Exercises

Although the focus of this chapter is the body of a workout, instructors should also be aware of techniques for flexibility exercise, specifically static stretching. Proper technique for static stretching is necessary in instances where muscle imbalance correction is the goal. Performing a stretch without perfect form can result in exacerbating movement dysfunction. Common static stretches addressing overactive muscles include: gastrocnemius, hip flexor complex, adductors, latissimus dorsi, pectorals, and upper traps.

Exercise Technique

Though every exercise differs in execution and technique, there are common guidelines that can be followed to emphasize safety and effectiveness. Working from bottom up, the feet should be pointing straight ahead and, when appropriate, knees and feet should be in alignment. When standing, knees should be soft and extended, in line with the second and third toe. The lumbo-pelvic-hip-complex should remain neutral with abs and glutes engaged. Moving up, the back should also be neutral without thoracic rounding. Shoulders should be back and down, while the cervical spine should remain neutral. Finally, the arms should be extended when stretched out, and, like the knees, should remain soft and not locked. Wrists should be straight and in a neutral position.

Providing Modifications

Modifications offer class participants the choice between two or more exercises to match individual needs, fitness goals, and daily preferences. Progression, a form of modification, offers incremental increases in exercise intensity or difficulty to help participants with aggressive or specific performance goals attend group fitness classes and get the challenge they desire. Regressions offer step-by-step decreases in exercise intensity or difficulty to help participants who are new or have lower levels of fitness feel successful in class. See **Table 6.1** for systematic progressions or regressions.

Progression

An option that allows the fitness class participant to increase complexity, impact, or intensity of a movement or movement patterns.

Regression

An option that allows the fitness class participant to decrease complexity, impact, or intensity of a movement or movement patterns.

Modifications

Adaptions to movements in order to accommodate specific requests, making moves possible for individuals with specific needs.

Table 6.1

The Proprioceptive Progression Continuum			
Proprioceptive Challenge	**Base of Support**	**Lower Body**	**Upper Body**
Foundational ↓ **Advanced**	Floor	Two-legs stable	Two-arm
	Sport beam	Staggered-stance stable	Alternating arms
	Half foam roll	Single-leg stable	Single-arm
	Foam pad	Two-leg unstable	Single-arm with trunk rotation
	Balance disc	Staggered-stance unstable	
	Wobble board	Single-leg unstable	
	BOSU ball		

Fitness has evolved to incorporate more balance training, sometimes communicated by instructors as *functional training*. Increasing proprioception in exercise movements and workouts can be helpful for participants, but they should always be done safely—and only within the limits of what a participant can safely control while still feeling challenged.

Strength-based Exercises

Strength-based exercises emphasize compound movements to achieve specific goals (strength increase, endurance, etc.). When selecting strength exercises, an instructor should keep in mind larger muscle groups; exercises using more than one muscle group are considered more functional.

Effective cueing can be tricky in the group environment due to the wide variety of participant goals and abilities. It is a good idea to start with the least challenging version of an exercise and then progress appropriately for the group. Once an advanced exercise is introduced, the instructor should re-visit the easier version or modification for those who are not ready to advance. It is even trickier to control what the participants think they should be doing. It is important to find ways of encouraging those who should advance without discouraging those who should not. A phrase such as, "if you are sensing fatigue, you are working at the perfect level; if not, try adding this variation" may help to encourage all class participants. Instructors should avoid cues that are not inclusive, negative, or overly aggressive, like "come on, you can do it; no pain, no gain."

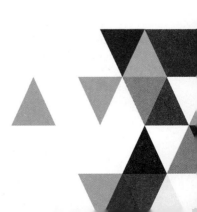

Planks (prone iso-abs)

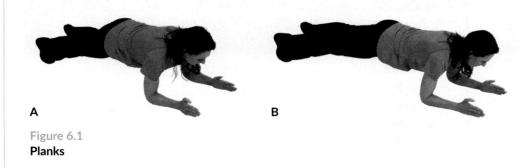

A   B

Figure 6.1
Planks

Primary Format(s)	Strength & Resistance, HIIT & Interval, Boot Camp
Progressions	Single leg iso-ab Iso-ab with arm reach Iso-ab to push-up position Iso-ab to rotation
Regressions	Iso-ab on knees Iso-ab on wall Reduce time holding
Common Form Mistakes	Pelvis dropping Excessive arch in low back Head dropping forward Shoulders elevated Holding breath Hips too high Hands clasped together Legs together
Cues to Correct	Engage core and glutes before starting exercise. Make the body rigid (like a board) from ears to knees. Depress shoulder blades and protract shoulder girdle. Keep forearms parallel. Legs and feet stay hip-width apart to prevent adductor assistance. Breathe normally.

Squat to Press

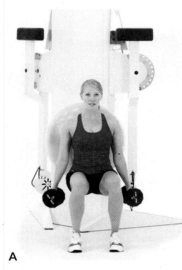
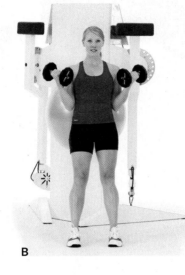
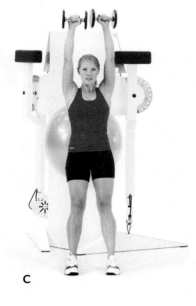

A

B

C

Figure 6.2
Squat to Press

Primary Format(s)	Strength & Resistance, Boot Camp, HIIT & Interval
Progressions	Increase external resistance Squat, curl to one-arm overhead press
Regressions	Squat to curl Standing curl to one-arm overhead press
Common Form Mistakes	Not completing each movement fully before starting the next Swinging hips for momentum
Cues to Correct	Keep chest tall and above hips, with back parallel to shins. Avoid swinging weight during curl. Focus on form over amount of weight lifted. Complete each movement individually before staring the next.

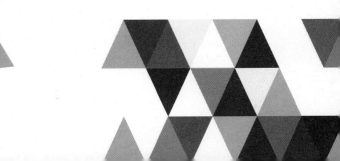

Push-ups

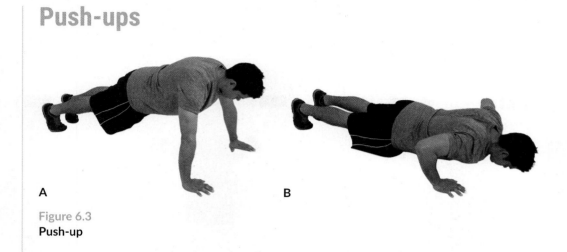

A   B

Figure 6.3
Push-up

Primary Format(s)	Strength & Resistance, HIIT & Interval, Boot Camp
Progressions	Elevate feet for decline push-up Perform on one leg Shift body-weight to one arm Slow down eccentric portion Wear weight vest
Regressions	Perform on knees Perform on wall Perform on bench
Common Form Mistakes	Low back arch Head dropping Not protracting shoulders at top of push-up
Cues to Correct	Engage glutes and abs. Maintain neutral cervical spine. Protract by pushing at the top.

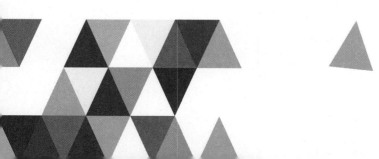

Scaption

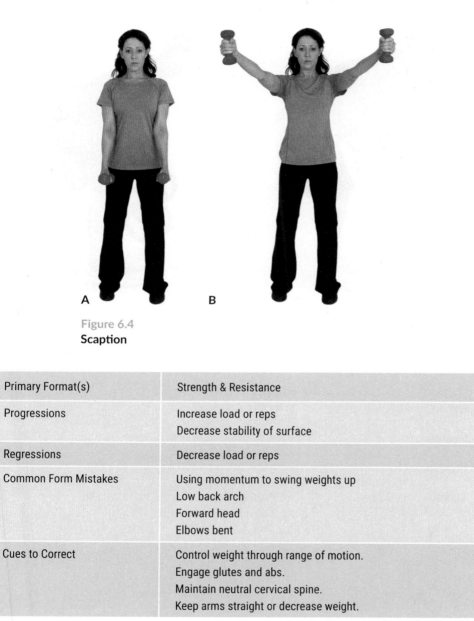

A   B

Figure 6.4
Scaption

Primary Format(s)	Strength & Resistance
Progressions	Increase load or reps Decrease stability of surface
Regressions	Decrease load or reps
Common Form Mistakes	Using momentum to swing weights up Low back arch Forward head Elbows bent
Cues to Correct	Control weight through range of motion. Engage glutes and abs. Maintain neutral cervical spine. Keep arms straight or decrease weight.

Bent Over Row

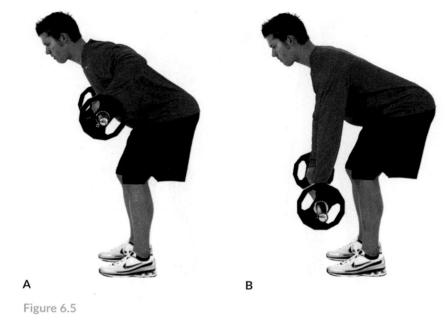

A

B

Figure 6.5
Bent Over Row

Primary Format(s)	Strength & Resistance
Progressions	Increase load or repetitions
Regressions	Decrease load or repetitions
Common Form Mistakes	Not maintaining neutral spine and looking up Not keeping shoulders down Rounding low back
Cues to Correct	Engage abs. Maintain neutral cervical spine. Tip forward at the hips like taking a bow.

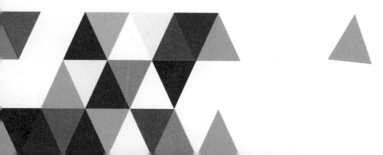

Renegade Rows

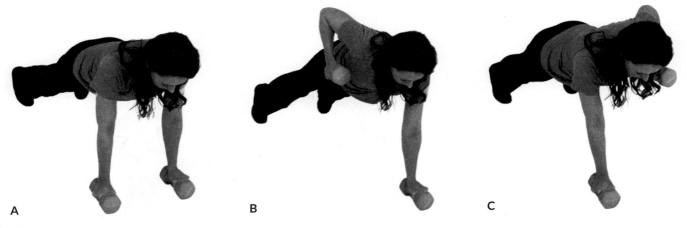

A   B   C

Figure 6.6
Renegade Rows

Primary Format(s)	Boot Camp, Strength & Resistance
Progressions	Increase load Add push-up between rows Perform single-leg
Regressions	Decrease or eliminate load Perform on knees Lay prone on stability ball
Common Form Mistakes	Shifting side-to-side Low back arch Retracting and winging scapula of stabilization arm Dropping head
Cues to Correct	Engage glutes and abs. Stabilize hips to prevent shifting from side to side. Engage shoulder muscles of down arm and protract scapula. Maintain neutral cervical spine with eyes looking directly at floor.

Lunges

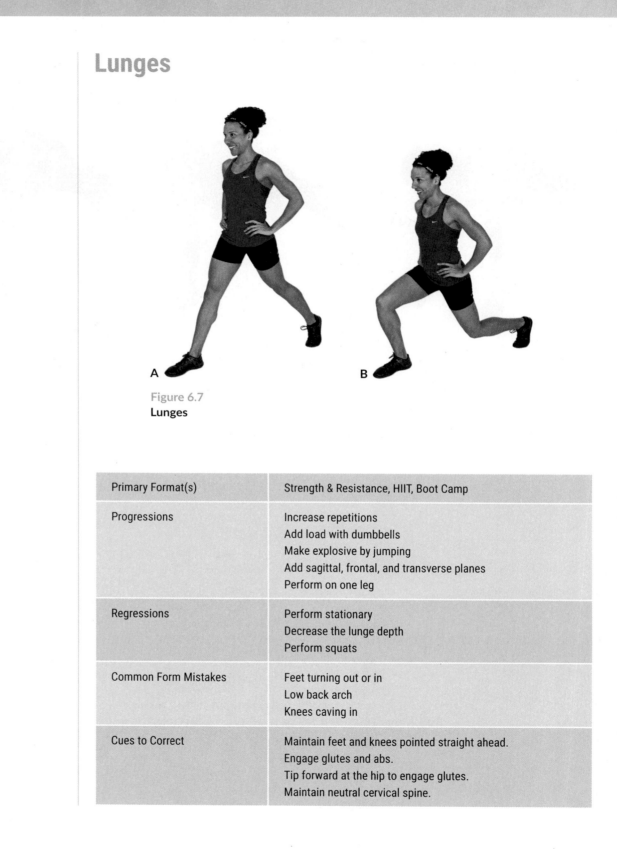

A   B

Figure 6.7
Lunges

Primary Format(s)	Strength & Resistance, HIIT, Boot Camp
Progressions	Increase repetitions Add load with dumbbells Make explosive by jumping Add sagittal, frontal, and transverse planes Perform on one leg
Regressions	Perform stationary Decrease the lunge depth Perform squats
Common Form Mistakes	Feet turning out or in Low back arch Knees caving in
Cues to Correct	Maintain feet and knees pointed straight ahead. Engage glutes and abs. Tip forward at the hip to engage glutes. Maintain neutral cervical spine.

Single-leg Squat

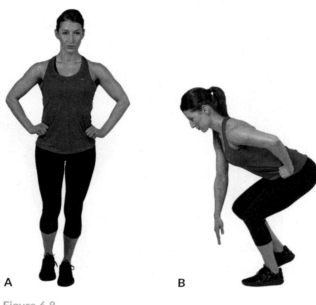

A

B

Figure 6.8
Single-leg Squat

Primary Format(s)	Strength & Resistance
Progressions	Squat lower Add small weight to reaching arm
Regressions	Reduce range of motion Put floating foot down for better control
Common Form Mistakes	Performing exercise to quickly Knee caving in Rotating at the trunk
Cues to Correct	Pick a spot on floor and keep eyes on it. Only squat as low as you can maintain perfect form. Sit back like you're seating yourself in a chair.

Single-leg Romanian Deadlift

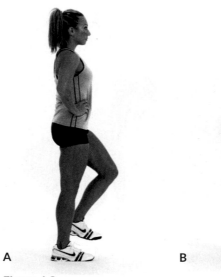

A   B

Figure 6.9
Single-leg Romanian Deadlift

Primary Format(s)	Strength & Resistance
Progressions	Add weight
Regressions	Reach to knee Reach to shin Use floating leg for light balance
Common Form Mistakes	Thoracic rounding Not hip hinging Locked knees Trouble balancing
Cues to Correct	Push your glutes back and bend at the hips. Soften the knees. Pick a spot on floor and keep eyes on it.

Tube Walking

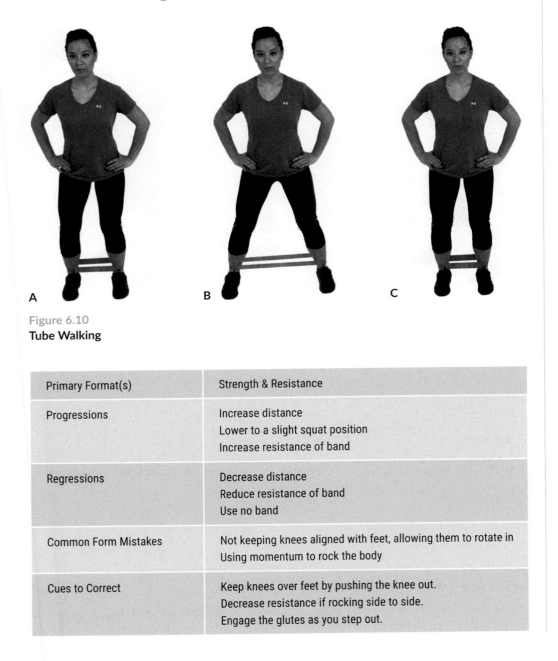

Figure 6.10
Tube Walking

Primary Format(s)	Strength & Resistance
Progressions	Increase distance Lower to a slight squat position Increase resistance of band
Regressions	Decrease distance Reduce resistance of band Use no band
Common Form Mistakes	Not keeping knees aligned with feet, allowing them to rotate in Using momentum to rock the body
Cues to Correct	Keep knees over feet by pushing the knee out. Decrease resistance if rocking side to side. Engage the glutes as you step out.

Kettlebell Swings

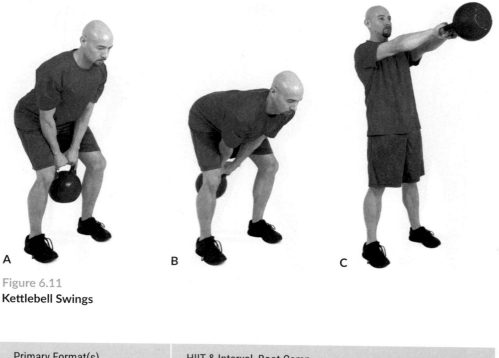

A   B   C

Figure 6.11
Kettlebell Swings

Primary Format(s)	HIIT & Interval, Boot Camp
Progressions	Increase load or repetitions
Regressions	Decrease load or repetitions
Common Form Mistakes	Not maintaining alignment or stability in the spine or shoulders
Cues to Correct	Engage glutes and abs. Engage lats.

Cardio-based Exercises

Cardio-based exercises emphasize higher-intensity exercises that are often high impact. The exercises maximize caloric burn and will sometimes incorporate strength-based movements. When selecting cardio exercises, it is important to remember participants will often seek regressions and progressions. These should be planned in advance; regressions should focus on reducing impact.

The ultimate goal of cardio is to push both the aerobic and anaerobic systems. Alternating brief periods of high-intensity work with low-intensity recovery periods (commonly referred to as intervals) results in overloading both energy systems. It is important to understand during steady state exercise, sufficient oxygen is supplied to, and used by, the working muscles. Hence, there is a balance between oxygen available for the body's use and the intensity level of the activity.

However, as the exercise intensity is increased to the point oxygen demands can no longer be met, anaerobic metabolism contributes to the energy requirements of the activity.

An example of this would a participant performing a series of high-intensity power moves for 3 minutes followed by 1 minute of body conditioning work combined with low- intensity squats. Continually incorporating this type of work-to-rest program into any workout will enable participants to reap the benefits of cardio training.

Burpees

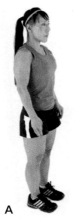
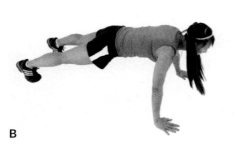
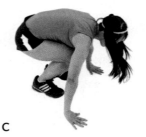
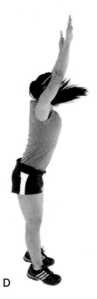

A   B   C   D

Figure 6.12
Burpees

Primary Format(s)	HIIT, Interval, & Boot Camp
Progressions	Increase tempo or reps Increase jump height Perform two push-ups Add a tuck jump
Regressions	Push-up from knees Use bench Do not perform jump Step legs out one at a time
Common Form Mistakes	Low back arch Turning feet out during squat Allowing head to fall forward and shoulders to elevate during push-up
Cues to Correct	Maintain feet in-line with knees. Engage glutes and abs. Maintain neutral cervical spine. Keep shoulder blades down.

Army Crawl

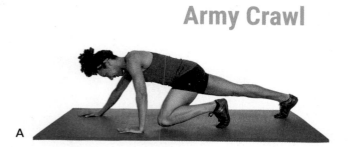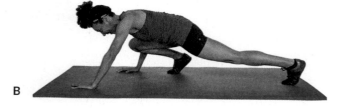

Figure 6.13
Army Crawl

Primary Format(s)	Boot Camp & HIIT
Progressions	Increase distance, time, or speed
Regressions	Reduce distance, time, or speed
Common Form Mistakes	Lifting hips too high while moving forward
Cues to Correct	Engage glutes and abs. Decrease speed.

Jack Push Climb

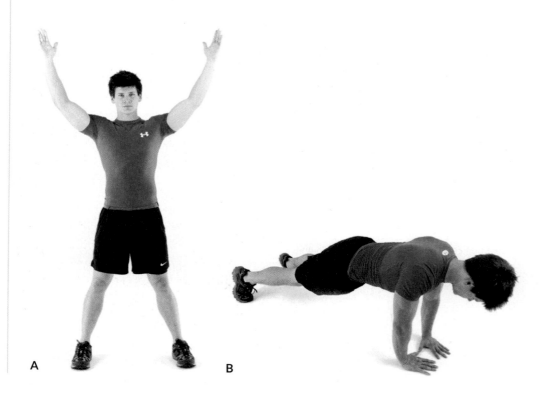

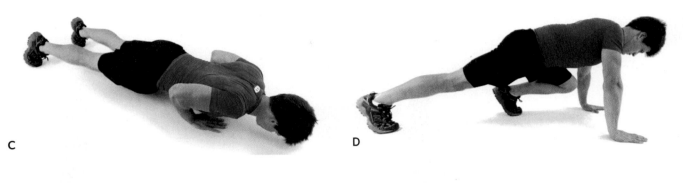

C

D

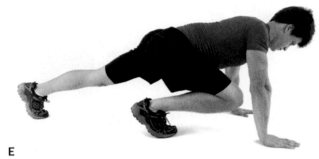

E

Figure 6.14
Jack Push Climb

Primary Format(s)	Boot Camp, HIIT & Interval
Progressions	Increase speed while maintaining form
Regressions	No arms overhead for jumping jack Stand up straight instead of jumping jack Plank instead of push-up Hold plank instead of mountain climber
Common Form Mistakes	Lack of core stability Head drop during plank and push-up
Cues to Correct	Slow down. Engage glutes and abs. Stabilize strong when kicking feet out behind you. Tuck chin in push-up and mountain climber.

Tuck Jumps

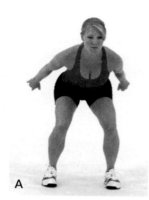

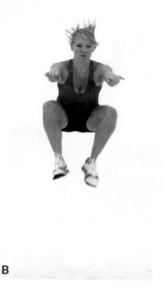

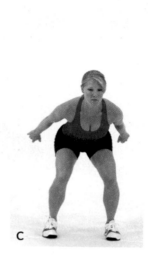

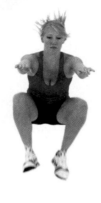

A   B   C   D

Figure 6.15
Tuck Jumps

Primary Format(s)	Boot Camp, HIIT, & Interval
Progressions	Increase repetitions
Regressions	Decrease repetitions Double squat in between Decrease the intended height of the knee drive Prisoner squat
Common Form Mistakes	Not keeping feet pointed straight head Allowing knees to cave inward Low back arch Looking down or looking up
Cues to Correct	Maintain feet in-line with knees. Maintain neutral cervical spine.

Speed Skaters

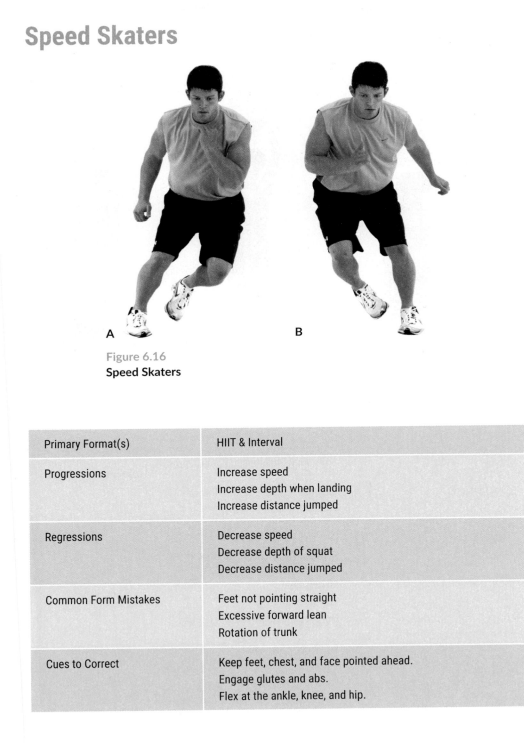

A   B

Figure 6.16
Speed Skaters

Primary Format(s)	HIIT & Interval
Progressions	Increase speed Increase depth when landing Increase distance jumped
Regressions	Decrease speed Decrease depth of squat Decrease distance jumped
Common Form Mistakes	Feet not pointing straight Excessive forward lean Rotation of trunk
Cues to Correct	Keep feet, chest, and face pointed ahead. Engage glutes and abs. Flex at the ankle, knee, and hip.

Overhead Medicine Ball Throw Downs

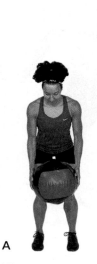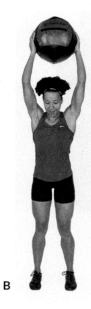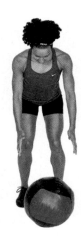

A   B   C

Figure 6.17
Overhead Medicine Ball Throw Downs

Primary Format(s)	Strength & Resistance, Boot Camp
Progressions	Increase reps and rate of throws Increase weight of MB
Regressions	Decrease load Decrease reps or rate of throws
Common Form Mistakes	Elbows bent Low back arch Not reaching completely overhead
Cues to Correct	Emphasize lats by keeping elbows extended and following through. Engage glutes and abs. Pick a spot on the floor to aim your throw.

Inch Worms

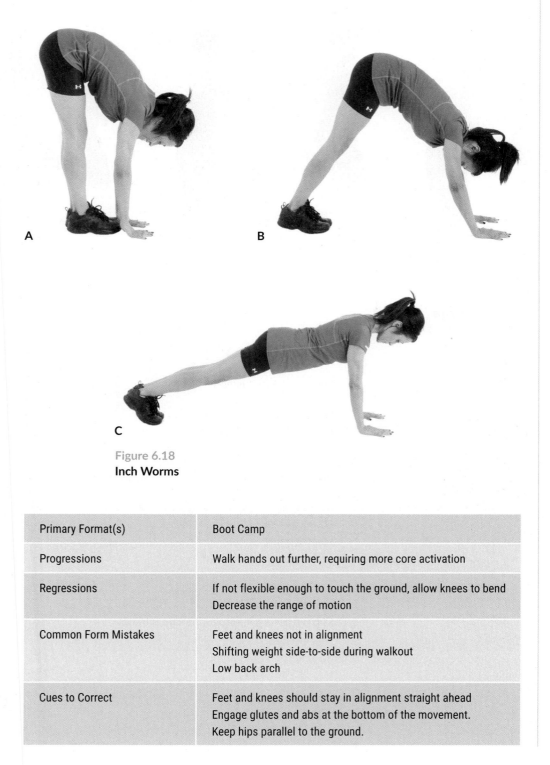

A

B

C

Figure 6.18
Inch Worms

Primary Format(s)	Boot Camp
Progressions	Walk hands out further, requiring more core activation
Regressions	If not flexible enough to touch the ground, allow knees to bend Decrease the range of motion
Common Form Mistakes	Feet and knees not in alignment Shifting weight side-to-side during walkout Low back arch
Cues to Correct	Feet and knees should stay in alignment straight ahead Engage glutes and abs at the bottom of the movement. Keep hips parallel to the ground.

Butt Kick Jumps

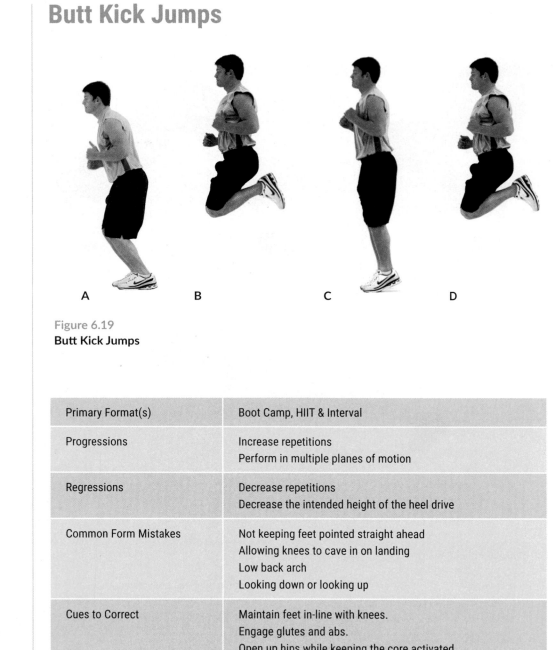

A   B   C   D

Figure 6.19
Butt Kick Jumps

Primary Format(s)	Boot Camp, HIIT & Interval
Progressions	Increase repetitions Perform in multiple planes of motion
Regressions	Decrease repetitions Decrease the intended height of the heel drive
Common Form Mistakes	Not keeping feet pointed straight ahead Allowing knees to cave in on landing Low back arch Looking down or looking up
Cues to Correct	Maintain feet in-line with knees. Engage glutes and abs. Open up hips while keeping the core activated. Maintain neutral cervical spine.

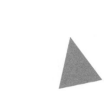

Crab Walk

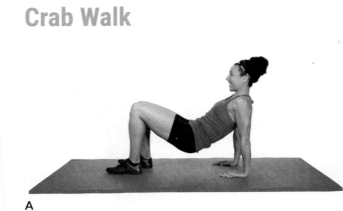
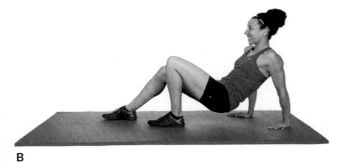
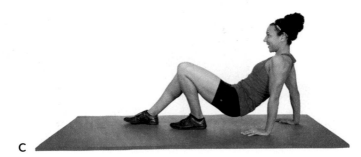

Figure 6.20
Crab Walk

Primary Format(s)	Boot Camp
Progressions	Increase distance, time, or speed
Regressions	Reduce distance, time, or speed
Common Form Mistakes	Feet too wide Hips too high Not maintaining shoulder depression Side-to-side "waddling" motion Rounding of the spine
Cues to Correct	Maintain feet in alignment with knees and hips/shoulders, with feet pointing straight ahead. Keep shoulder blades depressed by "sliding" scapula toward your back pockets. Engage glutes and abs.

Jump Lunges

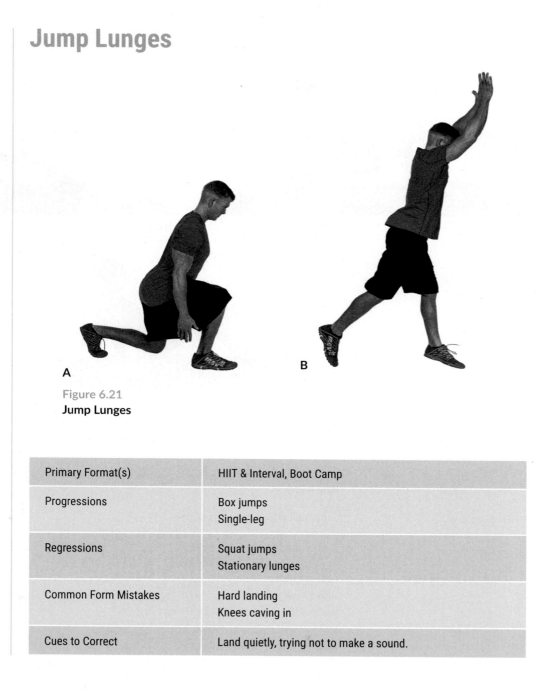

A

B

Figure 6.21
Jump Lunges

Primary Format(s)	HIIT & Interval, Boot Camp
Progressions	Box jumps Single-leg
Regressions	Squat jumps Stationary lunges
Common Form Mistakes	Hard landing Knees caving in
Cues to Correct	Land quietly, trying not to make a sound.

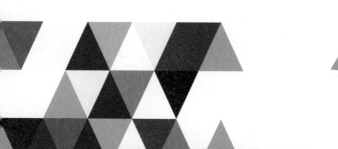

Yoga-based Exercises

Yoga exercises can serve a variety of purposes, such as flexibility, balance, core, and meditative purposes. When selecting exercises, consider the intention of the session with a strong emphasis on cueing.

There are a variety of styles for teaching yoga that center around the efforts and practice of several masters from India who came to the West over past years. The Iyengar method focuses on precision and alignment, which is typically a good foundation Bikram teachers use heat and repetition as a method for measuring progress. Satchadinanda attempts to integrate the various components of yoga practice—asana, chant, breathing, relaxation, meditation—to achieve a feeling of completion. Ashtanga focuses on the fitness principle of overload.

Camel Pose

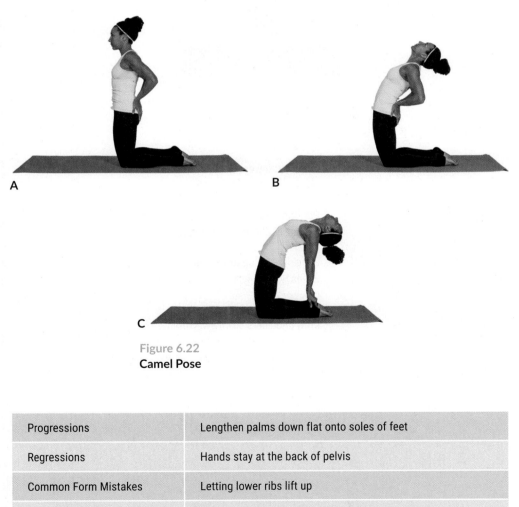

A

B

C

Figure 6.22
Camel Pose

Progressions	Lengthen palms down flat onto soles of feet
Regressions	Hands stay at the back of pelvis
Common Form Mistakes	Letting lower ribs lift up
Cues to Correct	Draw ribs in, lift up through chest.

Chair Pose

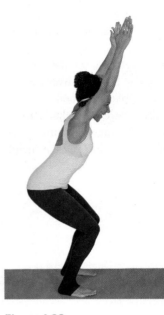

Figure 6.23
Chair Pose

Progressions	Lift heels, lower buttocks to heels, extend arms forward Place a block between thighs
Regressions	Perform pose near a wall so, in lowered position, tailbone just touches wall, offering support
Common Form Mistakes	Shoulders lift up toward ears Knees not aligned Low back arch
Cues to Correct	Draw shoulders down away from ears. Draw knees evenly together. Lengthen spine and draw navel toward spine. Engage and lengthen through arms.

Crow Pose

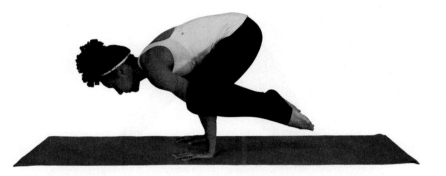

Figure 6.24
Crow Pose

Progressions	Squeeze legs against arms, straighten elbows Draw inner knees up near armpits
Regressions	Bring just one foot off floor at a time
Common Form Mistakes	Gaze directed back rather than forward
Cues to Correct	Look slightly forward, not back. Where eyes go, body follows. Elbows over wrists.

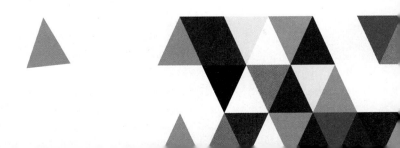

Downward-facing Dog Pose

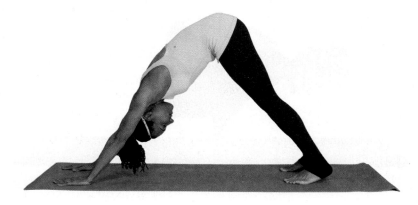

Figure 6.25
Downward-facing Dog Pose

Progressions	Perform on one leg and opposite arm
Regressions	Drop to knees
Common Form Mistakes	Gaze forward Back arched Weight in hands
Cues to Correct	Draw shoulders away from ears. Press through palms. Press through heels. Lift up through sits bones. Draw thighs toward back wall. Shift weight back into hips.

Eagle Pose

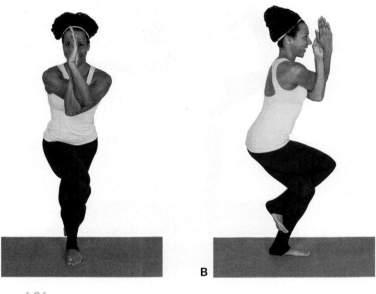

A   B

Figure 6.26
Eagle Pose

Progressions	After pointing toes downward, press foot back and hook top of foot behind lower right calf
Regressions	Use a wall for balance
Common Form Mistakes	General misalignment
Cues to Correct	Stack shoulders over hips and elbows over knees.

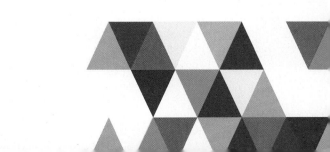

Standing Bow Pose

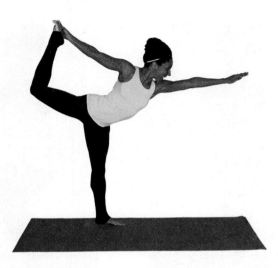

Figure 6.27
Standing Bow

Progressions	Use both hands when grabbing
Regressions	After grasping lifted foot, remain in this position Use a wall for balance.
Common Form Mistakes	Bending standing leg
Cues to Correct	Engage leg through quadriceps

Side Angle Pose

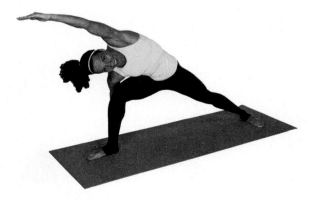

Figure 6.28
Side Angle Pose

Progressions	Bring right palm flat on floor Bring right thigh parallel to floor
Regressions	Rest right hand on block Decrease bend in right knee
Common Form Mistakes	Back heel lifts as front knee bends
Cues to Correct	As front knee bends and torso lowers to side, press strongly into back heel as though pressing back wall away. Press through outside of back heel.

Warrior III Pose

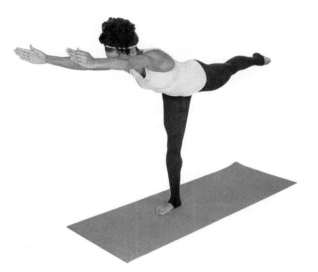

Figure 6.29
Warrior III Pose

Progressions	Draw arms back, palms down
Regressions	Balance on one foot with body upright Balance on one foot with hands by sides
Common Form Mistakes	Chest sinks down Back leg sinks down Hips are uneven
Cues to Correct	Lift through chest and draw shoulders back away from ears. Engage back leg. Press through heel and point toes to floor. Lower hip of lifted leg to align with other.

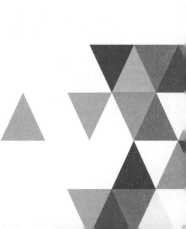

Wheel Pose

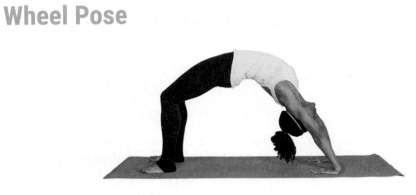

Figure 6.30
Wheel Pose

Progressions	Lift heels, press tailbone toward ceiling. Walk feet closer to hands.
Regressions	Support hands or feet on blocks
Common Form Mistakes	Knees and feet turning out
Cues to Correct	Press tailbone toward ceiling. Chest forward. Keep feet and knees in line with hip.

Wild Thing Pose

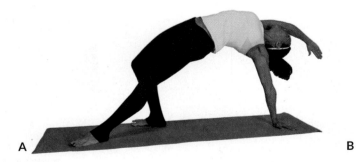
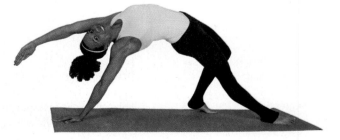

A   B

Figure 6.31
Wild Thing Pose

Progressions	Bring left palm to floor, coming into upward bow pose
Regressions	Lesser backbends
Common Form mistakes	Dropping hips Not fully extending arm
Cues to Correct	Lift up through hips, extend through fingertips.

Cycle-based Exercises

Cycle-based exercises emphasize athletic movements that could be used on a bicycle in a fast-paced environment. Indoor cycling has gained popularity through its appeal to all ages and levels of fitness within a non-impact, non-competitive environment. The lack of complicated choreography and the ability to individually control intensity attracts individuals who have previously found traditional cardiorespiratory classes too technical and strenuous. Indoor cycling also allows for competitive athletes, fitness enthusiasts, seniors, and special populations to ride side-by-side while obtaining their personal fitness and training goals. Many exercises in cycle can be progressed or regressed by increasing or decreasing resistance or speed, respectively; standing exercise can be regressed by having the participant sit back down.

The benefits of indoor cycling are:

▼ it strengthens heart and lungs.

▼ it increases muscle tone in lower body.

▼ it decreases stress and anxiety levels, resulting in better sleep.

▼ it increases bone density.

▼ it improves cholesterol and triglyceride levels.

▼ it increases energy levels.

▼ it is easy to learn.

▼ it is highly individualized.

Seated Flat

Performance Technique	1. Sitting in saddle (seat), riders pedal with moderate resistance at a cadence range between 80–100 RPM. 2. Hands in comfortable position with slight bend in elbows and proper alignment of neck and spine. 3. Upper body should be relaxed without over-gripping handlebars.
Common Form Mistakes	Hips bouncing in seat Knees bowing to outside Arms overstretched to end of bars Shoulders tense and raised toward ears Toes pointing down
Cues to Correct	Increase resistance until hips are no longer bouncing. Check bike set-up and draw knees in line with hips and ankles. Place hands on handlebars, close enough that it doesn't feel like reaching. Relax shoulders and open chest. Lower heel at top of pedal stroke and point toes forward.

Standing Flat

Performance Technique	1. Standing out of saddle (seat), riders pedal with enough resistance to support body weight at a cadence range between 80–100 RPM. 2. Spine should be neutral and hips should be stable, flexed forward, and aligned over pedals. 3. Hands should be comfortably placed slightly farther out on bars to improve stabilization, with a slight bend in elbows and proper alignment of neck and spine. 4. Slight side-to-side motion of torso is natural.
Common Form Mistakes	Inadequate resistance to maintain control or support body weight Hips unstable Hips too far forward without any flexion Excessive weight placed in hands/upper body or locked elbows Excessive neck and shoulder tension
Cues to Correct	Add enough resistance to maintain control. Stay strong through hips while allowing natural movement. Keep a slight bend at hips. Keep work in legs and use upper body for stabilization, slightly bending elbows. Avoid leaning on handlebars, keep neck and shoulders relaxed.

Seated Climb

Performance Technique	1. Sitting in saddle (seat), riders pedal with heavy to very heavy resistance at a cadence range between 60–80 RPM. 2. Hands in a comfortable position with a slight bend in elbows and proper alignment of neck and spine. 3. Upper body should be relaxed without over-gripping handlebars. 4. Hips may be slightly further back in saddle.
Common Form Mistakes	"Mashing" pedals (pushing hard straight down to bottom of pedal stroke) Excessive resistance Over-gripping handlebars Arms overstretched to end of bars Shoulders tense and raised toward ears
Cues to Correct	Use a full pedal stroke by engaging gluteus maximus and hamstrings. Add enough resistance so pedaling at 60 RPM is challenging but attainable. Relax hands and upper body, focus on legs. Place hands on handlebars, close enough that it doesn't feel like reaching. Relax shoulders and open chest.

Standing Climb

Performance Technique	1. Standing out of saddle (seat), riders pedal with heavy to very heavy resistance at a cadence range between 60–80 RPM. 2. Spine should be neutral and hips should be stable, flexed forward, and aligned directly over pedals. 3. Hands should be comfortably placed slightly farther out on bars to improve stabilization, with slight bend in elbows and proper alignment of neck and spine. 4. Slight side to side motion of torso is natural.
Common Form Mistakes	Inadequate resistance to meet objective Excessive resistance Hips too far forward without any flexion Excessive weight placed in hands/upper body or locked elbows Excessive neck and shoulder tension
Cues to Correct	Add enough resistance so pedaling out of seat at 60 RPM is challenging but attainable. If it is too hard to pedal at least 60 RPM or knee pain is felt, decrease resistance. Keep hips flexed and centered over pedals. Keep work in legs. Use upper body for stabilization with a slight bend in elbows. Avoid leaning on handlebars; keep neck and shoulders relaxed.

Seated Speed Drills

Performance Technique	1. Pedaling seated with light to medium resistance. 2. Increase cadence to 110–120 RPM for short durations (e.g., a set of 30–60 second or shorter speed pickups while maintaining same resistance).
Common Form Mistakes	Hips bouncing in seat Knees bowing to outside Arms overstretched to end of bars Shoulders tense and raised toward ears Toes pointing down
Cues to Correct	Add enough resistance to maintain control. Draw knees in line with hips and ankles. Place hands comfortably on handlebars, so it doesn't feel like reaching. Relax shoulders and open chest. Lower heel at the top of pedal.

Sprints

Performance Technique	1. Pedaling seated with moderately heavy to heavy resistance. 2. Stand up and accelerate hard to increase leg speed to 100–120 RPM. 3. Then sit for 10–20 seconds.
Common Form Mistakes	Not starting with enough resistance before standing into acceleration Not using enough resistance, resulting in bouncing in saddle Toes pointing down through pedal stroke Leaning on handlebars
Cues to Correct	Increase resistance until standing is necessary to maintain. Resistance should be heavy enough that it can only be maintained at a high speed for a few seconds. Keep the foot flat through front of pedal stroke. Keep body weight in legs.

Attacks

Performance Technique	1. While pedaling seated with moderately heavy to heavy resistance (60–80 RPM), stand and accelerate leg speed by 10–20 RPM out of saddle for short period of time. 2. Return to saddle and slow leg speed while maintaining resistance. 3. Perform in a series of 3–5 for approximately 15–30 seconds per "attack."
Common Form Mistakes	Not using enough resistance to stand up with control Using too much resistance to effectively accelerate Excessive body weight (leaning) on handlebars
Cues to Correct	Increase resistance until it is easier to stand than sit. Use enough resistance that it feels hard, but leg acceleration is still possible. Keep weight in the legs, not arms (hands).

Jumps

Performance Technique	1. Starting in seated position, keeping leg speed (RPM) constant, lift hips out of saddle for a short period of time. 2. Return to saddle. 3. Repeat alternating sequence of sitting to standing to sitting.
Common Form Mistakes	Using too little resistance "Slamming" down on saddle Putting too much weight in handlebars and "hoisting" up with upper body
Cues to Correct	Use enough resistance to maintain stabilization in and out of saddle. Use control and sit back lightly. Keep transitions smooth. Use handlebars for stability and balance but keep weight in legs and lift from hips.

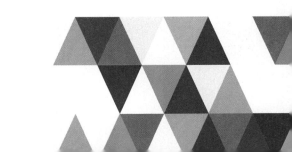

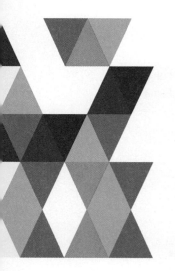

Summary

Familiarity with a variety of formats is valuable in helping a Group Fitness Instructor be adaptive and flexible. Understanding exercise technique is critical for effective instruction. Maintaining a focus on the five kinetic chain checkpoints, starting from the feet and moving up, will provide a systematic way of evaluating form for every movement. Progressions and regressions create an inclusive experience so a variety of participants can attend. Common regressions for prone exercises involve becoming more vertical through putting knees on the floor or hands on a bench. Common regressions for impact exercises such as squat jumps involve performing the exercise as a squat with no impact.

Chapter in Review

- ▼ Flexibility: static stretching
- ▼ Check points
  - ▪ Foot/ankle
  - ▪ Knees
  - ▪ LPHC
  - ▪ Shoulder girdle
  - ▪ Head
- ▼ Modifications: provide options for participants to meet skill, goal, preference
  - ▪ Progressions: increase intensity or difficult
  - ▪ Regressions: decrease intensity or difficult
- ▼ Strength-based exercises
  - ▪ Outcomes
    - ❖ Strength
    - ❖ Endurance
    - ▪ Target larger muscle groups or multiple muscle groups
- ▼ Cardio-based exercises
  - ▪ Higher intensity
  - ▪ Higher impact
  - ▪ Maximize caloric burn
- ▼ Yoga-based exercise
  - ▪ Flexibility
  - ▪ Balance
  - ▪ Core
  - ▪ Mind-body
- ▼ Cycle-based exercises
  - ▪ Athletic movements on bicycle
  - ▪ Fast-paced
  - ▪ Modifications
    - ❖ Alter resistance
    - ❖ Alter speed

Chapter 7
Class Planning and Preparation

 Learning Objectives

7.1. **Develop** a distinct class vision, outcome, and objective.

7.2. **Select** equipment based on class outcome.

7.3. **Identify** appropriate music to complement class objectives.

7.4. **Design** modifications that adhere to class outcome.

Class vision

A clearly defined intention of a class experience from the participant perspective that drives the outcome and components of a complete class.

The Importance of Planning

Planning the group fitness experience begins with a defined vision of the intent of the class. A class vision guides what is needed to support outcomes and objectives. The class *outcome* is derived from a defined class goal, whereas *objectives* are the milestones that lead up to and support that overall goal. The class vision is realized by the instructor's selection of movement order, music planning, equipment, prepped exercise modifications, and overall teaching style.

At the heart of group offerings are the participants, who deserve advanced planning and a motivational experience. Planning also helps the instructor:

▼ Create safe and effective workouts

▼ Maintain variety

▼ Maximize use of time

▼ Engage participants of all types

▼ Incorporate class "performance"

▼ Create reusable experiences

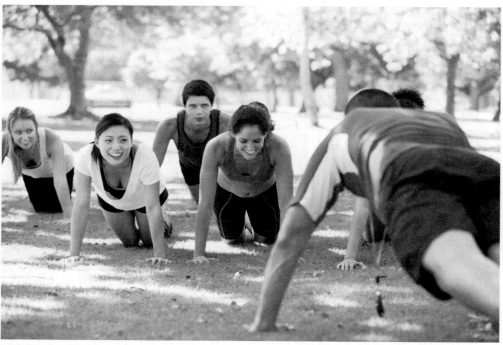

© Monkey Business Images/Shutterstock

Identifying Class Outcomes and Objectives

In order to identify outcomes and class objectives, instructors should ask themselves:

▼ What do participants expect to get out of this class, based on the title and description?

▼ What type of movement supports this outcome?

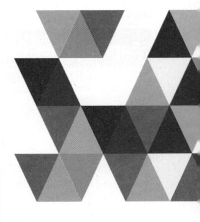

- ▼ What equipment is available?
- ▼ How much time is available to achieve the class vision?
- ▼ How can I manipulate intensity to accomplish the class goals?
- ▼ How should I arrange or sequence the class elements?

Once the outcome and objectives have been identified, an instructor can use a checklist (**Table 7.1**) or class template form (**Table 7.2**).

Table 7.1

Group Fitness Class Checklist	
Pre-class Planning	• Design class blueprint.
Intro	• Greet participants. • Be available before class to orient participants. • Have background music on or cued up when class starts. • Provide equipment recommendations. • Formally introduce self and class format. • Quickly explain options for modifications.
Movement Prep	• Begin general or specific movement prep. • Demonstrate movement selection with proper technique. • Transition movement prep into body of workout.
Body of Workout	• Build movement sequences logically, gradually, and progressively. • Use all three planes of motion and balance muscle groups. • Monitor intensity using training zones, the talk test, or RPE scales.
Transition	• Create a motivating and educational atmosphere. • Conduct the transition with body awareness exercises.
Outro	• Specific praise to group on effort and progress. • Invite participants to come back again. • Request feedback or questions after class.

Table 7.2

Sample Class Planning Sheet

Class Name	Strong
Vision	Moderate-intensity resistance training-based class designed to improve strength, cardiorespiratory fitness, burn calories, and leave participants feeling accomplished and empowered to do more.
Format	45 Minute Strength and Resistance
Music	High-energy radio hits: 130 BPM
Equipment Needs	Gliding discs, medicine balls, and medium dumbbells (8–12 lb)
Pre-class set-up	Participants will have independent set-up—no stations
Intro	Provide overview of class outcome (strength, cardio, and calorie burn). Identify equipment needed and provide overview of proper use. Offer motivating phrase to start.
Movement prep	• SMR pre-class • Static stretch: hip flexors, chest, lats • Planks (3 sets, progressing each time) • Floor bridges (2 sets of 12) • Floor crunches (1 sets of 12) • Single-leg squat, all planes of motion (1 set of 15 each) Time: 5–7 minutes (minimal rest in between sets)
Body of Workout	All exercises will be performed in varying tempos of 2/2, 3/1, and 1/1. Three exercises will be performed one after the other before moving onto the next set. No rest. 1. Squat Curl to Press: 16 reps 2. Lunge to Balance (sagittal, frontal, transverse): 16 reps 3. Push-ups: 16 reps 4. Lunge with Rotation: 16 reps 5. Squat to Press: 16 reps 6. Single-leg Squat: 16 reps per leg 7. Single-leg Squat Touchdown: 12 reps 8. Push-up with Rotation: 8 reps per side Time: 35–40 minutes, 1 set at each tempo for a total of 3 sets.
Transition	Participants do SMR on their own. Static stretch piriformis, biceps femoris, pecs. Time: 3–5 minutes.
Outro	Provide congratulations on completing 72 push-ups and almost 200 lunges total today. Rest, drink water, and foam roll. Time: <1 minute.

Teaching Method Considerations

A Group Fitness Instructor should consider the class delivery method to plan for pre-choreographed, pre-designed, or freestyle teaching.

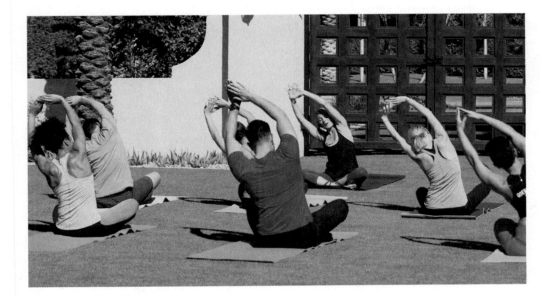

Pre-choreographed

Pre-choreographed classes offer instant credibility with participants because of brand or format consistency. Therefore, it is important to maintain a uniform experience throughout class planning and execution, which will require time to learn, rehearse, and master choreography with recommended cues. Pre-choreographed classes require an initial investment of time (and sometimes money), but they can be reused for weeks or months.

Considerations for pre-choreographed classes include:

▼ Time for initial learning, rehearsing, and memorization
▼ A schedule to learn and execute new choreography (e.g., 4 hours, once per month)
▼ All experience components (e.g., music, moves, equipment, cueing style)

Pre-designed

An initial time investment is needed to know and practice the pre-designed class structure, as typically seen in the form of an additional qualification. Then the instructor creates interchangeable

INSTRUCTOR TIP 👍

Pre-designed classes take less time for initial learning but will require a constant effort to add and update movements that fit the structure.

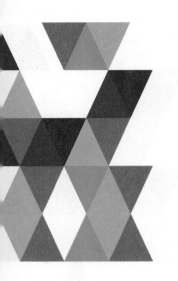

modules to bring variety and progression, while still maintaining continuity to the pre-designed structure. The teaching method considerations for pre-designed content include:

▼ An initial time and financial investment

▼ Ongoing time to update movement toolkit

▼ Only a few new moves introduced each class

Freestyle

An instructor designs and plans every aspect of a freestyle class which, despite its name, should have a concise structure centered around a meaningful class vision. The teaching method considerations for freestyle content include:

▼ Design of a class vision to ensure a connected and effective experience

▼ Use of movement patterns that have been previously taught with success

▼ Extra time needed for creating entirely new class experiences

▼ Creativity used sparingly to avoid overwhelming a group

Music Selection and Planning

A key factor that differentiates group fitness from other exercise is the use of music. Group Fitness Instructors use music to set pace, drive timing of verbal cues, enhance motivation, and support the overall outcome. Music also supports the desired mood or atmosphere and helps participants feel emotionally invested in the workout.

Many studies have concluded that music plays a significant role in exercise performance and adherence. Exercise performance is better and it offers physiological and psychological benefits[1,2]:

▼ *Dissociation*: Diverting the mind from feelings of fatigue and lowering perception of effort.

▼ *Synchronization*: Moving to music results improves movement efficiency.

▼ *Motor learning*: Music replicates forms of human locomotion.

The overall benefit to the participant is improved exercise performance and experience. Music can also assist instructors in creating, planning, teaching, and organizing class content.

INSTRUCTOR TIP 👍

Group Fitness Instructors can use music created by fitness music companies (such as Yes! Fitness Music® And Power Music®). These companies produce properly licensed music specifically engineered to enhance fitness activities.

⊘ **Check It Out**

Music can support the goal of a specific class component. Up-tempo (fast) music helps participants push harder without a corresponding increase in RPE, whereas down-tempo (slow) music promotes a faster heart rate recovery and reduced blood lactate levels.[3]

Music can be used to save time and increase efficiency and can help instructors track time and reps, create new choreography and movement patterns, provide performance fuel, and cue properly.

Musical Structure

Music starts with the beat. The beat of a song is the audible, metrical division that occurs within the foundational layer of music. The beat is the foundation upon which everything else works together to create sonic experiences.

Typically, beats are grouped together to form measures or bars. The downbeat is the first beat of a measure. Often, when someone is "off the beat," he or she missed the downbeat and did not start a movement on count 1.

Measures are grouped together to form phrases. In 8-count phrasing, there is an audible emphasis every 8 counts. In 32-count phrasing, a common musical structure used in group fitness, there is audible emphasis every 32 counts. This audio emphasis starts a few counts before the 32nd beat ends, creating a signal for an upcoming count "1" to begin a new 32-count phrase.

Using 32-count Phrasing

The musical structure in 32-count phrasing provides steady, clear, and distinct beats that are easy to follow. By creating movement patterns that are 32 counts, movements feel connected and complete for both the instructor and the participants. In addition, 32-count phrasing can also be used to count or track reps. At 128 BPM (a common tempo for group fitness), one 32-count phrase will take about 15 seconds to complete.

Tempo and Rhythm

Tempo and rhythm have different roles in the way music sounds and makes one feel. Musical tempo is the speed or pace of a piece of music and is denoted by beats per minute (BPM).

Rhythm is a pattern of repeated movement or sound. This repeated pattern structures the count.

Song Components

Most songs applicable to group fitness will follow a formula of components, or sections, that primarily include the verse, pre-chorus (i.e., build up), and the chorus. The verse is usually made up of lyrics and is the story or emotions as expressed by the writer. Each verse is different and supports the chorus in some way.

Beat

The audible, metrical division that occurs within the foundational layer of music.

Downbeat

The first beat of a measure.

32-count phrasing

A common musical structure used in group fitness where there is an audible build up and closure every 32 counts.

Beats per minute (BPM)

The number of beats in one minute.

Rhythm

A pattern or repeated movement or sound.

CAUTION ⚠️

With the ability to shift tempo, it can be easy to go too fast, which compromises movement patterns and increases risk for injury. Always test movements with the planned tempo to ensure a full range of motion can be performed safely. Many music apps will allow you to adjust the tempo for safety and enjoyment.

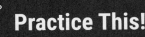

Practice This!

Find some 32-count music and start counting to hear and learn the phrasing; see if this style of music can enhance your teaching skills. Since 32-count fitness music is marketed as such, it is easy to find by searching online for "32-count fitness music."

INSTRUCTOR TIP 👍

To quickly find the tempo of your music, you can tap the number of beats you hear in 10 seconds and multiply that number by six. There are also various apps and digital tools that read and adjust tempo.

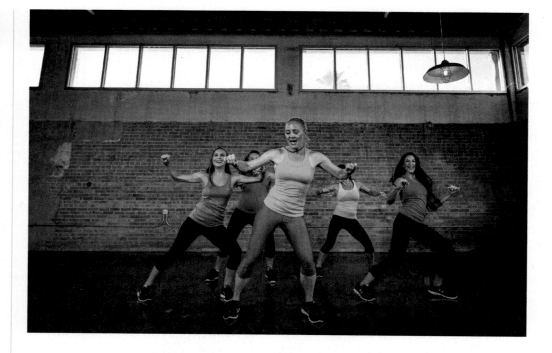

The pre-chorus sounds like a "build" with an obvious increase in intensity, which transitions to a dramatic release with the chorus. The chorus then hooks everything together and is repeated and emphasized throughout the song.

Tempo and Movement Safety

Tempo is important to promote safe movement patterns. It should allow proper time for a full range of motion of the intended movement (**Table 7.3**).

Table 7.3

Recommended Music Tempo (BPM) for Common Formats	
Class Format	**Recommended BPM Range**
Resistance Training	125–135 BPM
High-Intensity Intervals/Tabata	150–160 BPM
Boot Camp	130–140 BPM
Step	128–132 BPM
Barre, Pilates	124–128 BPM
Kickboxing	140–150 BPM
Aqua/Water/Seniors	122–128 BPM

If the music plays a central role in movement cueing and exercise selection, it is foreground music. If the music is not central to the movement, and is used to support the atmosphere (yoga, Boot Camp, etc.), it is background music.

Background music may be used in yoga, boot camps, or any other setting where music is beneficial to enhance a mood. Sometimes Group Fitness Instructors will use music as both a foreground and a background tool. For example, in a group strength class, some movements may be choreographed to the musical tempo, while other movements may ignore the beat, as it may be too fast or too slow for a specific exercise.

Music Selection

Instructors should select music appropriate for the tone and outcomes of the class. It is also important to consider the style. The musical genres and styles in **Table 7.4** work well for common class formats, because the sounds, rhythms, and lyrical structure often support the objective of the class.

With music, instructors should consider the following:

▼   *Tempo*—Is the music the right tempo for the class?

▼   *Non-stop mix*—Does the music need to be non-stop to keep movement continuous, or does it need gaps?

▼   *Style*—Is the music the right genre/style to support the activity?

Foreground music

Using tempo, lyrics or song components to drive the movements.

Background music

Using music to set the mood and support the atmosphere.

Musical style

A subset of a genre or classification of music from certain eras or cultures.

Table 7.4

Recommended Genres/Styles for Common Class Formats	
Class Format	**Recommended Genres/Style**
Weight-training or Sculpting	Top 40 Pop, Alternative, Classic Rock, Deep House, Progressive House
High-Intensity Intervals/Tabata	Electronic (House, Techno), Fast Top 40 Pop, Alternative, Indie Rock
Boot Camp	Dubstep, Alternative, Indie Rock
Cardio Dance/Latin	Latin, Dance, Pop, Hip-hop, R&B
Step	Pop, Thematic or Decade Compilations
Barre, Pilates	Tropical House, Classical, Jazz, Soul, Soft Rock
Kickboxing	Techno, Progressive House, Dubstep
Aqua/Water/Seniors	Oldies, Motown, Dance, Top 40 Pop
Yoga	Down-tempo (exotic or ambient), World, Indie or Alternative

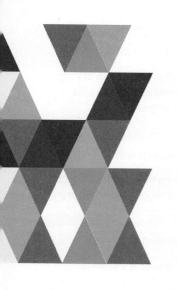

▼ *Energy*—Does the music energy support the intended movement

▼ *Variety*—Does the music match the variety of participants attending the class?

▼ *Audience*—Is the music appropriate for the audience and their interests? Does the music engage participants by using music they requested or have provided feedback on?

Modality and Equipment Considerations

Equipment, also known as an *exercise modality*, is a form or mode of exercise that creates a challenge to its user by presenting a specific stress to the body. It is important for instructors to be familiar with the various modalities, know how to best incorporate various modalities into a workout regimen, and understand when a given modality is most valuable. When planning for a class, equipment types and recommendations on resistance should be documented in advance. This gives the instructor a record of which equipment and settings were used, which is helpful information if the workouts revolve around use of the same modalities.

There are several factors which may determine what modalities are incorporated. The best choices will depend on class vision and participant-related factors such as:

▼ Age

▼ Fitness level

▼ Fitness goals

▼ Personal preference

Instructors should focus on modalities that align with the class vision, intended outcome, and the needs of the participants. Understanding the history of a modality, along with developing knowledge of its benefits, risks, and correct implementation, will enable the group instructor to make educated decisions about the proper use and integration of it into different exercise programs.

Modifications are critical in teaching; therefore, potential progressions or regressions of an exercise may directly affect the choice to implement a new modality for a participant. An instructor may not have access to certain modalities, so familiarity with a variety of equipment will assist an instructor in adapting to unforeseen circumstances.

Modalities for Group Fitness

There are 10 exercise modality categories commonly used in the group fitness setting. They include the following:

▼ Bodyweight training is one of the simplest and most basic exercise modalities, because no equipment is needed to perform exercises (Figure 7.1). It leverages a participant's bodyweight and position to create an exercise challenge, with a wide variety of movements and positions from which to choose. For example, it can be used for strength, balance (single-leg squat), plyometrics (speed-skaters), and yoga (crow pose).

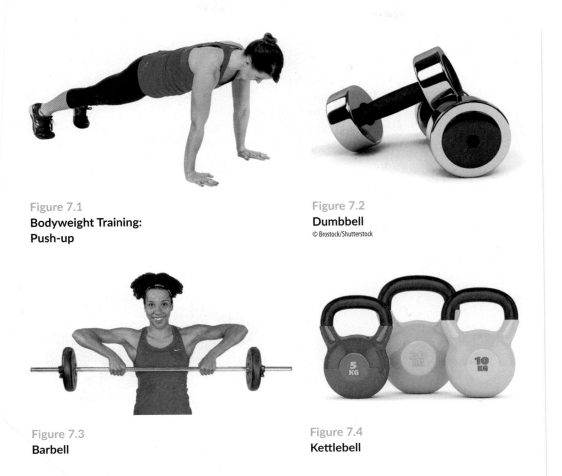

Figure 7.1
**Bodyweight Training:
Push-up**

Figure 7.2
Dumbbell
© Brostock/Shutterstock

Figure 7.3
Barbell

Figure 7.4
Kettlebell

▼ **Weighted Equipment:** (dumbbells, barbells, kettlebells, medicine balls, weighted bars, and others)

    a.   A dumbbell is a short, handheld bar with a weight at each end, typically used in pairs for group exercise (Figure 7.2).

    b.   A barbell is a long bar with fixed segments at each end that allow for placement of combinations of weight plates and a spring or collar lock (Figure 7.3).

    c.   A kettlebell is a rounded, cannonball-like free weight that has an arched handle and a flat bottom (Figure 7.4).

    d.   A medicine ball (Figure 7.5) is a weighted ball that can be used as a weight (e.g., Russian twist), as a balance tool (e.g., unstable push-up), or as a reactive power-training tool (e.g., throws and slams). Medicine balls are common tools used for power training.

▼ **Elastic Resistance** (bands, tubing, figure-8 tubes, looped bands): Resistance bands and tubing are either rubber or synthetic latex bands that provide a resistance to the body when stretched (Figure 7.6).

    a.   A band is a flat piece of elastic that may be in a loop or in long segments that can be held, cut, or tied to customize the band for a specific activity.

    b.   A tube is a hollow, circular elastic material that usually has handles.

Power trai

A for

p

CAUTION ⚠️

Incorporating a plyometric component to a group session can be a great way to add variety to a routine. However, plyometric exercises should be chosen with caution, as they require higher levels of athletic conditioning to safely perform, specifically on the deceleration of movement.

✓ Check It Out

While used for many similar exercises, medicine balls are different from *slam balls*, and it may be confusing to remember the uses for each. A medicine ball is typically covered in leather or rubber material, and will usually bounce back when thrown against a wall, floor, or hard surface. A slam ball is usually sand-filled, supple, and will not bounce back when thrown, forcing the participant to pick up the ball between each repetition.

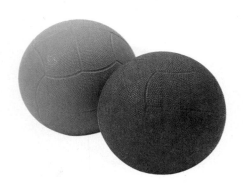

Figure 7.5
Medicine Ball
© Mark Herreid/Shutterstock

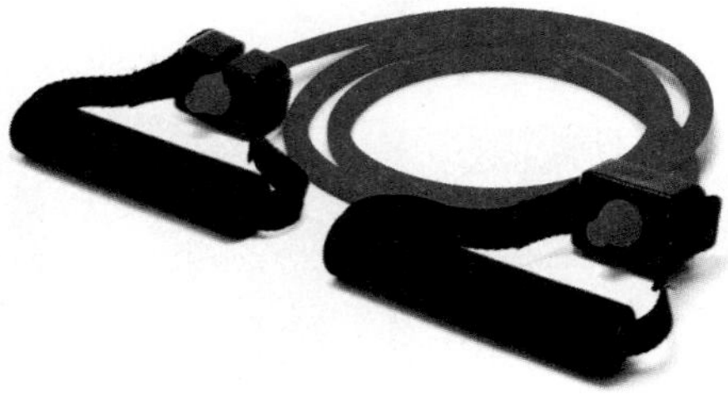

Figure 7.6
Elastic Resistance Band
© John Kasawa/Shutterstock

▼ **Balance** (stability balls, balance devices sliding discs)

   a. A stability ball is a large, inflated exercise ball that can be used for various forms of integrated training (Figure 7.7).

   b. Balance devices (i.e., half-dome balls) may be used to create instability through various types of movements from push-ups to squats.

   c. Sliding discs are pieces of equipment that glide along a relatively stable base of support.

▼ **Reactive, SAQ, and Power** (battle ropes, boxes, ladders, cones, dots, etc.): Many tools fit within this modality category, including various types of balls, ropes, boxes, ladders, cones, dots, and hurdles. Plyometric boxes are square or rectangular boxes used in plyometric training. Some of these modalities can be classified into more than one category.

▼ **Self-Myofascial Release** (foam rollers, Figure 7.8; rolling sticks; massage balls): Self-myofascial release (SMR) is a flexibility technique that focuses on the body's neural and fascial systems by decreasing excitation of receptors and releasing the tension of muscles.[4]

▼ **Suspension Training** (fixed straps, portable straps): The combined use of straps and the body's weight to place a stress load on the neuromuscular system (Figure 7.9).

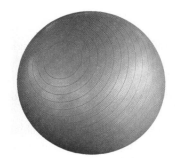

Figure 7.7
Stability Ball
© Paul Maguire/Shutterstock

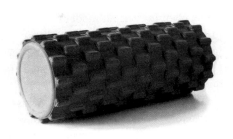

Figure 7.8
Foam Roller
© Givens87/Shutterstock

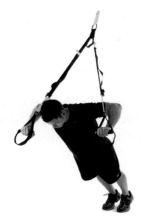

Figure 7.9
Suspension Trainer

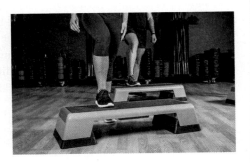

Figure 7.10
Step bench
© David Pereiras/Shutterstock

▼ **Aquatic** (belts, noodles, webbed gloves, paddles, water dumbbells)

   a. Aquatic belts are used in deep water workouts to keep participants afloat and challenge the core.

   b. Webbed gloves or water dumbbells are designed to increase drag, viscosity, and overall resistance in the water.

   c. Noodles are used for floatation and support during traveling movements.

▼ **Mind–body** (mats, blocks, straps)

   a. Yoga mats are anti-slip mats that vary in thickness, designed to support yoga postures and provide cushion, comfort, and support.

   b. Yoga blocks and straps are small tools that provide postural support for certain yoga poses, or when flexibility, strength, and range of motion are limited and need extra support or modifications.

▼ **Skill Mastery** (cycle bikes, step benches, mini-trampolines, ballet barres, boxing gloves, kick/punch bags): Specific pieces of equipment used for longer periods of time (e.g., an entire class) that require mastery of a skillset include stationary bikes, step benches (Figure 7.10), mini-trampolines, ballet barres, boxing gloves, punch/kick bags, and other format-specific equipment options.

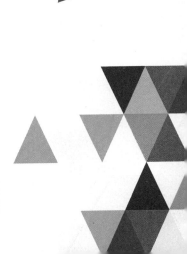

Modality Logistics

When planning various modalities in a class, it is important to include options that vary in weight or resistance level to allow for adjustments in size or intensity. A good practice is to set up the instructor station in the same way the participants will set up their stations. As class participants enter the room, they will have a visual of what is needed, and the instructor will be available for questions or support.

Equipment comes with specific usage guidelines and safety requirements, with which all instructors should be familiar and have practiced prior to using. To minimize the risk of injury among participants, an instructor must ensure the equipment is available in sufficient quantities for all participants and check that it is in good working order prior to starting any class.

Planning Movement Modifications

Even though a class may be carefully planned, new participants from unexpected demographics may show up at any time. An instructor should be prepared to provide modifications, progressions, and regressions for all movements that will be used in class. This may seem a daunting task for new instructors, but it becomes much easier as they build a mental library of exercises.

In any class format, guidelines regarding modifications for intensity and complexity should also be included in workout planning. Modifications offer class participants a choice of two or more exercises to better match individual skill sets, fitness goals, and daily preferences.

Class Rehearsal

After planning is done, the next step is to practice the movements for a logical flow that aligns with the science and safety of integrated fitness. Instructors should rehearse the components that are new and untested. In this way, time is managed efficiently and the instructor can provide a polished, finished presentation that leaves participants feeling energized, successful, and happy after class.

Memorizing Choreography

Instructors might be required to memorize choreography and can implement the following helpful tips:

- Verbal rehearsal—Play the music and practice saying the verbal cues for the choreography, without doing them.

- Mirroring rehearsal—Stand in front of a mirror and perform the movements as they should be performed in class, but on the opposite side.

- Test rehearsal—Use a family member or friend as your test participant.

Testing and Practicing

Some classes do not require detailed choreography but have sequences or patterns that may require a run-through to make sure they work in a real group setting. The other common area that requires testing and practicing is the intended tempo. An instructor may plan a circuit class

---

INSTRUCTOR TIP 👍

Plan class modifications, progressions, and regressions one class at a time, to keep class planning effective. With experience comes more efficient planning and teaching skills!

at 140 BPM, but may realize during testing and rehearsal that the movements cannot possibly be performed at that speed, and therefore change the tempo to 125 BPM. Testing prior to class reduces the risk of injury and keeps class flow moving in a positive direction. Instructors should practice in real time—play the music at the planned tempo and verbally cue and physically practice the exercise sequences. If it feels rushed, it is better to adjust the desired performance to a slower pace.

Other ways to test and implement new class content include:

▼ Offering free demo classes when testing or refining new content or teaching skills.

▼ Launching the new content in conjunction with a promotional event or giveaway.

▼ Kicking off a new class with a team presentation. For example, a program director may choose to pair a popular class with a new class in a "double-header" format.

Summary

Planning is the culmination of applying principles of integrated training, all workout components, and flawless exercise technique for an effective, engaging class experience. Classes with a clear vision, a detailed plan, and sound rehearsal provide a polished, positive experience for participants, while selections in music, equipment, and movements play an integral role in providing the most effective workout. Making an effort to plan quality classes in advance is a habit that pays off over the lifespan of a career. Additionally, thoughtful preparation and planning can contribute to a more successful implementation of class outcomes.

Chapter in Review

▼ Planning for teaching methods
   ▪ Pre-choreographed
   ▪ Pre-designed
   ▪ Freestyle

▼ Music selection
   ▪ BPM
      ❖ Resistance: 125–135 BPM
      ❖ HIIT/ Tabata: 150–160 BPM
      ❖ Boot Camp: 130–140 BPM
      ❖ Step: 128–132 BPM
      ❖ Barre/Pilates: 124–128 BPM
      ❖ Kickboxing: 140–150 BPM
      ❖ Aqua/ Seniors: 122–128 BPM
   ▪ Style
      ❖ Strength: alternative, classic rock, house
      ❖ HIIT: house, techno, pop, alternative
      ❖ Boot Camp: dubstep, alternative, indie rock
      ❖ Cardio dance/Latin: latin, dance, pop, hip-hop, R&B
      ❖ Step: Pop, thematic compilations
      ❖ Barre/Pilates: House, classical, jazz, soul, soft rock
      ❖ Kickboxing: techno, house, dubstep
      ❖ Aqua/Seniors: oldies, Motown, dance, pop
      ❖ Yoga: exotic or ambient, world, indie, alternative
   ▪ Musical structure
   ▪ 32-count

▼ Equipment selection

▼ Planning modifications

▼ Rehearsal and testing

References

1. Bacon CJ, Myers TR, Karageorghis CI. Effect of music-movement synchrony on exercise oxygen consumption. *J Sports Med Phys Fitness*. 2012;52(4):359–365.

2. Karageorghis C, Priest D. Music in sport and exercise: an update on research and application. *Sport J*. 2008;11(3). Accessed http://thesportjournal.org/article/music-sport-and-exercise-update-research-and-application/.

3. Lee S, Kimmerly DS. Influence of music on maximal self-paced running performance and passive post-exercise recovery rate. *J Sports Med Phys Fitness*. 2016;56(1-2):39–48.

4. Curran PF, Fiore RD, Crisco JJ. A comparison of the pressure exerted on soft tissue by 2 myofascial rollers. *J Sports Rehabil*. 2008;17(4):432–442.

© Syda Productions/Shutterstock

Chapter 8
Adapting to Class Dynamics

 Learning Objectives

8.1.   **Identify** methods for responding to unexpected variables in the classroom.

8.2.   **Explain** methods for assessing and ensuring movement quality in participants during workouts.

8.3.   **Identify** general safety, emergency response, and environmental considerations, and mitigations for risk.

Introduction to Class Dynamics

Even with perfect preparation, there will be unexpected situations that require a Group Fitness Instructor to make quick decisions or changes to the overall plan for the class. The ability to understand these dynamics will help the instructor quickly resolve or adapt to these situations. By implementing some general procedures on the day of class, instructors can also work to circumvent unforeseen circumstances.

Pre-class Set-up

On-site class preparation includes organizing the room, cueing the music, checking the microphone, and arranging participants as they come in. Being aware, organized, and prepared will set the tone for class and make the transition into the workout seamless, giving participants confidence in their instructor.

Generally instructors should arrive 15 minutes early to prepare for class, allowing time to evaluate equipment, ensure the sound system is working properly, and resolve any apparent technical difficulties. It is common for classes to be scheduled back to back, which means instructors must make the best use of time just before and right after class.

Music Set-up

Instructors should

- Test music
- Test music volume (not to exceed 85 dB)
- Play music to set tone and create excitement
- Set tempo to appropriate BPMs
- Silence any mobile devices
- Bring backup music

Microphone Check

Microphones allow the instructor to deliver instruction that can be heard over music without straining the voice. The following are a few tips to ensure the microphone is ready for class:

- Check the battery life
- Use a windscreen (i.e., foam cover)
- Check mic volume to ensure instructor and music can be heard clearly
- Position mic correctly on the body

⊘ Check It Out

Many gyms have different sound or microphone equipment, and sometimes things go wrong with the equipment available. To prevent some easily avoidable issues that could delay the class, maintain an "instructor kit" with the following items:

- Auxiliary cord with a ¼-inch adaptor
- Batteries (AA, AAA, and 9-volt are most common)
- Back up CD with usable class music
- Charger for digital music device
- Instructor microphone belt
- Windscreen
- Disposable ear plugs for participants who may be sensitive to sound

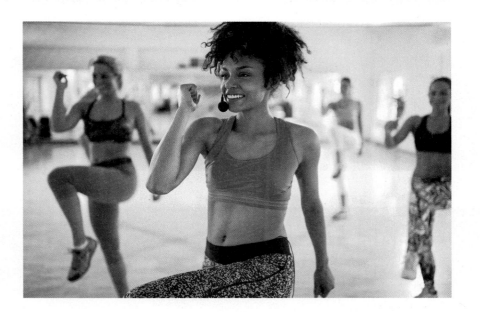

Equipment Needs

Informing participants of what they need as they are coming into the room allows them to set up their stations before class. Setting up equipment before class will build rapport and optimize the arrangement of participants. This works best when everyone is using the same equipment.

It is important to evaluate equipment to be used in class to look for any obvious signs of deterioration or dysfunction. Common signs of equipment deterioration include tears, chips, fraying, or peeling. Additionally, it is important to look for broken pedal clips on cycles, cracks in step platforms, and holes or tears in yoga mats. Remove any broken or dysfunctional items from the floor, if possible, or indicate the malfunctioning equipment with appropriate signage. Instructors should follow up with the facility staff to report any broken or malfunctioning equipment. All equipment should be moved out of the workout space when not in use to prevent accident or injury.

In formats like cycling, where large equipment is necessary, bikes or other equipment should be spaced far enough apart to ensure safe mounting and dismounting. Participants will need to adjust the equipment to fit their needs once they arrive.

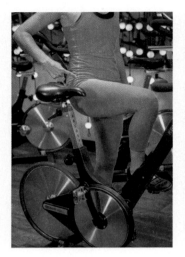

Figure 8.1
Proper Seat Height

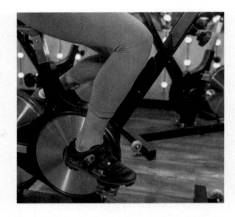

Figure 8.2
Proper Knee and Toe Alignment

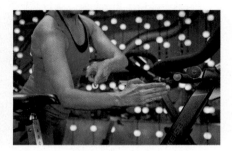

Figure 8.3
Proper Seat and Handlebar Distance

⊘ Check It Out

Bike seats should be adjusted to come up against the participant's hip (**Figure 8.1**); the seat should be moved to locate the knees over the toes once seated (**Figure 8.2**), and handlebars should be set at an appropriate height and distance to ensure a neutral spine (**Figure 8.3**).

🏃 Practice This!

Practice setting up your bike using these standard guidelines.

1. Sit comfortably on saddle, move one crank forward and down until perpendicular to floor with pedal parallel to floor.
2. Place heel on pedal with foot parallel to floor—knee should demonstrate a relaxed, extended position (7° flexion). Adjust seat height accordingly.
3. Sit comfortably on saddle, move one crank forward until it is parallel to floor.
4. Place ball of foot directly over the pedal spindle (middle portion). The bump just below the kneecap (tibial tuberosity) should align directly over the spindle. Adjust forward and rear position of seat accordingly.
5. Sit comfortably on saddle and place hands on most comfortable portion of handlebars with spine as neutral as possible. Adjust handlebar height and travel until weight is evenly distributed between rear-end and wrists.

Participant Arrangement

The arrangement of participants is important for the safety and success of class. Group Fitness Instructors should consider spacing needs of participants to ensure the arrangement is safe for movement in the workout. Proper technique is essential for participant safety, so the Group Fitness Instructor should be in a position to both see all participants and be seen by them. Some of the most effective arrangements include staggered (Figure 8.4), row (Figure 8.5), circuit (Figure 8.6), and circle (Figure 8.7).

▼ **Staggered**: Allows the instructor to teach from the front of the room while being able to view all participants. This may create some obstructed views of demonstrations. It is important to ensure adequate space to be attentive through the various lines.

▼ **Row**: Allows instructors to move through the room to coach participants using large equipment. This may have some space limitations, and individuals at the ends may feel excluded. It is important to remember to visit those on the ends and ensure adequate space.

▼ **Circuit**: Allows the instructor to move from station to station, coaching specific to the exercise at each one. This arrangement can create space and equipment constraints and may reduce the quality of feedback if multiple exercises are being performed simultaneously.

▼ **Circle**: Allows circular jogging, as well as forward and backward movement toward the center of the room. This arrangement requires an instructor's back to be turned to participants at times, which can complicate explanations and demonstrations. Additionally, it can create unwanted competition or poor role modeling between participants watching one another. Instructors may have difficulty navigating among participants.

> **INSTRUCTOR TIP** 👍
>
> Staggered arrangements are helpful for classes heavy in instructor demonstration, while classes with large equipment might benefit from a row or circuit arrangement.

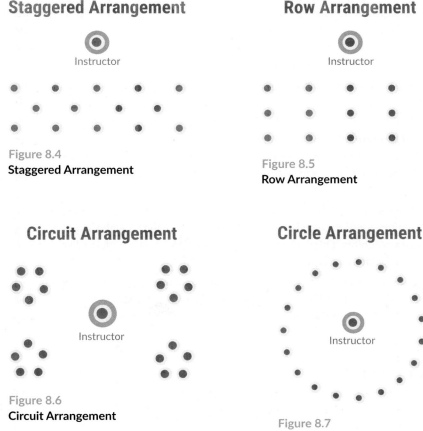

Staggered Arrangement

Figure 8.4
Staggered Arrangement

Row Arrangement

Figure 8.5
Row Arrangement

Circuit Arrangement

Figure 8.6
Circuit Arrangement

Circle Arrangement

Figure 8.7
Circle Arrangement

> ### ✓ Check It Out
>
> If the class is interrupted, get your class back on track as soon as possible with the following tips:
> - Give participants a task or exercise while you address the interruption.
> - Use the interruption to prompt participants to grab a drink or check their heart rates.
> - Make the interruption go away as quickly as possible!
> - Give the class instructions first, and then attend to individual needs.
> - Assign a participant to count reps and time while you address the problem.

On-the-Spot Considerations

A good instructor has the ability to adapt to the conditions of each class. Even if a class is planned well, the workout space, equipment, or participants can create unexpected situations.

- ▼ **Unexpected participants:** Sometimes, a set list of participants is created due to limited space or equipment. The best way to address an unexpected participant is to talk to the person one-on-one before class starts or after class to avoid disrupting others.

- ▼ **Space limitations:** When space becomes an issue, movements and equipment will need to be adjusted to make sure all participants are able to safely execute exercises. Instructors can have participants perform exercises standing in place to reduce the risk of running into or tripping up another participant. On some occasions, there will be no option but to turn participants away.

- ▼ **Equipment changes:** Facilities will often change equipment inventory over time. Instructors must practice with this equipment in advance before use. Planning backups for equipment (both audio and exercise) will help instructors mitigate these types of issues.

- ▼ **Timing challenges:** Instructors running late on a previous class or at the beginning of class can limit the time available for the workout. In these cases, the instructor should adjust the least important or most time-consuming portion of class to accommodate the loss of time.

- ▼ **Managing conflict:** The best way to manage the conflict is dealing with it right away. Common conflicts include new participants occupying a regular's spot or limited equipment availability. Offer suggestions that make both participants feel valued, such as asking a regular participant to show the new participant how class works.

- ▼ **Managing participants:** Participants who gravitate toward the front row typically seek attention, while those in the back rows tend to shy away from the spotlight. It is important for instructors to manage these personalities appropriately to engage everyone effectively.

Monitoring

Monitoring is the act of observing movements to ensure proper form and functioning of the kinetic chain. Monitoring should be done throughout class:

- ▼ *During bilateral movements*—Teach the move on the right, then monitor on the left.
- ▼ *After a new or starting movement cue*—Once participants have been properly cued and are moving, focus on watching the class execute movements.
- ▼ *After a timed sequence starts*—When doing a move for 30 seconds, an instructor can cue the move, say "start", then walk around and monitor the movements more closely.
- ▼ *During simple movements*—An instructor may cue a simple move like "jog in place," then walk around or jog with the class with a focus on monitoring effort, execution, and energy.
- ▼ *During countdowns*—An instructor may start a countdown, then walk around and monitor during the remaining reps.

INSTRUCTOR TIP 👍

New participants often need time to work through the learning curve. Allow room for new participants to learn and experiment before transitioning or correcting.

Types of Monitoring

There are two main types of monitoring: physical and emotional. *Physical monitoring* is the act of monitoring everything about the physical movement. Physical signs that may show a participant is in need of assistance, extra cueing, or motivation include:

- ▼ not performing a full range of motion.
- ▼ low effort.
- ▼ poor form.
- ▼ talking to neighbors.
- ▼ excessive breathing, gasping.
- ▼ putting the equipment down.
- ▼ stopping completely.

Emotional monitoring is the act of monitoring the participant's emotional response to the workout. Signs that show a participant is in need of assistance, extra cueing, or motivation include:

- ▼ looks of confusion or frustration.
- ▼ looking at the clock or door.
- ▼ avoiding eye contact with the instructor.
- ▼ poor posture.
- ▼ heavy sighs.
- ▼ going extra fast or particularly slow.
- ▼ excessive stopping.

Assessing and Ensuring Movement Quality

Understanding possible muscle imbalances and limitations allows an instructor to give cues for correcting movement in class. Instructors can do a light assessment before and during class with the following in mind.

Postural distortion patterns

Common postural malalignments and muscle imbalances that individuals develop based on a variety of factors.

Pronation distortion syndrome

A postural distortion syndrome characterized by foot pronation (flat feet) and adducted and internally rotated knees (knock knees).

Lower crossed syndrome

A postural distortion syndrome characterized by an anterior tilt to the pelvis (arched lower back).

Upper crossed syndrome

A postural distortion syndrome characterized by a forward head and rounded shoulders.

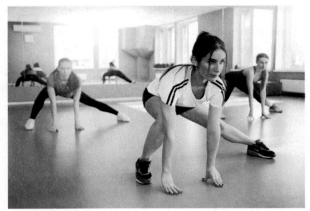
© Basyn/Shutterstock

The Importance of Posture

Proper postural alignment helps produce effective and safe movement. Good posture ensures the muscles of the body are aligned at the proper length–tension relationships necessary for efficient functioning of muscles around a joint. Proper posture is essential in maximizing strength and power gains.[1–4]

Muscle Imbalances and Injury

When observing posture, instructors are evaluating participants for muscle imbalances. In general, when muscle imbalances are present, a certain muscle (or muscles) associated with a joint (or joints) may be in a shortened state while other muscles are in a lengthened state, affecting the position of the joint. Over time, this can lead to injury or pain.

Postural Assessments

Posture is often viewed as being static. However, posture is constantly changing to meet the demands placed on the kinetic chain. The observation process should search for any movement distortions that may lead to injury.

Static Postural Assessment

Static posture provides a snapshot of the body's alignment and may warn of potential problems. Poor posture highlights overactive or shortened muscles and muscles that are underactive or lengthened, which affect the way a participant moves and responds to exercise. Posture provides information for the instructor to cue the participant into the correct exercise technique or offer modifications.

Postural distortion patterns are common postural malalignments and muscle imbalances individuals develop based on a variety of factors (e.g., lifestyle, occupation). Three common distortion patterns have been identified: pronation distortion syndrome, lower crossed syndrome, and upper crossed syndrome[5]:

▼ *Pronation distortion syndrome*—A postural distortion syndrome characterized by foot pronation (flat feet) and adducted and internally rotated knees (knock knees) (Figure 8.8; **Table 8.1**).

▼ *Lower crossed syndrome*—A postural distortion syndrome characterized by an anterior tilt to the pelvis (arched lower back) (Figure 8.9; **Table 8.2**).

▼ *Upper crossed syndrome*—A postural distortion syndrome characterized by a forward head and rounded shoulders (Figure 8.10; **Table 8.3**).

Table 8.1

Pronation Distortion Syndrome Summary

Short Muscles	Lengthened Muscles	Altered Joint Mechanics
Gastrocnemius Soleus Peroneals Adductors Iliotibial (IT) band Hip flexor complex Biceps femoris (short head)	Anterior tibialis Posterior tibialis Gluteus medius/maximus	Increased: Knee adduction Knee internal rotation Foot pronation Foot external rotation Decreased: Ankle dorsiflexion Ankle inversion

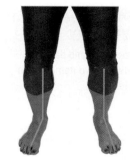

Figure 8.8
Pronation Distortion Syndrome

Table 8.2

Lower Crossed Syndrome Summary

Short Muscles	Lengthened Muscles	Altered Joint Mechanics
Gastrocnemius Soleus Hip flexor complex Adductors Latissimus dorsi Erector spinae	Anterior tibialis Posterior tibialis Gluteus maximus Gluteus medius Transverse abdominis	Increased: Lumbar extension Decreased: Hip extension

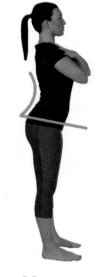

Figure 8.9
Lower Crossed Syndrome

Table 8.3

Upper Crossed Syndrome Summary

Short Muscles	Lengthened Muscles	Altered Joint Mechanics
Upper trapezius Levator scapulae Sternocleidomastoid Scalenes Latissimus dorsi Teres major Subscapularis Pectoralis major/minor	Deep cervical flexors Serratus anterior Rhomboids Mid-trapezius Lower trapezius Teres minor Infraspinatus	Increased: Cervical extension Scapular protraction/elevation Decreased: Shoulder extension Shoulder external rotation

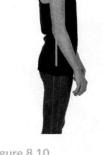

Figure 8.10
Upper Crossed Syndrome

Symmetry

Proportion and balance between two items or two sides.

Key Points to Remember When Observing Static Posture

In general, when assessing a static posture, the Group Fitness Instructor is checking for proper alignment of the kinetic chain checkpoints, symmetry, and specific postural distortion patterns. The instructor should not scrutinize the participant, but instead look for gross deviations in overall posture; any postural deviations seen should be obvious and naturally occurring.

Postural assessments require observation of the kinetic chain. The use of the five kinetic chain checkpoints allows the Group Fitness Instructor to systematically view the body in an organized fashion. The kinetic chain checkpoints are as follows:

▼ Foot and ankle

▼ Knee

▼ Lumbo-pelvic-hip complex (LPHC)

▼ Shoulders

▼ Head and cervical spine

A static postural observation could assess an individual's posture from the front (anterior), side (laterally), and from behind (posterior).

General Safety Considerations

It is the instructor's responsibility to make the workout environment and the exercises as safe as possible to prevent injury.

▼ **Equipment Safety:** A participant using equipment inappropriately could be at risk of injuring themselves or another participant. This might include improper bike fit, incorrect form when using weights, poorly stacked step platforms, or incorrectly fastened straps.

▼ **Overexertion:** Overexertion can be dangerous. Stopping the class, attending to the participant, and referring him or her for medical attention is a priority.[6] Some signs a participant could be at risk include:

■ Abnormally rapid heart rate

■ Fever

■ Nausea and vomiting

■ Disorientation or confusion

▼ **Dehydration:** An instructor should seek help for a participant immediately if they show the following signs of dehydration[7]:

■ Confusion

■ Rapid heart rate

■ Rapid breathing

■ Passing out

- Lack of sweating
- Extreme thirst

▼ **Fatigue:** If a participant shows the following signs, the instructor should halt the class and seek medical help for the participant immediately[8]:

- Shortness of breath
- Chest pain
- Irregular or rapid heartbeat
- Dizziness or feeling lightheaded
- Severe abdominal, pelvis, or back pain

▼ **Temperature:** The recommended air temperature for a facility is 68–72°F (20–22°C) when participating in most group fitness formats. Some specialty formats are performed in a heated environment, where additional education and qualifications are required.

▼ **Sound Volume:** Sound/noise levels are measured in decibels (dB). The permissible exposure is 85 dB averaged over an 8-hour period.[9] Instructors will want to balance the volume of the music with the volume of their voice to avoid yelling and possibly damaging their voice permanently. If participants are having trouble following the music, consider turning up the bass, so they can *feel* the beat while still hearing instructor cues.

▼ **Clothing and Footwear:** Instructors usually cannot advise participants prior to the first class, but they can discuss the best options in class and offer modifications for next time.

▼ **Flooring:** Wood flooring is soft enough for impact and smooth enough for movement. Some locations have other types of flooring such as carpeting, rubber, or cement, which make movements more difficult and increase the risk of injury. Flooring should be taken into consideration when selecting exercises.

▼ **Contraindicated Exercises:** Some exercises are not recommended for the general population because of risk for injury:

- Straight-leg deadlifts
- Hurdler stretch

CAUTION ⚠

The louder the music, the shorter amount of time it takes for noise-induced hearing loss to occur. Make sure you know your decibels and consider the long-term hearing of yourself and your participants before you crank up the volume.

⊘ Check It Out

How long will your shoes last? It is estimated that 25% of shock absorption is lost after 50 miles in running, 33% is lost after 100–150 miles, and after 250–500 miles shoes retain less than 60% of their original ability to absorb shock. In general, high-impact shoes have about a 500-mile life span, which translate roughly into 100 hours of high- or low-impact classes or 3-6 months of regular use. Other factors that can reduce the longevity of shoes include a heavier body weight, poor construction quality, and a rough flooring or outdoor exercise surface.

- Straight-leg sit ups
- Overhead kettlebell swings
- Good mornings
- Specific exercises not recommended for special populations (women, seniors, children)

Introduction to Emergency Situations and Response

The contents that follows are *for reference and review purposes only*, as instructors must remain within their scope of practice. It is the instructor's responsibility to react correctly and efficiently while waiting for emergency services to arrive.

Group Fitness Instructors need to be competent in emergency response protocol for participants. This is accomplished through training and certification in cardiopulmonary resuscitation (CPR) and operation of the automated external defibrillator (AED) device.

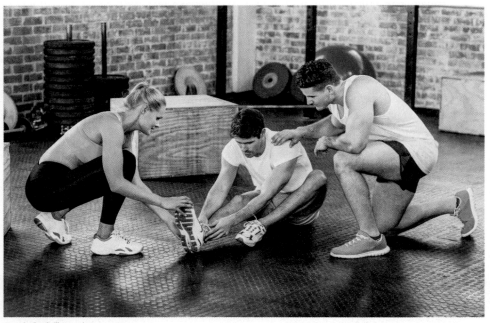

© wavebreakmedia/Shutterstock

Group Fitness Instructors should be familiar in emergency response topics, including:

▼ Recognizing an emergency
▼ Disease and injury prevention

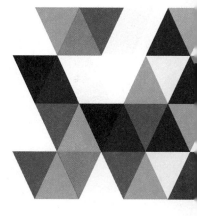

- ▼ CPR/AED/First Aid
- ▼ Blood-borne pathogen training
- ▼ Emergency preparedness

Recognizing and Responding to an Emergency

The most important step in minimizing the effect of a medical emergency is recognizing it as early as possible. An initial survey of the area gives the responder an idea of the circumstances and potential condition of individuals, as well as hazards to anyone in the immediate area.

Next, one should look for any signs which may indicate the individual is in trouble, which may include the following:

- ▼ Position of the individual (standing, seated, crouching, doubled over, or supine)
- ▼ Skin color
- ▼ Bleeding
- ▼ Level of consciousness
- ▼ Pain or discomfort
- ▼ Distress

As soon as both the individual and the situation have been surveyed and assessed, emergency medical personnel should be notified by calling 9-1-1. If the affected individual is unresponsive or if there is an absence of breathing or pulse, the responder must begin CPR/AED efforts while another party places the call (if no other person is available, the responder should call 9-1-1 first, then begin resuscitation). Even in situations where a pulse and respiration are present, 9-1-1 should be contacted.

In situations where the individual has not lost consciousness yet remains in distress, after calling 9-1-1, the instructor should progress to the next part of the assessment phase: communication. Communication is the most important phase in assessing an individual's condition and will direct the next phase of the assessment process. Ask a few concise direct questions, such as:

- ▼ What happened?
- ▼ How are you feeling?
- ▼ Where is the pain?

If the individual's health history is unknown, ask if they have any medical conditions that may exacerbate the emergency.

Each fitness facility should have a prearranged emergency response activation plan; employees should familiarize themselves with these protocols. First responders may be responsible for calling emergency services, providing details on the injury or illness, and directing emergency services to the scene while also diverting bystanders away from the area. Each facility may have protocols in place for recording and reporting situational details after the event for liability purposes.

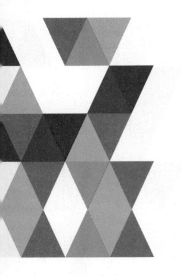

The Exercise Environment

One variable often overlooked is the environment of an exercise class; most of the time, classes will be in an indoor, temperature-regulated room controlled centrally by the fitness facility. However, opportunities sometimes allow for Group Fitness Instructors to teach classes outdoors.

Temperature

A reasonable temperature for an exercise class is around 68–72°F (20–22°C), although participants living in different climates will have different levels of temperature acclimation. Age and gender also factor into an individual's hot or cold tolerance.[10]

Should inclement weather or temperature make exercise outdoors dangerous, instructors should be prepared to do the following:

▼ Move class to a climate-controlled space

▼ Minimize time in extreme weather

▼ Actively alter exercise sessions if signs of weather-related stress are observed

▼ Have appropriate emergency equipment available (e.g., ice, cold water, cold packs, mobile phone)

Exercise in the Heat

During exercise, the human body expends about 70–80% of the energy produced as heat.[10] This makes heat injury (*hyperthermia*) a serious threat for anyone taking part in physical activity in

INSTRUCTOR TIP 👍

It is important instructors look to maintain the comfort for the class as a whole and avoid responding to individual requests that may not reflect the larger group's comfort.

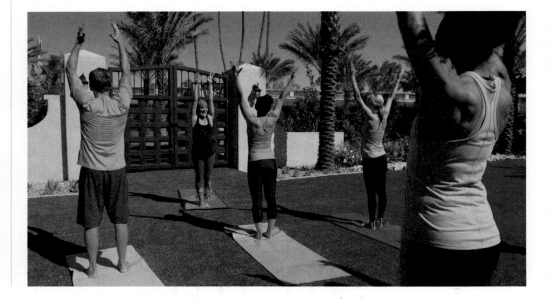

hot conditions. If core temperature rises above 102°F (38.9°C), heat exhaustion can occur. Heat exhaustion is characterized by[11]:

- ▼ profuse sweating.
- ▼ pale skin.
- ▼ dizziness.
- ▼ hyperventilation.
- ▼ rapid pulse.

As core temperature pushes over the 104°F(40°C) mark, the dangerous condition of heat stroke can occur, with symptoms including[11]:

- ▼ sudden collapse and unconsciousness.
- ▼ flushed, hot skin.
- ▼ reduced sweating.
- ▼ shallow breathing.
- ▼ further increased heart rate.

Death can occur if core temperature rises to 107°F (41.7°C).[11]

Humidity

Humidity can affect the way the body cools itself. If the air is humid, the water in sweat does not evaporate into the surrounding air readily, lowering sweat's ability to remove heat from the body. High levels of caution should be taken when exercising in hot and humid conditions.

Exercise in the Cold

Exercising in colder environments presents its own set of physiological and safety concerns. When exercising in temperatures below freezing, always make sure skin is adequately covered. Wind chill should also be taken into consideration. For this reason, it is highly recommended to dress in multiple thin layers of clothing that can be progressively removed (outer garments first), or placed back on, throughout the duration of a cold-weather exercise session to maintain comfort and safety. Head covering is also recommended, as it can be removed or replaced easily to accommodate the temperature.

Hypothermia (lowering of the core body temperature to 95°F/35°C or lower) can occur any time environmental conditions are colder than internal body temperature. As temperature drops, shivering occurs; however, shivering will cease as core temperature drops below 85–90°F (29.5–32.2°C), followed by death if core temperature falls below 85°F/29.5°C.[11] Symptoms of hypothermia include:

- ▼ shivering.
- ▼ pale skin.
- ▼ bluing of the lips, hands, and feet.

> ### ⊘ **Check It Out**
> Air quality can have an adverse effect on individuals with asthma. These individuals typically keep a bronchodilating inhaler at hand for use prior to exercise or at the onset of symptoms; however, breathing through the nose or with pursed lips may reduce or dissipate symptoms of asthma.

When this occurs, the instructor should remove the participant from exercising and get them into a warm, dry space to recover. If the participant stops shivering while out in the cold, medical attention should be sought right away. Advanced stages of hypothermia may also see the affected individual become confused, lose coordination, and potentially lose consciousness. Additionally, cold environments can increase blood pressure through generalized vasoconstriction, which may exacerbate issues for those with hypertension.[12]

Altitude

As altitude increases, atmospheric pressure decreases and the concentration of oxygen molecules is thereby also reduced. This means the same breath of air at high altitude will contain less oxygen than one at low altitude, and red blood cells become less saturated with oxygen. The heart therefore must pump more liters of blood per minute to maintain oxygenation; for example, $\dot{V}O_{2max}$ has been shown to be reduced by up to 27% at 4,000 meters of elevation.[10]

Air Quality

Poor air quality affects outdoor exercise by reducing oxygen levels as well. Ozone has been shown to decrease $\dot{V}O_{2max}$ and other respiratory function, while sulfur dioxide can cause issues of bronchoconstriction for people with asthma; carbon monoxide binds hemoglobin, thus reducing oxygen transport in a manner similar to altitude.[10] Dust and smoke are also highly irritating to the cardiorespiratory system.

The U.S. Environmental Protection Agency (EPA) developed the Air Quality Index (AQI), with values ranging from good to hazardous (**Table 8.4**).[13] Exercise should not take place in environments where the AQI is higher than 150, with those sensitive to air pollution avoiding exposure to values over 100.

Managing Risk

Risk of an injury or other emergency in the group fitness classroom can never be fully avoided; however, a number of best practices and training techniques can be implemented to ensure participants are exercising in the safest environment possible.

Participants can be safeguarded from risk when instructors design classes that emphasize injury prevention. This is accomplished through the progressive application of integrated fitness, specifically during the movement preparation segment of a class. Strains, sprains, and other non-contact injuries can be further avoided by matching the movement prep to the higher-intensity main body workout to ensure the body will be ready.

Table 8.4

EPA Air Quality Index		
Air Quality Index(AQI) Values *When the AQI is in this range:*	**Levels of Health Concern** *...air quality conditions are:*	**Colors** *...as symbolized by this color:*
0 to 50	Good	Green
51 to 100	Moderate	Yellow
101 to 150	Unhealthy for Sensitive Persons	Orange
151 to 200	Unhealthy	Red
201 to 300	Very Unhealthy	Purple
301 to 500	Hazardous	Maroon

Note: Values above 500 are considered beyond the AQI. Follow recommendations for the Hazardous category.[13]

Summary

Whether reacting to a change in group attendance, equipment, or location, or responding to a classroom emergency, it is the Group Fitness Instructor's responsibility to act calmly and effectively to handle the situation in the best way possible. Through planning and classroom set-up, the risks of accidents or injuries are reduced. Keeping participants safe and informed is paramount to building trust and rapport with participants, so by continuously monitoring the classroom and participants, everyone in the group fitness space will be able to maximize their experience and enjoyment.

Chapter in Review

- ▼ Classroom set-up and preparation
  - ▪ Microphones
  - ▪ Participant arrangement
  - ▪ Equipment
- ▼ Unexpected elements
  - ▪ Equipment changes
  - ▪ Space

- ▪ Time available
- ▪ Conflict
- ▼ Monitoring
  - ▪ Physical
  - ▪ Emotional
- ▼ Postural assessments
  - ▪ Pronation distortion syndrome

- Lower crossed syndrome
- Upper crossed syndrome
- General safety
  - Dehydration
  - Temperature
  - Volume
  - Clothing and footwear
  - Flooring
- Emergency response
  - Protocol
  - Reducing risk
- Exercise environment
  - Temperature and weather
  - Altitude
  - Air quality

References

1. Neumann D. *Kinesiology of the Musculoskeletal System: Foundations for Rehabilitation*. 2nd ed. St. Louis, MO: Mosby/Elsevier; 2010.
2. Powers CM, Ward SR, Fredericson M, Guillet M, Shellock FG. Patellofemoral kinematics during weight-bearing and non-weight-bearing knee extension in persons with lateral subluxation of the patella: A preliminary study. *J Orthop Sports Phys Ther*. 2003;33:677–685.
3. Sahrmann SA. Posture and muscle imbalance: Faulty lumbo-pelvic alignment and associated musculoskeletal pain syndromes. *Orthop Div Rev-Can Phys Ther*. 1992;12:13–20.
4. Sahrmann, SA. *Diagnosis and Treatment of Movement Impairment Syndromes*. St. Louis, MO: Mosby; 2002.
5. Janda V. Muscles and motor control in cervicogenic disorders. In: Grant R, ed. *Physical Therapy of the Cervical and Thoracic Spine*. St. Louis, MO: Churchill Livingstone; 2002.
6. La Forge R. Overexertion can cause serious harm. *IDEA Health & Fitness Source*. 2004;22(1):20–24.
7. Mayo Clinic. Diseases and Conditions: Dehydration. http://www.mayoclinic.org/diseases-conditions/dehydration/basics/symptoms/con-20030056. Accessed May 27, 2017.
8. Mayo Clinic. Symptoms: Fatigue: When to see a doctor. http://www.mayoclinic.org/symptoms/fatigue/basics/when-to-see-doctor/sym-20050894. Accessed May 27, 2017.
9. Occupational Safety and Health Administration (OSHA). *Occupational Noise Exposure*. https://www.osha.gov/SLTC/noisehearingconservation/. Accessed May 27, 2017.
10. Powers SK, Howley ET. *Exercise Physiology: Theory and Application to Fitness and Performance*. 7th ed. New York, NY: McGraw-Hill; 2009.
11. Prentice WE. *Essentials of Athletic Injury Management*. 10th ed. New York, NY: McGraw-Hill; 2016.
12. Castellani JW, Young AJ. Human physiological responses to cold exposure: Acute responses and acclimatization to prolonged exposure. *Auton. Neurosci*. 2016;196:63–74.
13. Environmental Protection Agency (EPA). Air Quality Index (AQI) Basics. https://airnow.gov/index.cfm?action=aqibasics.aqi. Accessed May 27, 2017.

Chapter 9
Communication and Learning Styles

Learning Objectives

9.1. **Identify** styles of learning.

9.2. **Describe** elements of basic communication relevant to group fitness instruction.

9.3. **Describe** various cueing techniques.

9.4. **Explain** strategies for providing feedback to and monitoring group participants.

9.5. **Describe** methods for building and improving rapport with class participants.

Understanding Learning

In the group fitness setting, there are typically three types of learners, and there is no single way in which all participants learn. Therefore, instructors should seek to implement a combination of teaching methods to adequately meet the learning needs of a diverse group.

Learning styles represent the way a learner *prefers* to learn, not necessarily the most effective way to learn. Styles may also change based on the task or as efficiency improves. Learning styles are best explained using the visual-auditory-kinesthetic (VAK) model. VAK asserts that people learn through three methods: seeing (i.e., *visual* learning), hearing (i.e., *auditory* learning), and moving (i.e., *kinesthetic* learning).

Visual Learning

Visual learners prefer to learn by seeing or watching. With movement, visual learners prefer to see things displayed and demonstrated and find value in the observation of body language. Instructors can accommodate visual learning through the demonstration of correct and incorrect movement in exercise and the use of gestures for direction (see Figures 9.1–9.13).

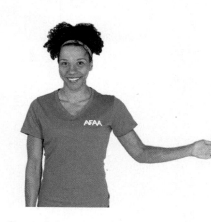

Figure 9.1
Indicating Direction: Right

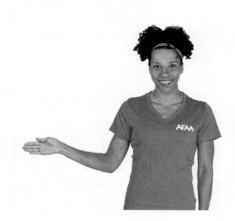

Figure 9.2
Indicating Direction: Left

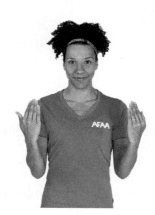

Figure 9.3
Move Forward

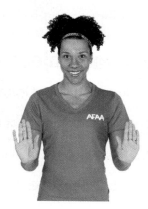

Figure 9.4
Move Back

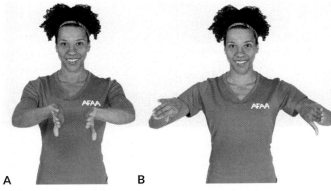

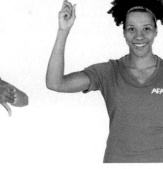

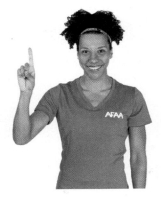

A   B

Figure 9.5
Spread Out

Figure 9.6
Turn Around

Figure 9.7
Counting (1, 2, 3)

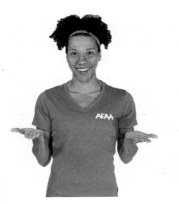

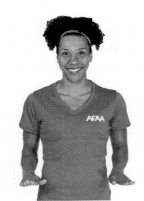

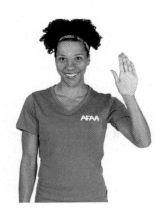

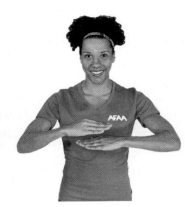

Figure 9.8
Higher

Figure 9.9
Lower

Figure 9.10
Stop

Figure 9.11
Faster

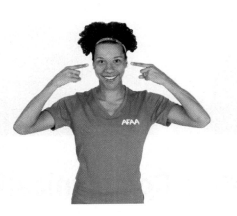

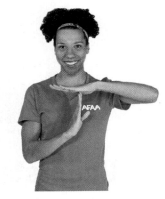

Figure 9.12
Watch Me

Figure 9.13
Time Out

> ### Practice This!
>
> Stand up and practice performing a lunge. While you do this, consider how you might deliver instructions to your participants on performing the lunge correctly. Practice a visual instruction by performing the lunge; a verbal instruction by describing or explaining it; and a kinesthetic through slow, step-by-step movement along with a description of how the body should feel.

Auditory Learning

Auditory learners prefer to learn by listening to clear, spoken, orderly directions. Avoiding unnecessary, wordy statements is an important skill. Verbal cues must be anticipated with precise timing. This means the information must be heard and understood by the class participants immediately before the movement occurs.

Kinesthetic Learning

Kinesthetic learners prefer to learn through movement or touch. Generally, these learners will be coordinated in their movement and react quickly to changes. Instructors can accommodate kinesthetic learning by demonstrating exercises for the class, especially those with complex movements, before asking everyone to execute them. For kinesthetic learners, the Group Fitness Instructor should encourage participants to try a few reps themselves before performing the move with intensity. Incorporating all three strategies for visual, auditory, and kinesthetic learners is important in creating a collective, compelling group fitness experience.

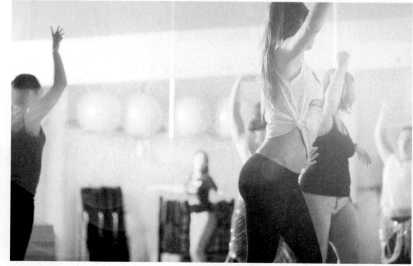

© nikitabuida/Shutterstock

Understanding Communication

Communication is the process of gathering inputs (such as sounds, signs, or behaviors) and interpreting them into a meaning. This meaning is conveyed through various methods of verbal and nonverbal communication. Instructors can facilitate safe and productive workouts for their participants by implementing communication best practices.

Verbal Communication

One of the most import verbal communication skills for a Group Fitness Instructor is the ability to speak clearly and succinctly. The effective use of voice in the classroom is a learned skill. Both what is cued and how it is cued are equally important. Through variations in how something is spoken, an instructor can alter the meaning of a message without changing the words themselves.

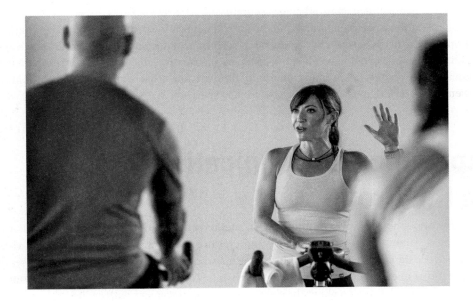

Supportive Word Choice

Because words represent an idea, concept, or object, each person can interpret them based on his or her personal contexts. Instructors should be careful to select words that avoid bias toward race, ethnicity, nationality, religion, gender, sexual orientation, age, class, or ability. Using supportive communication creates a climate of trust, caring, and acceptance.[1]

To facilitate supportive communication, Group Fitness Instructors can implement the following approaches[1]:

▼ Use "I" statements rather than "you" statements.

▼ Ask open-ended questions rather than critical statements.

▼ Work to understand how someone is feeling and engage with them.

▼ Avoid making rigid pronouncements by softening statements with qualifiers like, "You might want to consider . . ." or "Perhaps you could try . . ."

Supportive communication

Language that creates a climate of trust, caring, and acceptance.

▼ Work together and use "we" statements.

▼ Look to provide new approaches or solutions rather than focus on mistakes.

Nonverbal Communication

Nonverbal communication is communication other than written or spoken language that creates meaning for someone.[1] It may include facial expressions, emotions, eye contact, posture, gestures, and signals.

It is important to understand the ways in which nonverbal communication can alter intended meaning. First, nonverbal messages can communicate feelings and attitude through facial expressions or body positioning. Second, nonverbal messages are more believable than verbal ones—and they are critical to successful relationships. Instructors should work to coordinate verbal messaging with nonverbal messages to present an authentic message; by presenting welcoming body language and facial expressions, instructors can make a positive impression quickly, earning the trust of participants. Finally, nonverbal messages can substitute for verbal messages or complement, contradict, or reiterate verbal cues.[1]

One of the most powerful forms of nonverbal communication in the group fitness setting is the appropriate use of eye contact. Eye contact is a means of making participants feel acknowledged. Avoiding eye contact could give the impression an instructor is disinterested or inexperienced. Ultimately, eye contact helps build community through nonverbal communication and can help participants feel both present and engaged in the experience.[2]

Applying Communication in the Group

Both one-way and two-way communication methods are used in the group fitness setting. One-way communication occurs when a communicator (i.e., instructor) sends an audio, visual, or kinesthetic signal with no confirmation of receipt from the receiver. This occurs in classes due to the ratio of one instructor to multiple participants. One-way communication is appropriate when giving broad direction about the class, workout, or movement pattern; however, it should not be the primary type of communication from an instructor.

Two-way communication occurs when the communicator sends an audio, visual, or kinesthetic signal and the receiver communicates a response back to the sender. Participants will communicate in various ways, so it is important that instructors allow adequate time for two-way communication

Communication Expectations

Instructors with superior communication skills are much more likely to make positive connections with their classes. The following guidelines foster engaging, effective communication in the group setting.

Nonverbal communication

Communication other than written or spoken language that creates meaning.

One-way communication

When a communicator (instructor) sends an audio, visual, or kinesthetic signal with no confirmation of receipt from the receiver(s).

Two-way communication

When a communicator (instructor) sends an audio, visual, or kinesthetic signal and the receiver communicates a response back to the sender.

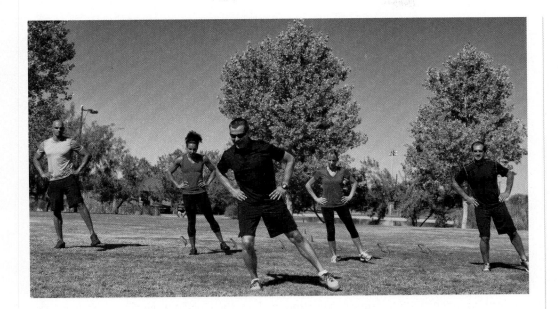

Be Specific

Specific, straightforward communication encourages positive change and empowers participants to move correctly. In a diverse group setting there will likely be one participant who is new or inexperienced; it is best for instructors to practice consistent specificity, and explain exactly what to do and how it should feel.

Avoid Conflicting Messages

Due to the dynamics of having multiple fitness levels in a single class, it is easy for an instructor to send conflicting messages. It becomes important to focus on one message at a time: Do the participants need to work harder? Do they need correction? Do they need motivation? Instructors should focus on one area of improvement before moving on to another; telling the class how to fix it or to continue their positive actions.

Own Your Message

Group Fitness Instructors should try to use the phrases "I" and "my" instead of "the club" or "you should." Instructors disown their messages when they do not take personal responsibility for them. Participants want to know that their chosen instructor is qualified and confident before they incorporate the instructor's education and methods into their own daily lives.

Deliver Messages at the Time of Occurrence

When Group Fitness Instructors see participants performing incorrect or dysfunctional movements, specific feedback should be provided immediately. This allows the participant to better understand and comprehend the change, as well as reduce the risk for injury. It is better to take a few seconds to quickly fix an improper movement, than let a participant neurologically process or learn improper patterns they then have to *unlearn* later.

INSTRUCTOR TIP

To implement two-way communication, try this: "I'm going to count our burpees down from ten. When we get to five, join in to let me know you're on board with finishing strong!"

> **⊘ Check It Out**
>
> In order to make sure comments, corrections, and feedback are received in supportive and positive manner, try the following formula:
> 1. Start with a positive observation: "I love your energy!"
> 2. Communicate the correction: "Bring your arms up to shoulder level" (Add a smile, a tap to the shoulder, or a nod).
> 3. Conclude with a positive statement: "That's where I need you to be! Your shoulders should be feeling good."

Be Positive and Supportive

Engaging communication should never come in the form of threats, negative comparisons, sarcasm, or judgment. Sarcasm can sometimes lighten the mood and work in a group setting, but only when the instructor has established rapport and knows each participant. Threats may seem fun, such as "every one of you has to give me 10 more push-ups or we start over!" but can quickly alienate participants who do not have the capacity to keep up with group expectations.

Attitude

Instructors should make a conscious effort to have a positive, inviting attitude in the group fitness setting. Some of the best ways for instructors to demonstrate this attitude is to:

▼ be open for feedback or criticism.

▼ remind themselves, and the class, they are there for the participants' benefit—not their own.

▼ be friendly.

▼ be a leader.

▼ look the part.

Demonstrating Value

Demonstrating value is a form of two-way communication that helps participants feel welcome, understood, and cared for. If an instructor wants to see a participant again, building value-based connections should be part of his or her teaching toolbox. Instructors should practice this through:

▼ *Punctuality*—Arriving early, starting class on time, and ending on time.

▼ *Learning and using the names of participants*—Setting a goal to meet (and remember) someone new each class.

▼ *Being available*—Making time before or after class to answer questions.

▼ *Equipment preparation*—Making sure equipment is accessible and ready for class.

▼ *Class environment*—Making sure the temperature and sound are at levels appropriate for the class format and demographic.

▼ *Cater to the classroom*—Helping participants locate equipment, towels, or water quickly, and giving struggling individuals positive attention.

▼ *Minding manners*—Being polite and courteous in all communication.

▼ *Clear communication*—Openly explaining class objectives and equipment needed at the beginning of class.

Building Rapport

Rapport-building is fostered before class and in the opening, continues throughout class, and may be reinforced as participants are leaving. Some examples of rapport-building activities include:

▼ meeting participants and learning their goals.

▼ making eye contact with participants in conversation and during class.

▼ learning and using participants' names.

▼ taking an interest in participants' lives and families.

▼ taking music or exercise requests.

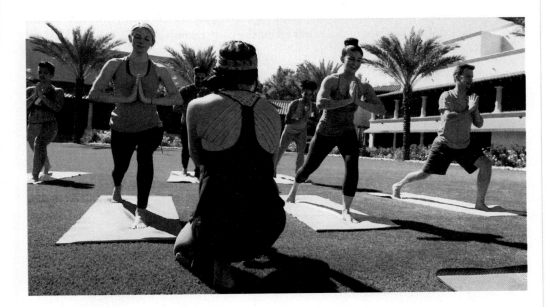

Two of the most crucial times for more focused connection, preparation, and recognition are before participants start moving and as the class comes to an end. Participants are most focused on the instructor during these times. It is also an opportunity for the instructor to use a more conversational tone rather than short coaching cues.

Teaching

Teaching—the act of showing or explaining how to do something—is a key component of effective instruction, but it is only a piece of the whole process. When participants can integrate a movement outside of class that improves the overall function of their daily lives, then successful instruction has occurred.

Styles of Teaching

There are various styles of teaching that instructors may use during a class to create a learning environment for the participant. Teaching styles may change by class format, participant demographics, class objectives, or by an instructor's personal strength in a certain style. Many group fitness classes benefit from a combination of teaching styles within a single class period, which helps an instructor connect with the various learning needs of a diverse class.

There are five main styles of teaching[3]:

▼ **Cue-based teaching** is focused on continuous, reliable, and precise verbal cues that occur simultaneously with movement.

▼ **Visual teaching** is focused on demonstrating correct form and technique while providing a comprehensive view of the movement or pattern from start to finish.

▼ **Mirroring**—or, mirror imaging—is an instruction technique in which instructors teach their class or sections of their class facing the participants (Figure 9.14)

Cue-based teaching

Use of continuous, reliable, and precise verbal cues that occur simultaneously with movement.

Visual teaching

Demonstrating aspirational form and technique while providing a comprehensive view of the movement or pattern from start to finish.

Mirroring

Teaching technique in which instructors face their participants and perform movements as if they are the participants' reflection in a mirror.

INSTRUCTOR TIP 👍

It's professional standard to be able to mirror image the class. Instructors should learn, thoroughly practice, and master this important teaching technique.

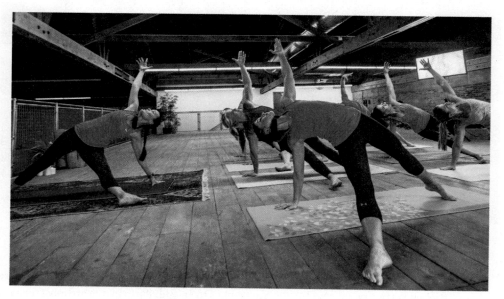

Figure 9.14
Mirror Imaging

Practice This!

To start practicing mirror imaging, face an open room or wall and try cueing everything you do on the opposite side. Want to, for example, perform bicep curls with a lunge to the instructor's right? Remember to cue it as "okay, let's do bicep curls with a lunge to the left." After a few practice sessions in an empty room, try it in the classroom. If you need the class to move right, raise your left hand, point to the left, and move to *your* left (their right).

▼ Reflective imaging is a technique in which an instructor faces the same direction as the participants and uses a mirror's reflection to teach or cue movements.

▼ Timed coaching is a technique in which an instructor is focused on verbal coaching and motivational phrasing in order to push participants through timed movement sequences.

Teaching Methods

Various methods for teaching exercise combinations are commonly used in the fitness classroom. Among these methods, the following may assist the foundational instructor in cueing his or her participants:

▼ *Part-to-Whole*: This method teaches one move or exercise in a combination (repeating as necessary) before teaching the second move (repeating as necessary). Then, the instructor cues participants to add the second move to the first. This is repeated with the rest of the combination.

▼ *Repetition-Reduction*: This method teaches a combination of moves by first teaching the move and repeating it until participants have it mastered. This is repeated with each additional move. Then, the instructor returns to the starting move and reduces the number of repetition with each move.

▼ *Simple-to-Complex (Layering)*: This method teaches a combination of movements at a basic level, and then adds additional movements, range, or intensity to build upon each movement for more complexity.

▼ *Slow-to-Fast (Half-time)*: This method teaches an exercise or combination of exercises at a slower rate or at half the speed at which it will be performed. Once mastered, the instructor cues the participants to speed up to the appropriate tempo.

Cueing Techniques

When spoken cues become repetitive, participants may lose the connection between the words and the movements. To provide an optimal learning environment and meaningful workout experience, instructors should use a variety of cueing techniques.

Three-dimensional Cueing

Three-dimensional cueing incorporates cues that speak to the visual, auditory, and kinesthetic needs of the various types of learners. Three-dimensional cueing should be used in most group fitness classes, as it allows instructors to communicate with the most participants possible.

> ## ✓ Check It Out
>
> Instructors can appeal to all learners through the *Show, Tell, Do* method.
> - Show: Demonstrate what you're expecting participants to do.
> - Tell: Tell participants what you'd like them to do, and how.
> - Do: Give participants the opportunity to perform the action themselves.

Remember that:

▼ A *visual learner* is most likely to think: "*Show* me what to do, and I will follow." These types of learners learn best by seeing a demonstration of the movement.

▼ An *auditory learner* is most likely to think: "*Tell* me precisely how to do it, and I will follow." These types of learners require a clear, concise verbal description of the movement.

▼ A *kinesthetic leaner* is most likely think: "Tell me *where* and *how* I should *feel* it, and I will follow." These types of learners connect with words like *sense, pretend, imagine, feel*, and *touch*.

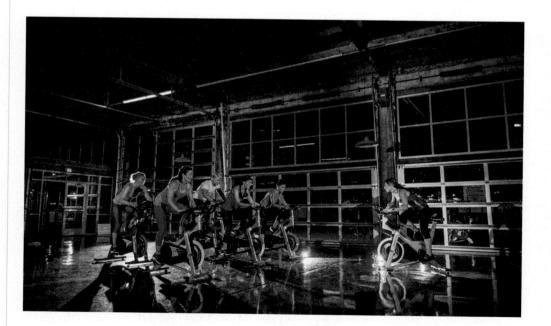

Types of Cues

There are many types of cues that can be used during a group fitness class to meet the needs of individual participants, build community, create connections, and improve the overall experience

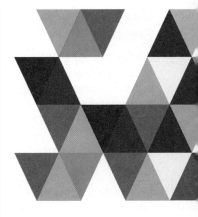

of exercise for the participant. Instructors should use a variety of cues throughout each class. Options that work well in the group fitness setting include:

- ▼ **Personal**: a short, personal anecdote disconnected from class purpose; builds community and rapport
- ▼ **Safety**: cues that reminds participants of proper technique and correct improper movement
- ▼ **Motivational/inspirational**: positive cues about performance, effort, or ability to complete the exercise
- ▼ **Alignment**: descriptions of body set-up or execution
- ▼ **Respiration**: cues reminding participants when and how to breathe
- ▼ **Rhythmical**: cues related to timing of movements or upcoming timing changes
- ▼ **Informational/educational**: explanations of the reason for and potential benefit of a movement
- ▼ **Numerical**: communications of the numbers for sets, repetitions, and other counted portions of movement
- ▼ **Anatomical**: explanations of the muscles or body parts involved
- ▼ **Directional**: cues indicating direction of movement, such as left, right, front, and back
- ▼ **Empowering**: cues to help participants understand how movement empowers their lives beyond the gym
- ▼ **Spatial**: cues that reference one's body in relationship to other participants, equipment, or both
- ▼ **Movement**: cues to describe the movement or pattern to be performed

Some participants respond well to hands-on cueing. Kinesthetic learners may find this type of guidance helpful, but instructors must **always** obtain permission from participants before offering this type of corrective feedback and understand the best practices of using hands-on cueing techniques. For participants who are not receptive to a hands-on cue, instructors can either show them the correction on the instructor's body or verbally cue them to move towards the instructor's hands so the participant makes contact with the instructor only upon reaching the correct position; either method may ease their discomfort by giving them control.

Hands-on cueing

A movement correction technique that requires the instructor to redirect the participant through the use of touch.

INSTRUCTOR TIP

Redundant cues that are not attached to any particular behavior or participant can become inefficient and irrelevant. Work at being mindful when calling out cues, paying attention to what is being said, how often, and at what volume.

✓ Check It Out

Some research recommends using the same verbal cue up to three times per class, and then changing from what would become a *habitual cue* to an *inspirational cue*.[4] A habitual cue is one used repeatedly and commonly. Switching from a habitual cue to inspirational cue (or another type of cue) instantly commands attention, as it sounds and feels very different.

Pre-cue

Used to technically set up the movement or movement pattern in a timely, efficient, clearly stated way.

Main Movement Cue

Explains the intended movement, often as the instructor is simultaneously demonstrating proper form of the movement.

Nonverbal Cue

Uses expression, gestures, posture, or other nonverbal forms of communication to keep the class engaged.

Motivational Cue

Used to encourage participants during challenging movements or to keep them going when fatigue affects performance.

Positive-based Cueing

(also known as positive cueing) Choosing words that cue to the solution rather than the problem.

Autonomy-supportive Cueing

Coaching practice focused on creating an environment that emphasizes self-improvement, rather than competing against others.

Timing of Cues

The best cues are short and to the point, yet detailed enough to ensure participant success. The following sequence can be effective in helping participants understand expectations:

1. Pre-cue—used to set up the exercise. These cues must be fast, efficient, clear, and offer information necessary to perform the movement before it begins.

2. Main Movement Cue—explains the intended movement as the instructor is demonstrating proper form. These cues encourage safety, instruct proper technique, cue correct body positioning, and describe precise form when executing movements.

3. Nonverbal Cue—After providing a pre-cue and a movement cue, mirror image participants, smile, make direct eye contact, nod your head, clap your hands, or emphasize the energy and beat of the music.

4. Motivational, Educational, or Personal Cue—breaks up the monotony of "do this" instruction and helps participants realize the benefits that may come as a result of their time and effort in class.

Positive-based Cueing

Positive-based cueing means an instructor chooses words that cue to the solution rather than the problem. In positive cueing, the instructor speaks only to the behavior desired so all participants hear, understand, process, and immediately implement the correction, saving time and avoiding any possible injury.

Positive cueing relies on the fact that the brain cannot process a negative thought without first positively understanding all words used in the sentence or command. For example, if an instructor tells a participant, "Don't hold your hand weights wrong so your wrist bends backwards," the words focus on the negative and emphasize an incorrect movement. To process the thought and convert the words into movement, the brain must positively identify a movement that corresponds to the *opposite* of the command—which still might not promote the correct movement. Holding the hand weights with wrists bent forward, for example, would be just as incorrect as holding them so the wrists bend backward, yet it is a reasonable response to the negative command. The positive command that gets the correct result would be, "Keep your wrists in a neutral position to help you activate muscle engagement."

Autonomy-supportive Cueing

Autonomy-supportive cueing is a positive cueing practice recommended by sport and exercise psychologists. This style of coaching focuses on creating an environment that emphasizes self-improvement, rather than competition[3,5]:

▼ Providing choices within limits

▼ Offering rationales for activity structures

▼ Avoiding overt control and criticism

▼ Providing informational feedback

▼ Limiting participants' ego involvement throughout their program (i.e., focus on self-improvement instead of comparing to others)

Musical Cueing

The beat of the music can help the instructor cue on time and assist the participants to anticipate upcoming changes. Because movements are typically changed or started on the downbeat (count 1 of an 8-count phrase), instructors can use *4-beat* or *2-beat cueing* to help participants perform movements with proper form and technique.

4-beat cueing is when an instructor counts down from 8 and provides verbal or visual cues on counts 4-3-2-1. For example, "8, 7, 6, 5, squat, to, the, right" (which would be spoken over counts 4, 3, 2, 1), then the participant is able to squat to the right on the downbeat (first beat) of the next phrase.

2-beat cueing is when an instructor provides verbal/visual cues on the last two counts of a phrase, right before the downbeat hits. For example, "8, 7, 6, 5, 4, 3, squat, right!"

Participant-centered Teaching Approaches

Instructors who effectively integrate all three learning styles in their teaching create more engaging experiences. This participant-centered approach places the needs of the group above the desires of the instructor. Through rapport building, effective communication, and positive interaction, instructors create value for their participants.

Participant-centered instruction can be facilitated in the following ways:

▼ To connect with participants verbally, instructors should use words that *include,* rather than *exclude,* the greatest number of participants.

▼ To visually engage all participants in class in the most meaningful way, instructors may wish to use frequent eye contact, provide visual reassurance (such as thumbs-up), and walk around the room.

▼ To engage all participants in class in a kinesthetic way, instructors may wish to use language that focuses on how movement should feel or encourage participants to imagine scenarios that help facilitate the intended behavior.

Providing Feedback

The ability of a Group Fitness Instructor to provide various forms of positive feedback helps participants find new confidence, motivation, education, and empowerment during exercise. It is important for the instructor to learn how often to provide feedback as well as how and when to make corrections.

Applying Positive-based Correction Techniques

Combining visual, auditory, and kinesthetic techniques for positive-based correction becomes the main goal in providing feedback. When a correction is necessary, this means trying to elicit a corrective change in participants' behavior in the most encouraging manner possible. Instructors should give feedback in a non-threatening, inclusive way.

INSTRUCTOR TIP 👍

In a class setting, participants stay motivated and seem to learn better when they hear counts going DOWN.

4-beat cueing

Counting down from 8 and providing verbal and/or visual cues on counts 4-3-2-1.

2-beat cueing

Counting down from 8 and providing verbal and/or visual cues on counts 2-1, or the last two counts of a phrase.

Participant-centered Instruction

Movement selection that offers options in intensity and complexity for a variety of skill and fitness levels.

Positive-based correction

(also known as positive correction) Using various forms of verbal and nonverbal feedback to elicit a corrective change in the most encouraging manner possible.

Table 9.1

Positive-based Correction Examples	
Common Negative Cues	**Positive Correction**
"Don't forget to breathe."	"Keep breathing."
"Don't go that way."	"Go right."
"Don't let your shoulders round in."	"Pull your shoulders back and down."
"Don't let your hips sag in plank position."	"Raise your hips up."
"Don't stop."	"Keep going!"

See **Table 9.1** for some positive-based correction examples.

Post-workout Feedback and Questions

After class, participants may request specific feedback on their performance or answers to their questions about fitness. Instructors should only respond to questions that fall within their scope of practice and the limits of their expertise. In general, instructors should try to keep questions related to the completed class. If questions are of a health or medical nature, the participant should be referred to a licensed medical professional.

Summary

Effective instruction is more than just shouting verbal cues; it is a comprehensive approach to teaching, monitoring, and motivating large groups of people with various goals, fitness levels, and capabilities. When participants walk away from a group fitness class in a better place than before it began—physically, emotionally, or functionally—then successful instruction has taken place.

Chapter in Review

- ▼ Learning styles
  - ▪ Visual
  - ▪ Auditory
  - ▪ Kinesthetic
- ▼ Effective communication
  - ▪ Verbal

- ▪ Non-verbal
  - ❖ Eye contact
- ▼ Communication expectations
- ▼ Customer service expectations
- ▼ Building rapport
- ▼ Teaching styles

- ▪ Cue-based
- ▪ Visual
- ▪ Mirroring
- ▪ Reflective imaging
- ▪ Timed coaching
- ▼ Teaching Methods
  - ▪ Part-to-Whole
  - ▪ Repetition-Reduction
  - ▪ Simple-to-Complex
  - ▪ Slow-to-fast
- ▼ Cueing techniques
  - ▪ Three-dimensional
  - ▪ Types & timing
  - ▪ Positive
  - ▪ Autonomy supportive
  - ▪ Musical
- ▼ Participant-centered instruction

References

1. Beebe SA, Beebe SJ, Ivy DK. *Communication: Principles for a Lifetime.* 5th ed. New York, NY: Pearson; 2015.
2. Hall N, Fishburne GJ. Mental imagery research in physical education. *J Imagery Res Sport Phys Activ.* 2010;5(1). https://doi.org/10.2202/1932-0191.1045.
3. Conroy DE, Coatsworth JD. Assessing autonomy-supportive coaching strategies in youth sport. *Psychol Sport Exerc.* 2007;8(5):671–684.
4. Eckmann T. *101 Brain Boosters.* Monterrey, CA: Healthy Learning; 2013.
5. Wilson PM, Rodgers W. The relationships between autonomy support, exercise motives, and behavioral intentions in females. *Psychol Sport Exerc.* 2004;5:229–242.

Chapter 10
Inclusive Instruction for Special Populations

Learning Objectives

10.1. **Explain** the influence common chronic conditions may have on group fitness participation.

10.2. **Identify** common considerations for participants belonging to special populations groups.

10.3. **Identify** appropriate modifications for participants belonging to special populations groups.

© Rawpixel.com/Shutterstock

Introduction to Inclusive Instruction

Because most group fitness classes include participants with varying degrees of ability, instructors must strive to teach multi-level classes accessible to all. This participant-centered approach focuses on the delivery of information that provides options for intensity and complexity of movements for a variety of fitness levels. Instructors should create a consistent, engaging experience for each participant and empower them with the opportunity to make decisions about personal movement selection.

Fitness professionals are not qualified to diagnose or treat any medical condition and must remain within their scope of practice when working with special populations. Individuals should openly discuss their exercise habits, training regimen, and goals with their physician, and instructors should be prepared to share detailed information about the class design with both parties.

CAUTION ⚠

Fitness professionals must remain within their scope of practice when working with participants who have serious medical conditions.

Chronic Conditions

The likelihood of encountering individuals with a variety of chronic health conditions is high. Instructors must be well-informed about the associated risks and know how to adapt class design, exercises, instruction, and class programming (**Table 10.1**).

Table 10.1

Chronic Conditions

Chronic Condition	Definition
Obesity	Individuals with a BMI of 30 or above.
Hypertension	Chronically high blood pressure as defined by a systolic pressure above 140 mm Hg and/or a diastolic blood pressure above 90 mm Hg.
Coronary heart disease	Coronary arteries of the heart become narrowed due to fatty build-up along the walls of the arteries.
Congestive heart failure	A complex condition defined by impairment of the heart.
Atherosclerosis	Narrowing of the arteries due to a build-up of plaque along their walls.
Peripheral artery disease	Condition in which blood flow to the extremities is reduced due to the narrowing of arteries.
Stroke	An acute condition in which blood supply to the brain or areas of the brain is greatly reduced or interrupted; individuals who have suffered a stroke may be left with chronic paralysis or physical dysfunction.
Cancer	Abnormal, invasive growth of cells within the body.
Osteoporosis	Bones become thin, fragile, and prone to fracture.

Hypertension

Hypertension—or, high blood pressure—is a common chronic condition for which exercise is recommended for prevention and reduction.[1–6] Cardiorespiratory exercise reduces blood pressure and risk of hypertension as it increases stroke volume and heart rate,[7] although caution is warranted to avoid excessive increases in blood pressure. Resistance training, once considered something hypertensive patients should avoid,[4,5] has been found to be useful as a supplement to cardiorespiratory exercise in order to improve functional capacity; it does not exacerbate high blood pressure.

Table 10.2 shows some basic exercise guidelines and acute variables for individuals suffering from high blood pressure.[5]

Obesity

Overweight and obese participants may need alterations to general exercise, especially those with medical conditions that often coexist with overweight and obesity, including hypertension, hyperlipidemia, type 2 diabetes, and osteoarthritis.[8–11] Most affected individuals recognize their limitations and will use the modifications provided.

Cardiorespiratory exercise is an important component of fitness programs for obese participants, because it can decrease the risk of cardiorespiratory disease and increase caloric expenditure.[12]

Table 10.2

Basic Exercise Guidelines for Participants with Hypertension	
Mode	Classes such as indoor cycling, low-impact cardiorespiratory activities, dance, group rowing.
Frequency	3–7 days per week.
Intensity	50–85% of maximum heart rate.
Duration	30–60 minutes per day.
Special Considerations	Avoid heavy lifting and Valsalva maneuvers; make sure the participants are breathing normally. Modify tempo to avoid extended isometric and concentric muscle action. Avoid lying down. Allow participants to stand up slowly to avoid possible dizziness.

⊘ Check It Out

Factors to consider when teaching to obese individuals:
- Provide options for bodyweight exercises.
- Provide options that don't involve rapid transitions from seated or lying to standing.
- Provide options that reduce range of motion.
- Provide options that reduce speed of motion.
- Provide options that reduce impact on joints.

Dyspnea

Difficulty or troubled breathing.

Heart palpitations

Heart flutters or rapid beating of the heart.

Table 10.3 outlines some basic exercise guidelines for obese individuals.[12]

Cardiovascular Disease

Coronary heart disease, congestive heart failure, atherosclerosis, and peripheral artery disease are conditions that impair physical function, increase risk of mortality, and are a leading cause of disability for both men and women. Exercise, in the proper doses, can improve cardiorespiratory and muscular fitness, decrease morbidity and mortality, positively influence risk factors such as obesity and hypertension, and enhance overall quality of life.[13–16]

Light to moderate cardiorespiratory exercise can provide individuals with cardiovascular disease an appropriate level of stress to the cardiovascular system, resulting in improved function.[15] Resistance training complements cardiorespiratory exercise because improved muscular fitness contributes to the ability to perform and sustain exercise. An individual who exhibits dyspnea (i.e., difficulty or troubled breathing) during exercise should take longer breaks and train with reduced loads. Exercise must be ceased immediately if chest pain, nausea, dizziness, or heart palpitations result.

Table 10.4 shows some basic exercise guidelines and acute variables for individuals suffering from cardiovascular diseases.[15]

Table 10.3

Basic Exercise Guidelines for Participants Who Are Obese	
Mode	Classes such indoor cycling, dance, resistance, or aquatics.
Frequency	At least 5 days per week.
Intensity	60–80% of maximum heart rate; if needed the ranges for training can be adjusted to 40–70% of maximum heart rate.
Duration	40–60 minutes per day or 20- to 30-minute sessions twice each day of cardiorespiratory training.
Special Considerations	Make sure the participant is comfortable. Exercise should be performed in a standing or seated position when possible. The participant may have other chronic diseases. In these cases a medical release should be obtained from the individual's physician.

Table 10.4

Basic Exercise Guidelines for Participants with Cardiovascular Disease	
Mode	Classes such as indoor cycling (carefully monitored), low-impact cardiorespiratory activities, or dance formats.
Frequency	3–5 days per week.
Intensity	40–60% of peak work capacity.
Duration	Work up to 20–45 minutes.
Special Considerations	Upper body exercises cause increased dyspnea and must be monitored. Allow for sufficient rest between sets.

Table 10.5

Basic Exercise Guidelines for Participants Recovering from Stroke	
Mode	Large muscle group activities.
Frequency	3–7 days per week
Intensity	50–80% of maximum heart rate
Duration	20–60 minutes per session
Special Considerations	Be sure that the participant can balance for the appropriate exercise. Standing or seated exercises are advised. Movement patterns should be progressed before weight.

Stroke

Stroke often leads to a sedentary lifestyle, physical inactivity, low fitness levels, and post-stroke functional limitations.[17] Muscle weakness after a stroke also affects ability to perform daily activities.[17,18] Special attention should be given to stability, which may be compromised until balance and coordination improve.

Table 10.5 shows some basic exercise guidelines and acute variables for individuals who have suffered a stroke.[19]

Cancer

Cancer-related fatigue commonly interferes with normal functioning and contributes to muscle wasting, declines in cardiorespiratory fitness, negative changes in body composition, and depression.[20,21] Research has shown cardiorespiratory exercise and resistance training may counteract many of the side effects of cancer treatments.[21–27] Exercise should be avoided during periods of increased infection, ataxia, dizziness, or during wound recovery from surgery.[23]

Table 10.6 shows some basic exercise guidelines and acute variables for individuals being treated for cancer.[23,24,21]

Osteoporosis

Osteoporosis is a skeletal condition of decreased bone mass and increased risk of fracture. Exercise has been shown to reduce bone mass loss and increase bone mineral density.[28,29] For those with osteoporosis, exercise can be a valuable tool for improving physical function, decreasing risk of falls and fractures, and improving quality of life.[30]

The greatest exercise risk for those suffering from osteoporosis is bone fracture, either caused by excessive weight or falls during exercise. Instructors should do all they can to help prevent a fracture from occurring.[31]

Table 10.7 shows some basic exercise guidelines and acute variables for individuals with osteoporosis.[28–30]

Ataxia

The loss of control of body movements.

Table 10.6

Basic Exercise Guidelines for Participants with Cancer	
Mode	Classes such as low-impact cardiorespiratory activities, circuit-style classes with plenty of options provided, balance, and core training classes.
Frequency	3–5 days per week.
Intensity	50–70% of maximum heart rate.
Duration	15–30 minutes per session.
Special Considerations	Avoid heavy lifting in initial stages of training. Allow for adequate rest intervals, and progress the participant slowly. Only use SMR if tolerated by the participant. Avoid SMR for participants undergoing chemotherapy or radiation treatments. There may be a need to start with only 5 minutes of exercise and progressively increase, depending on the severity of conditions and fatigue.

Table 10.7

Basic Exercise Guidelines for Participants with Osteoporosis	
Mode	Stationary or recumbent cycling, aquatic exercise, or low-intensity yoga.
Frequency	2–5 days per week of moderate activities or 3 days per week of vigorous activities.
Intensity	40–85% of $\dot{V}O_2$ peak.
Duration	20–60 minutes per day or 8- to 10-minute bouts.
Special Considerations	Progression should be slow and well monitored. Exercises should be progressed toward free sitting (no support) or standing. Participants should breathe in a normal manner and avoid holding their breath as in a Valsalva maneuver. If a participant cannot tolerate SMR or static stretches due to other conditions, perform slow rhythmic active or dynamic stretches. Twisting motions should be performed slowly, if at all.

Special population

A group of people who have similar conditions or characteristics that require alterations to the general exercise plan.

Special Populations

A special population represents a group of people with similar conditions or characteristics that require unique alterations to an exercise program to ensure health, safety, and effectiveness. **Table 10.8** describes some of the special populations that Group Fitness Instructors may encounter.

Table 10.8

Special Populations	
Special Population	**Definition**
Youth	Children and adolescents between the ages of 5 and 18 years.
Older Adults	Individuals aged 65 years or older.
Prenatal	Individuals who are pregnant.
Postnatal	Individuals who have recently given birth.

Age

Most general exercise guidelines are designed specifically for healthy individuals between 18 and 65 years of age. Evidence exists on the benefits of exercise for youths and older adults, but participants in these populations may require some adaptations for safety and effectiveness.

Youth

Many studies on youth resistance training have found that resistance training results in improved muscular fitness, body composition, power, and motor coordination among children and adolescents, with relatively low risk of injury if the resistance training is age-appropriate and supervised.[32–37]

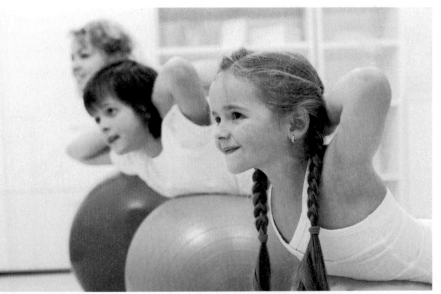

© Ilike/Shutterstock

Table 10.9 shows some basic exercise guidelines and acute variables for youth fitness programs.[32–37]

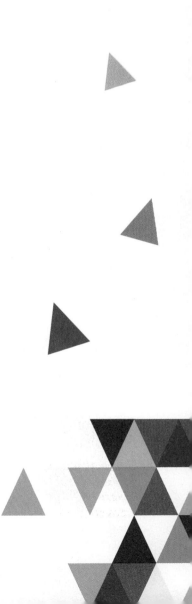

Table 10.9

Basic Exercise Guidelines for Youth Group Fitness Programs	
Mode	Circuit style classes with lots of variety and opportunity for individualization and interaction work well for youth. Most classes as deemed safe by motor control.
Frequency	5–7 days per week.
Intensity	Moderate to vigorous activities.
Duration	60 minutes per day.
Special Considerations	Progression for the youth population should be based on postural control and not on the amount of weight that can be used. Make exercising fun!

Older Adults

Older adults (65 years and older) can achieve life-altering improvements in muscular fitness if working out correctly and safely. Research supports the use of resistance training among older adults for increasing muscle mass, strength, function, and balance, enhancing power, and either improving bone mineral density or preventing bone mass decline.[38–43] Resistance training is a valuable tool for improving the health, fitness, and independence of older adults. Resistance training among older adults is highly productive, and the incidence of injury is extremely low.[38]

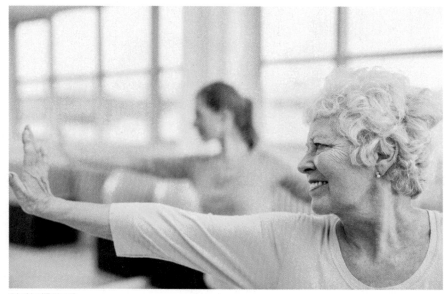

© Jacob Lund/Shutterstock

Table 10.10 shows some basic exercise guidelines and acute variables for older adults.

Table 10.10

Basic Exercise Guidelines for Older Adults	
Mode	Classes such as aquatics, chair-based resistance training formats, cycle, and basic or beginner yoga.
Frequency	3–5 days per week of moderate activity or 3 days per week of vigorous activity.
Intensity	40–85% of $\dot{V}O_2$ peak.
Duration	30–60 minutes per day or 8- to 10-minute bouts.
Special Considerations	Progression should be slow and well-monitored. Exercises should be progressed toward free sitting (no support) or standing. Participants should breathe in a normal manner and avoid holding their breath such as with the Valsalva maneuver. If a participant cannot tolerate SMR or static stretches due to other conditions, perform slow rhythmic active or dynamic stretches.

Instructors should ensure proper lifting techniques at very light loads and low volume. As the participant becomes accustomed to training, optimizes proper movement, and responds well, loads can gradually increase for progression. If certain exercises create pain or excessive discomfort in muscles, immediate alterations should be made to avoid injury. Pain or discomfort in the joints should also be avoided. Bodyweight exercise with the support of a chair or other device is a good starting point for many older adults.

Pregnancy

Group Fitness Instructors may encounter pregnant participants in class. Their participation should be encouraged (with physician consultation), as regular exercise before, during, and after pregnancy has a wide range of benefits for both the mother and the baby.[44–49] These benefits include:

- improved weight management.
- reduced incidence of gestational diabetes.
- decreased hypertension.
- enhanced body image.
- improved psychological well-being.
- decreased risk of premature labor.
- shorter delivery and hospitalization.
- improved fetal development.
- decreased risk of obesity in both the mother and child.

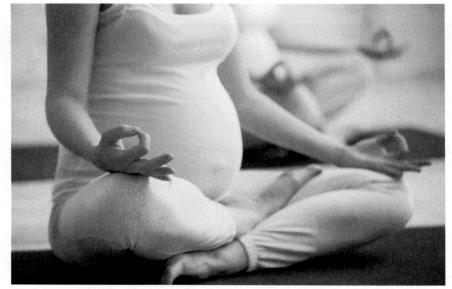

The Group Fitness Instructor should offer modifications to the exercise routine to account for the increased secretion of the hormone *relaxin*: which relaxes joints during pregnancy. As joints become less stable, loads must be controlled and proper exercise technique strictly adhered to. High impact, reactive exercises should be replaced with exercises that present less stress on the joints. Additionally, participants should be advised to avoid excessive range of motion in flexibility exercises.

Special attention should be paid to controlling body temperature during exercise; therefore, exercise in hot and humid environments should be limited. Resistance exercises selected should promote total-body fitness, with special emphasis on the core musculature to reduce low back pain and maintain posture.

Table 10.11 shows some basic exercise guidelines and acute variables for pregnant individuals.

Table 10.11

Basic Exercise Guidelines for Pregnancy	
Mode	Low-impact classes that avoid jarring motions such as indoor cycling, low-impact cardiorespiratory activities, light resistance, and aquatics. All activities should be cleared by the participant's physician.
Frequency	5–7 days per week.
Intensity	Light to moderate intensity; 13–14 on the Borg scale.
Duration	20–30 minutes per day.
Special Considerations	Avoid exercises in a prone or supine position after 12 weeks of pregnancy. Avoid SMR on varicose veins and areas of swelling. Plyometric movement is not advised in the second and third trimesters.

Postpartum exercise has garnered a great deal of attention in the research literature as well, showing significant benefits including[46]:

▾ Body fat loss

▾ Improved cardiorespiratory and muscular fitness

▾ Improved bone health

▾ Enhanced mood

The timing of return to exercise following delivery should be at the discretion of the individual in consultation with her primary care physician, but typically ranges from 6–12 weeks after delivery. Low-intensity resistance training can be added to focus on core and total-body muscular endurance, within the following guidelines:

▾ *Frequency*: 2–3 days per week

▾ *Volume*: 1–3 sets per exercise (no more than 8–10 exercises per session)

▾ *Repetitions*: 10–15 per set

▾ *Intensity*: Less than 50% of 1RM

Bodyweight exercises, combined with exercises performed while holding the baby, can be excellent choices to produce improvements in muscular fitness, stability, and muscle coordination immediately following pregnancy.

The Americans with Disabilities Act (ADA)

According to the United States Census Bureau, as of 2010, nearly 1 in 5 people in the U.S. had a disability.[49] Of the over 56 million people (approximately 19% of the population) affected, more than 50% of people with disabilities indicated they get no physical activity whatsoever.[50] The Americans with Disabilities Act (ADA) "prohibits discrimination against people with disabilities in employment, transportation, public accommodations, communications, access to state and local government's programs and services."[51]

Regardless of experience level with disability issues, opportunities exist to "remove the obstacles that traditionally get in the way of gym participation."[50] To be compliant with the law, fitness and recreational facilities must provide general access and reasonable accommodations for people with disabilities. Fitness professionals should adopt the following practices of inclusion[50]:

▾ *Show enthusiasm*—Creative opportunities for inclusion should be offered with positivity and energy without being condescending.

▾ *Make accommodations*—Even without special modifications, some programs and equipment can be adapted.

▾ *Keep activities age-appropriate*—Avoid perpetuating the myth that persons with disabilities are "different" by using child-like games, toys, or rewards. Whenever possible, participants with disabilities should "learn by the same rules as a person without disabilities."[50]

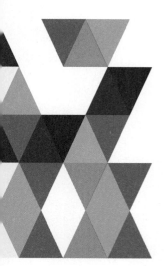

▼ *Other tips*:

■ Introduce yourself and make eye contact as you would with any other participant.

■ Connect and acknowledge the individual's presence.

■ Respond to all communicative attempts by observing body language.

■ Do not refer to an individual as "handicapped" or "disabled." He or she is a person *with* a disability or medical diagnosis.

■ Understand that a person's wheelchair or other mobility device is an extension of his or her body. Respect personal space and never move a wheelchair out of its user's reach.

■ Use clear and concise instructions and demonstrate whenever possible.

■ Encourage participants to keep working on tasks rather than rewarding "false wins."

Summary

Inclusive instruction requires the Group Fitness Instructor to understand the abilities, goals, and limitations of participants in classes and be prepared to provide modifications to help each feel successful. Participant- centered instruction requires an understanding of the complex behavioral factors that motivate or discourage individuals, and instructors can cue in a manner which is inclusive of all, regardless of race, gender, age, or ability.

Chapter in Review

▼ Common chronic conditions

■ Hypertension
  ❖ High blood pressure
  ❖ Cardio should be primary mode of exercise

■ Obesity
  ❖ >30 BMI
  ❖ Cardio should be primary mode of exercise

■ Cardiovascular diseases
  ❖ Including coronary heart disease, congestive heart failure, atherosclerosis, and peripheral arterial disease
  ❖ Light to moderate cardio

  ❖ Resistance training to help improve ability to perform and sustain activity

■ Stroke
  ❖ Can cause balance and coordination issues as well as muscle weakness
  ❖ Special focus on stability activities recommended

■ Cancer
  ❖ Causes fatigue, muscle wasting, and declines in cardio fitness
  ❖ Cardio and resistance training can counteract side effects of treatments

- Avoid exercise during periods of increased infection
  - Osteoporosis
    - Causes decreased bone mass, increasing risk of fracture
    - Activity can prevent bone mass loss and increase bone mineral density
    - High risk of bone fracture
- Special populations
  - Age
    - Youth: focus on resistance training improves muscular fitness, body composition, power, and motor coordination
    - Older adults: focus on resistance training improves muscle mass, strength, function, balance, power, and bone mineral density

- Pregnancy
  - During pregnancy
    - Relaxin relaxes joints, creating less stability
    - Avoid hot and humid environments
    - Emphasize core musculature during resistance activities
  - Post-partum
    - Return should be dictated by participant's physician
    - Bodyweight exercise recommended to improve fitness, stability, and coordination
- Individuals with disabilities (ADA)
  - Remove obstacles to help facilitate participation
  - Practice inclusion

References

1. Cornelissen VA, Fagard RH. Effect of resistance training on resting blood pressure: A meta-analysis of randomized controlled trials. *J Hypertens.* 2005;23:251–259.
2. Fagard RH. Exercise characteristics and the blood pressure response to dynamic physical training. *Med Sci Sports Exerc.* 2001;33(6 suppl):S484–S492.
3. Kelley GA, Kelley KS. Progressive resistance exercise and resting blood pressure: A meta-analysis of randomized, controlled trials. *Hypertension.* 2000;35:838–843.
4. Li Y, Hanssen H, Cordes M, Rossmeissi A, Endes S, Schmidt-Trucksäss A. Aerobic, resistance and combined exercise training on arterial stiffness in normotensive and hypertensive adults: A review. *Eur J Sport Sci.* 2015;23:443–457.
5. Wallace JP. Exercise in hypertension: A clinical review. *Sports Med.* 2003;33:585–598.
6. Whelton SP, Chin A, Xin X, He J. Effect of aerobic exercise on blood pressure: A meta-analysis of randomized, controlled trials. *Ann Intern Med.* 2002;136:493–503.
7. Le V-V, Mitiku T, Sungar G, Myers J, Froelicher V. The blood pressure response to dynamic exercise testing: A systematic review. *Prog Cardiovasc Dis.* 2008;51:135–160.
8. Balsalobre-Fernández C, Tejero-González CM. Effects of resistance training on the body fat in obese people. *Rev Int Med Cien Activ Fis Deporte.* 2015;15:371–386.
9. Barnes JT, Elder CL, Pujol TJ. Overweight and obese adults: Exercise intervention. *Strength Cond J.* 2004;26:31–33.

10. Strasser B, Siebert U, Schobersberger W. Resistance training in the treatment of the metabolic syndrome. *Sports Med.* 2010;40:397–415.

11. Vincent HK, Raiser SN, Vincent KR. The aging musculoskeletal system and obesity-related considerations with exercise. *Ageing Res Rev.* 2012;11:361–373.

12. Ismail I, Keating SE, Baker MK, Johnson NA. A systematic review and meta-analysis of the effect of aerobic vs. resistance exercise training on visceral fat. *Obes Rev.* 2012;13:68–91.

13. LaFontaine T. Resistance exercise for persons with coronary heart disease. *Strength Cond J.* 2003;25:17–21.

14. Roitman JL, LaFontaine T. Exercise, atherosclerosis, and the endothelium: Where the action is (part II). *Strength Cond J.* 2006;28:75–77.

15. Tran QT. Resistance training and safety considerations for chronic heart failure patients. *Strength Cond J.* 2005;27:71–72.

16. Brogardh C, Lexell J. Effects of cardiorespiratory-fitness and muscle-resistance training after stroke. *PM R.* 2012;4:901–907.

17. Morris SL, Dodd KJ, Morris ME. Outcomes of progressive resistance strength training following stroke: A systematic review. *Clin Rehabil.* 2004;18:27–39.

18. Gordon NF, Gulanick M, Costa F, et al. Physical activity and exercise recommendations for stroke survivors: An American Heart Association Scientific Statement from the Council on Clinical Cardiology. *Circulation.* 2004;109:2031–2041.

19. Dimeo F. Effects of exercise on cancer-related fatigue. Cancer. 2001;92:1689–1693.

20. Strasser B, Steindorf K, Wiskemann J, Ulrich CM. Impact of resistance training in cancer survivors: A meta-analysis. *Med Sci Sports Exerc.* 2013;45:2080–2090.

21. Cramp F, James A, Lambert J. The effects of resistance training on quality of life in cancer: A systematic literature review and meta-analysis. *Support Care Cancer.* 2010;18:1367–1376.

22. Hayes SC, Spence RR, Galvao DA, Newton RU. Australian Association for Exercise and Sport Science position stand: Optimizing cancer outcomes through exercise. *J Sci Med Sport.* 2009;12:428–434.

23. Lonbro S. The effect of progressive resistance training on lean body mass in post-treatment cancer patients—a systematic review. *Radiother Oncol.* 2014;110:71–80.

24. Meneses-Echavez JF, Gonzalez-Jimenez E, Ramirez-Velez R. Supervised exercise reduces cancer-related fatigue: A systematic review. *J Physiother.* 2015;61:3–10.

25. Puetz TW, Herring MP. Differential effects of exercise on cancer-related fatigue during and following treatment: A meta-analysis. *Am J Prev Med.* 2012;43:e1–e24.

26. Paramanandam VS, Roberts D. Weight training is not harmful for women with breast cancer-related lymphoedema: A systematic review. *J Physiother.* 2014;60:136–143.

27. Wilhelm M, Roskovensky G, Emery K, Manno C, Valek K, Cook C. Effect of resistance exercises on function in older adults with osteoporosis or osteopenia: A systematic review. *Physiother Can.* 2012;64:386–394.

28. Petranick K, Berg K. The effects of weight training on bone density of premenopausal, postmenopausal, and elderly women: A review. *J Strength Cond Res.* 1997;11:200–208.

29. Zhao R, Zhao M, Xu Z. The effects of different resistance training modes on the preservation of bone mineral density in postmenopausal women: A meta-analysis. *Osteoporos Int.* 2015;26:1605–1618.

30. Giangregorio LM, Papaioannou A, MacIntyre NJ, Ashe MC., Heinonen A, Cheung AM. Too Fit to Fracture: Exercise recommendations for individuals with osteoporosis or osteoporotic vertebral fracture. *Osteoporosis.* 2014;25:821–835.

31. Buranarugsa R, Oliveira J, Maia J. Strength training in youth: An evidence-based review. *Rev Portug Cienc Desport.* 2012;12:87–116.

32. Behringer M, Vom Heede A, Yue Z, Mester J. Effects of resistance training in children and adolescents: A meta-analysis. *Pediatrics.* 2010;126:1199–1210.

33. Schranz N, Tomkinson G, Olds T. What is the effect of resistance training on the strength, body composition and psychosocial status of overweight and obese children and adolescents? A systematic review and meta-analysis. *Sports Med.* 2013;43:893–907.

34. Peltier L, Strand B, Christensen B. Youth performing resistance training: A review. *J Youth Sports.* 2008;4:18–23.

35. Falk B, Tenenbaum G. (1996). The effectiveness of resistance training in children: A meta-analysis. *Sports Med.* 22:176–186.

36. Payne V, Morrow J, Johnson L, Dalton S. Resistance training in children and youth: A meta-analysis. *Res Q Exerc Sport.* 1997;68:80–88.

37. Baechle TR, Westcott W. *Fitness Professional's Guide to Strength Training Older Adults.* 2nd ed. Champaign, IL: Human Kinetics; 2010.

38. Cadore EL, Pinto RS, Bottaro M, Izquierdo M. Strength and endurance training prescription in health and frail elderly. *Aging Dis.* 2014;5:183–195.

39. Gomez-Cabello A, Ara I, Gonzalez-Aguero A, Casajus JA, Vicente-Rodriguez G. Effects of training on bone mass in older adults: a systematic review. *Sports Med.* 2012;42:301–325.

40. Peterson MD, Sen A, Gordon, PM. Influence of resistance exercise on lean body mass in aging adults: A meta-analysis. *Med Sci Sports Exerc.* 2011;43:249–258.

41. Stewart VH, Saunders DH, Greig CA. Responsiveness of muscle size and strength to physical training in very elderly people: A systematic review. *Scand J Med Sci Sports.* 2014;24:e1–e10.

42. Tschopp M, Sattelmayer MK, Hilfiker R. Is power training or conventional resistance training better for function in elderly persons? A meta-analysis. *Age Ageing.* 2011;40:549–556.

43. Fieril KP, Glantz A, Olsen MF. The efficacy of moderate-to-vigorous resistance exercise during pregnancy: A randomized controlled trial. *Acta Obstet Gynecol Scand.* 2014;94:35–42.

44. Hopkins SA, Cutfield, WS. Exercise in pregnancy: Weighing up the long-term impact on the next generation. *Exerc Sport Sci Rev.* 2011;39(3):120–127.

45. Larson-Meyer DE. The effects of regular postpartum exercise on mother and child. *ISMJ.* 2002;4:1–14.

46. O'Connor PJ, Poudevigne MS, Cress ME, Motl RW, Clapp JF. Safety and efficacy of supervised strength training adopted in pregnancy. *J Phys Act Health.* 2011;8:309–320.

47. Schoenfeld B. Resistance training during pregnancy: Safe and effective program design. *Strength Cond J.* 2011;5:67–75.

48. White E, Pivarnik J, Pfeiffer K. (2014). Resistance training during pregnancy and perinatal outcomes. *J Phys Act Health.* 11:1141–1148.

49. United States Census Bureau (USCB). Profile America Facts for Features: CB15-FF.10 25th Anniversary of Americans with Disabilities Act. *United States Census Bureau News*, 2015. https://www.census.gov/newsroom/facts-for-features/2015/cb15-ff10.html. Accessed May 29, 2017.

50. Spicer PM. Exercise is for everyone! *IDEA Pers Train.* 2004;2005(2). http://www.ideafit.com/idea-personaltrainer/2004/february/http://www.ideafit.com/idea-personal-trainer/2004/february/. Accessed May 29, 2017.

51. United States Department of Labor (USDOL). *Americans with Disabilities* Act. https://www.dol.gov/general/topic/disability/ada. Accessed May 29, 2017.

Chapter 11
Class Engagement and Motivation

Learning Objectives

11.1. **Explain** how to use themes, sounds, and variation for an engaging class experience.

11.2. **Describe** key motivation techniques.

11.3. **Identify** the traits of SMART goals.

11.4. **Describe** methods for building and engaging a fitness community.

Elements of Engaging Experiences

A successful instructor has the ability to make a compelling presentation. Instructors are performers who engage their audience (participants) and motivate them to achieve results and outcomes from the workout that keep them coming back.

Performance and Presence

Participants become more invested in class objectives when an instructor has a strong performance and presence. *Performance* is the ability to convey a message in a theatrical way to engage the most participants. Performance includes the way cues, movements, music, ambience, attire, volume, and attitude of the instructor make individuals feel. *Presence* refers to an instructor's ability to command attention by being confident, prepared, positive, and inviting. An instructor develops presence by demonstrating correct form, posture, and technique, dressing professionally, and behaving in a way that shows his or her emotional and energetic engagement. Instructors with presence are more successful at earning the confidence, trust, and compliance of their participants.

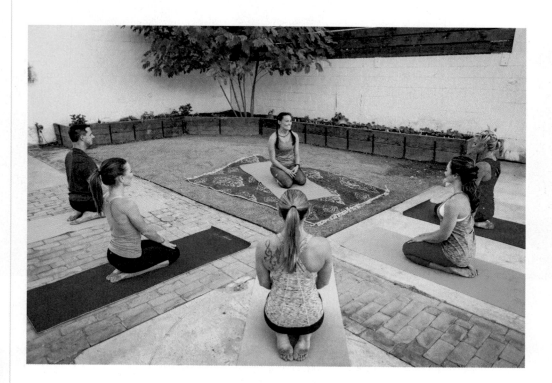

INSTRUCTOR TIP 👍

Attire makes a difference in engagement so dress for the class outcome and format (e.g., fitted attire for core conditioning, colorful attire for dance, hats or dark coloring for boot camp, and so on.).

Confidence

Confidence stems from a combination of expertise and behavior. Familiarity with material enables instructors to offer timely, helpful feedback and suggestions, which participants value; while behaviors such as eye contact, positive attitude, and supportive demeanor are just as

Practice this!

Practice delivering cues by recording yourself. Note how you sound but *also* how you look. Does your body language and eye contact match the cue? Do you seem natural or nervous? Keep practicing to increase confidence.

important when instructors offer guidance for specific movements.[1] Instructors can use some of the following tips to show confidence:[2]

▼ Use dynamic verbal, visual, and physical cueing during movement.

▼ Alternate between watching body movements and looking into participants' eyes if an instructor feels nervous.

▼ Practice enunciation, and vary the tone every third sentence. Being as clear as possible will help save one's voice so every word counts.

▼ Project one's voice from the diaphragm (the muscles felt when one places a hand over the abdomen and coughs).

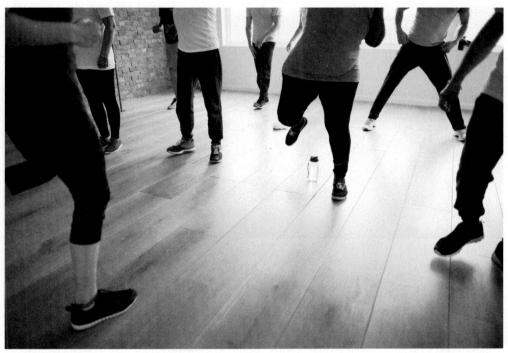

© Rawpixel.com/Shutterstock

Fostering Engagement with Music

Music is an essential tool that promotes mental and physical engagement. The lyrics and overall sound can work synergistically with the movements, performance of the instructor, and class ambience to create a comprehensive experience. Bold, forceful beats can help participants push

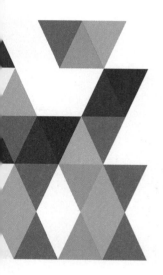

through difficult movements; while positive, empowering lyrics may motivate participants to rise to challenges. Music should support the class outcome. Instructors can follow a few simple guidelines and tips to help support class flow and overall energy:

▼ Use a variety of music types during class.

▼ Use trendy pop, dance, or hip-hop music or select well-known, popular "oldies" to foster a musical connection.

▼ Use dramatic segments, chorus, or downbeats in a song for visual, verbal, or motivational cues.

▼ Select music with lyrics that match the movements being performed.

▼ Stay on the beat, as appropriate for the format, and count reps or time by using song components.

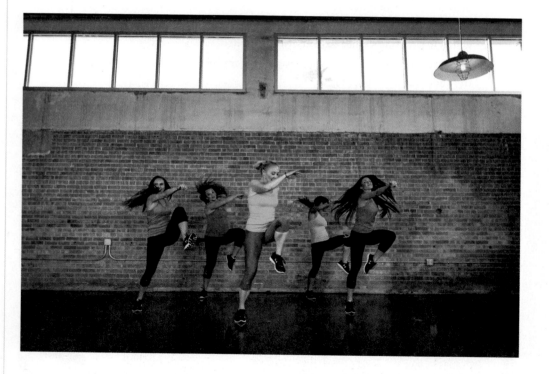

Fostering Engagement with Edutainment

Edutainment

The balanced combination of education and entertainment used to deliver an instructional experience in the most compelling way possible.

The word edutainment comes from the combination of *education* and *entertainment*. When an instructor balances the educational and entertainment needs of a diverse group, they are using edutainment to keep everyone engaged. An education-driven instructor may focus on verbal cues that tell participants what muscle they are working, how to make progressions and regressions, or what plane of motion they are using. Conversely, an entertainment-driven instructor may engage participants through humor, showmanship, lighting or volume changes, or the use of names and personal connections into their teaching style. Ideally, instructors learn to balance these two styles of teaching in order to create the most compelling group fitness experience.

Fostering Engagement with Variety

Scientific training principles, such as *overload* and *progression*, are rooted in the human body's primal need for change and variety. Additionally, variety works to alleviate boredom, generate interest in new challenges, and expand the participants' experiences and activities. Instructors can use the following tasks to incorporate more variety:

▼ Add a single new exercise or movement pattern.

▼ Add one new song to a favorite mix.

▼ Change the order of movements.

▼ Change the sets, reps, rest time, or interval ratio.

▼ Create a long-term plan for progression.

▼ Play a different genre of music.

Motivating Participants

During a group fitness class, it can be difficult for participants to track their own performance, progress, and movement quality. Thus, an effective Group Fitness Instructor must motivate the participants of each class in an effective, timely manner. The instructor should take ownership of accounting for and communicating the participants' achievements both in the short term (e.g., how many squats they performed in a class) and long term (e.g., how someone has improved over several classes) to help participants feel valued and more motivated.

Types of Motivational Cues

Group Fitness Instructors can utilize various types of motivational cues to teach more effectively. Motivational cues are helpful to keep participants focused when feeling tired or bored. Some of the motivational cues that work well in the group fitness setting include:

▼ *Time or Rep Countdown*—Telling them how much longer they have to "hold" or "push."

▼ *Performance*—Complimenting them to assist in finding the energy to push harder in good form.

▼ *Physical or emotional benefit*—Emphasizing the physical or emotional results of a movement.

▼ *Competition*—Using competitive elements (when appropriate or comfortable for participants).

Motivating through Intrinsic and Extrinsic Factors

People are motivated by many different kinds of rewards. Extrinsic motivation refers to a reward separate from the activity undertaken to obtain it. These extrinsic rewards can take numerous forms,

Extrinsic motivation

The performance of an activity to obtain a reward separate from the activity itself.

Intrinsic motivation

The performance of an activity for rewards directly stemming from the activity itself.

🏃 Practice this!

Imagine the participants performing a challenging 60-second plank. Try to call out the duration remaining every 15 seconds to help participants realize they only have 45, 30, or 15 seconds remaining before the challenge is over. Making it through a difficult task creates feelings of success and empowerment, likely bringing them back for more classes.

including money, prestige, status, trophies, or positive feedback from others. Conversely, intrinsic motivation refers to a reward directly related to the activity itself. Feeling a natural endorphin high, getting energized, and more alertness at work could be intrinsic motivations prompting participants to attend classes regularly. Other intrinsic motivating factors might include improvements in strength, reductions in body fat, sleeping better, and changing body measurements. One intrinsic reward is the inherent satisfaction of the activity itself—the simple enjoyment of performing the activity without any consideration of receiving anything additional for participation.

Being intrinsically motivated is valued because it has been associated with a sustained level of performance, participation, and a variety of positive outcomes including creativity, persistence, increased energy, autonomy, increased interest, and an enhanced sense of competence.[3,4] The latest research makes it clear that intrinsic and extrinsic motivation do not present an either/or situation, but rather exist on a continuum. When participants in group fitness have a combination of both intrinsic and extrinsic motivation factors, research suggests they are more likely to stay with an activity program for the greatest amount of time and success.[5] When participants have external, obtainable reasons to work out, they also will be more likely to put more effort into their intensity.[5]

See **Table 11.1** for examples of intrinsic and extrinsic motivation.

✓ Check It Out

There has been much debate whether extrinsic rewards undermine intrinsic motivation. In the business world, many believe extrinsic rewards do not negatively affect intrinsic motivation. Those in education believe extrinsic rewards are very damaging to the intrinsic motivation of school age children, while others believe it is merely the controlling factor of the reward that affects intrinsic motivation.

Think about how you have been rewarded in the past. What worked and what didn't?

Table 11.1

Examples of Intrinsic and Extrinsic Motivation

Intrinsic	Extrinsic
• "Think about how good you're going to feel when you're done with this." • "Think about all the things that brought you here today and congratulate yourself for showing up and working out with me." • "Fit people are happier people overall compared to sedentary people."[6]	• "If I burn 400 calories here, then I can have 400 calories more at dinner." • "This yoga class will help my joints feel better so I can run that marathon." • "Rosie loves going to this class, so I might as well go with her since we are going to lunch together after."

Table 11.2

Strategies for Enhancing Intrinsic Motivation
Strategies for Enhancing Intrinsic Motivation

- Provide positive feedback
- Seek input
- Create engaging class experiences

- Help make successful experiences
- Reiterate positive feelings associated with activities
- Provide information on accomplishments and progress

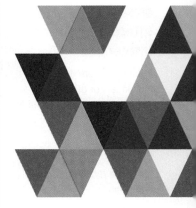

Enhancing Intrinsic Motivation

It is important for a Group Fitness Instructor to make regular exercise and participation in group fitness classes intrinsically motivating. Review the strategies and ideas in **Table 11.2** for increasing intrinsic motivation.

Influences on Human Behavior

Many factors influence the way individuals behave, including cognitive influences (e.g., self-efficacy, self-talk), affective influences (e.g., positive and negative emotions), interpersonal influences (e.g., group fitness classes, eating in groups), behavioral influences (e.g., positive reinforcement, self-monitoring), and sensation influences (e.g., pain associated with working out, feelings of hunger).

Cognitive Influences

An individual's way of thinking or "inner dialogue" can have a significant influence on behavior. Two important cognitive factors that influence behavior are confidence and self-talk, both of which are powerful motivating cognitive traits. Research has found self-efficacy—the belief in one's ability to execute a certain behavior—to be the strongest predictor of physical activity.[7]

Self-efficacy stems from several different sources Group Fitness Instructors can tap into to increase their participants' confidence[8]:

- ▼ *Performance accomplishments* are the strongest source of self-efficacy, as they focus on participants' personal task improvement and success, rather than on comparisons with others.

- ▼ *Modeling,* or watching other, similar individuals successfully perform the desired task, can increase a participant's self-efficacy in their ability to complete the task as well (e.g., "If she can do it, so can you!").

- ▼ *Verbal persuasion,* in which an instructor, coach, or friend encourages the participant to perform the task successfully, also supports self-confidence (e.g., "You got this!").

- ▼ *Imagery,* or imagining themselves performing a task, can increase participants' self-confidence in their ability to actually perform it.

In terms of exercise or nutritional goals, confidence can enhance adherence to a program.

Confidence

Feeling or belief of certainty.

Self-talk

One's internal dialogue.

Self-efficacy

The belief in one's ability to execute a certain behavior.

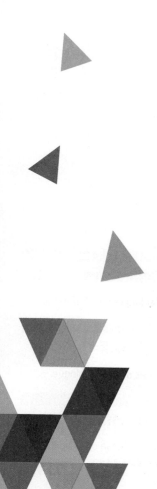

Interpersonal influences

Influences from those individuals or groups with whom one interacts regularly.

Affective influence

Influence resulting from emotions.

Sensation influences

Physical feelings an individual experiences as they relates to behaviors involved in establishing a healthy lifestyle.

Interpersonal Influences

An individual's motivation and behavior in relation to eating and exercise are influenced by a social support network. Social support includes companionship, encouragement, assistance, or information from friends, family members, and coworkers as well as tangible aid and advice, suggestions, and information from professionals.

Many group-oriented programs are effective because they offer enjoyment, social support, increased sense of personal commitment, and opportunities to compare progress and fitness with others. Being part of a group also fulfills the need for affiliation, which is one of the main reasons people give for why they exercise. Instructors can activate these interpersonal influences by inviting participants back and reminding them their presence is valued and their absence is noticed.

Affective Influences

Emotional states in the participant, or affective influences, also have an influence on behavior. Positive or negative emotions may change how (or whether) the participant adheres to an exercise or nutrition program. Conversely, the effects of exercising and eating on emotions can be just as important at changing emotional states; mental health professionals rate exercise as the most effective technique for changing a bad mood.[9] As Group Fitness Instructors work with their participants, they might be helping to enhance their participants' mood.

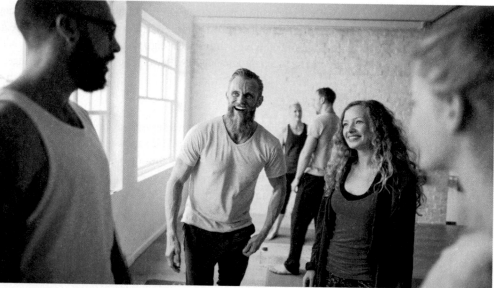

© Rawpixel.com/Shutterstock

Sensation Influences

Sensation influences are physical feelings individuals experience as they relate to behaviors involved in establishing a healthy lifestyle.

> ### ⊘ Check It Out
>
> A type of positive reinforcement called *premacking* was developed by psychologist David Premack and involves pairing an unlikely behavior with a likely one to reinforce the first. An example of this in group fitness would be an instructor creating an enjoyable, relaxing transition after the body of the workout. The idea of relaxing and stretching after a hard workout can reinforce the challenge of the intense body of the workout.[10]

Beginners just starting to work out will likely feel some physical discomfort following the first few classes. Therefore, instructors should try to ensure they do not overload new participants with too much too soon, as the pain may discourage them from returning to class. Conversely, because of the prevalent "no-pain, no gain" mentality, those new to exercise believe it is "supposed to hurt." Instructors can dispel this perception by encouraging participants to work at a level that will facilitate efficient improvements without excessive discomfort.

Behavior Influences

Behavior influences are those influences created as a result of an individual's behavior. Some behaviors elicit a positive feeling in the participant, making them more inclined to repeat the behavior. For example, if an individual starts tracking their activity to hit a movement goal, the tracking behavior will influence the person to walk more—which in turn might encourage continued tracking, resulting in a self-supporting feedback loop. Additionally, by implementing a system of self-monitoring, they may find they are more committed to their program and more capable to identify the patterns and behaviors that support or inhibit progress.

Positive Reinforcement

Positive reinforcement focuses on providing individuals with a reward for exhibiting a specific behavior, with the goal of increasing the likelihood of the desired behavior being repeated. Sport and exercise psychologists agree that the predominant approach should be positive reinforcement, although criticism is sometimes necessary.[11]

The Transtheoretical Model (Stages of Change)

Behavior change is seen as a process that occurs over time, as demonstrated by the Transtheoretical Model (Stages of Change).[12] The Transtheoretical Model (TTM) states that individuals progress through a series of stages of change, and movement through these stages is cyclical—not linear—because many do not succeed in their efforts at establishing and maintaining lifestyle changes

Behavior influences

Influences that are created as a result of an individual's own behavior.

Positive reinforcement

The practice of offering a reward following a desired behavior to encourage repetition of the behavior.

Transtheoretical Model (TTM)

States that individuals progress through a series of stages of behavior change, and that movement through these stages is cyclical—not linear.

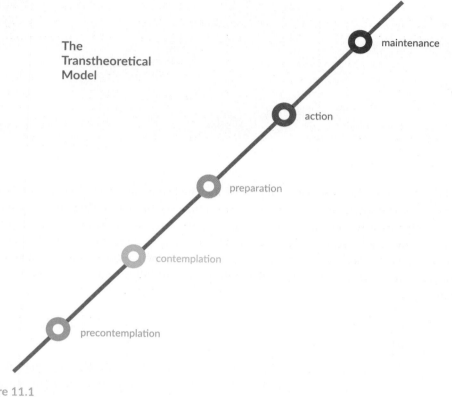

The Transtheoretical Model

Figure 11.1
Transtheoretical Model

Precontemplation stage

Stage of change in the Transtheoretical Model in which individuals do not intend to change their high-risk behaviors in the foreseeable future.

Contemplation stage

The stage of change in the Transtheoretical Model in which individuals are contemplating making a change within the next 6 months.

Preparation stage

The stage of change in the Transtheoretical Model in which individuals intend to take action in the near future, usually within the next month.

for the long term. The pattern of the TTM is shown in Figure 11.1 and comprises five stages: pre-contemplation, contemplation, preparation, action, and maintenance.

Precontemplation

In the precontemplation stage of the TTM, individuals do not intend to change their high-risk behaviors in the foreseeable future. In relation to exercise, this usually means the individual is not anticipating starting an exercise regimen in the next 6 months. Essentially, these individuals are non-exercisers. People in this stage tend to avoid reading, talking, or thinking about the behavior that needs to be changed.[13]

Contemplation

Individuals in the contemplation stage are thinking about making a behavior change within the next 6 months. They are typically aware of the pros of changing their behavior (e.g., the positive effects of exercise), but they are also acutely aware of the cons of this behavior change (e.g., more time away from the family).

Preparation

In the preparation stage of the TTM, individuals intend to take action in the near future, usually within the next month (e.g., "I plan on exercising three or more times a week for 20 minutes or longer"). In addition, these individuals usually have taken some significant action toward making the behavior change in the past year, such as joining a health club, contacting a physician, engaging in more activity, or buying a piece of exercise equipment. Most people in this stage have some sort of plan of action.

Action

Individuals in the action stage of the TTM have made specific, overt modifications to their behavior within the past 6 months. Individuals in this stage may exercise regularly but have been doing so for less than 6 months. Change in this phase is not stable, and it corresponds with the highest risk for relapse.

Maintenance

The maintenance stage of the TTM is the period from 6 months after the behavioral change has been made until a time point at which the risk of returning to prior behavior has been completely terminated. Individuals in this stage have been exercising regularly and have done so for more than 6 months. Once they have been engaged in this behavior for 5 years (for example), it is likely they will continue to maintain regular exercise throughout their life span, except in the event of injury or other unexpected health-related problems.

Connecting with Participant Goals

While working individually with each participant during class exceeds the responsibilities of Group Fitness Instructors, there may still be common goals for a class, or series of classes. In such instances, instructors should know how to set realistic goals for general groups. As instructors get to know regulars or field workout questions, they may start to learn about individual participant goals. In such situations, instructors should remind participants to ensure that, whatever their goals, they are *SMART goals* (Figure 11.2).

Action stage

The stage of change in the Transtheoretical Model in which individuals have made specific, overt modifications to their behavior within the past 6 months.

Maintenance stage

The stage of change in the Transtheoretical Model that begins 6 months after the criterion has been reached until a time point at which the risk of returning to the old behavior has been terminated.

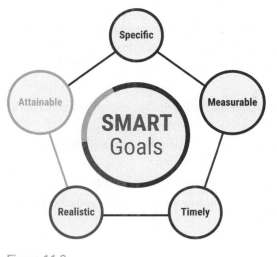

Figure 11.2
SMART Goals

Fitness message

A benefit statement or philosophy related to fitness.

Fitness mission statement

An informative statement about what an instructor does (or wants to do).

Fitness vision statement

An inspirational statement about what an instructor wants to be in the future.

Fitness community

An evolving, growing, and dedicated group of people who follow, trust, and regularly communicate with a Group Fitness Instructor.

INSTRUCTOR TIP 👍

To build a solid brand and fitness community, aim for consistency between all platforms and messages.

The acronym SMART—Specific, Measurable, Attainable, Realistic, and Time-oriented (Timely)—is widely used in health and fitness settings, as well as in business. It is a way of simplifying the goal-setting process to help individuals set more productive and realistic goals.

Examples of SMART Goals:

▼ We will do 30 pushups in the first 30 minutes of class today.

▼ I will attend 8 resistance classes and 8 cycle classes over the next 30 days.

Building a Brand and Fitness Community

Once a Group Fitness Instructor establishes successful methods of communicating with participants, a personal brand and dedicated following are built. A *fitness brand* evolves from the instructor's goals and philosophies on fitness, such as their fitness message, mission statement, and vision statement. These components drive the way an instructor prepares and teaches, self-promotes, and grows as a leader in the group fitness arena. Having a clear fitness brand helps an instructor focus on *what* to promote and *how* to promote it.

A fitness message is typically a *benefit* statement or philosophy; it is about what the instructor believes fitness can do for someone. It is an *informative* statement about *what an instructor does* (or wants to do). It comes from logical thinking and practical application. It should be short, catchy, and digestible.

A fitness vision is an inspirational statement or short paragraph about where an instructor plans to be in the future. A vision should be longer than a mission statement, with a bit more detail on the outcome, and also be more focused on inspiring people with positive opportunities.

Fitness Community

Instructors who invest time in building a brand and dedicated following actively develop a fitness community. This community evolves as more people begin to trust, follow, and interact with the instructor. There are a number of great ways to get started in building a fitness community, such as:

1. Giving specific, verbal feedback that objectively reflects the participant's form or execution.

2. Giving specific, verbal feedback that subjectively reflects the instructor's care and involvement with the participants.

3. Using first names or professions where possible to individualize the experience.

4. Engaging participants in conversation before and after class.

5. Hosting group outings.

✓ Check It Out

Start out with a consistent headshot/image that shows *your* fitness personality and resonates with your brand, message, mission, and vision. Use this same headshot/image across all media platforms as you get started to build a following and allow for instant identification with your brand. Once you have a following, you'll be able to swap out your imaging with other fun promotions and strategies down the road.

6. Aligning oneself with a charity or philanthropic outreach program in the community.
7. Facilitating friendly competition among participants.
8. Using social media, text messages, and email to communicate as appropriate.

Beyond Class Engagement

No discussion of the Group Fitness Instructor's responsibilities in relation to communication and cueing strategies would be complete without a comprehensive look at of the communication that can take place beyond the confines of the class setting.

Prior to class, there are opportunities to communicate and create long-lasting impressions, such as helping a participant who has her hands full as she walks into the club, arranging equipment, spending time in the locker room, or waiting outside of the studio for class to

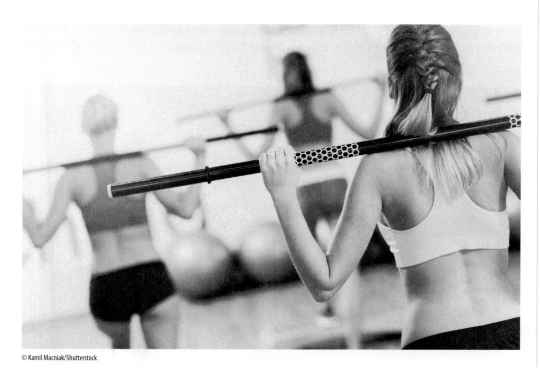

© Kamil Macniak/Shutterstock

Table 11.3

Initiating Engagement Before and After Class

Before Class	After Class
• "What are you hoping to work on today?" • "Were you sore after the last class?" • "Have any fun plans after class today?"	• "What did you like most about class today?" • "What was the most challenging part of class today?" • "What was your favorite song today?" • "Do you have any big plans for the weekend?"

start. The time between when class ends and the point where participants leave the gym or studio is one last opportunity to engage in face-to-face communication and leave a positive impression. Putting equipment back, being open and available to answer questions after class, and walking outside of the club are all good times to engage participants after class. The more engaged participants feel about their instructor's interest in their progress and overall experience, the more likely they are to return and recruit others to attend class as well.[14] The questions in **Table 11.3** are good examples for initiating two-sided communications with class participants.[15]

Using Social Media to Drive Engagement

Social media offers the Group Fitness Instructor multiple channels and platforms to communicate with students beyond the class setting. Social media also offers platforms to build community and recruit new participants and followers. Because certain demographics tend to use certain

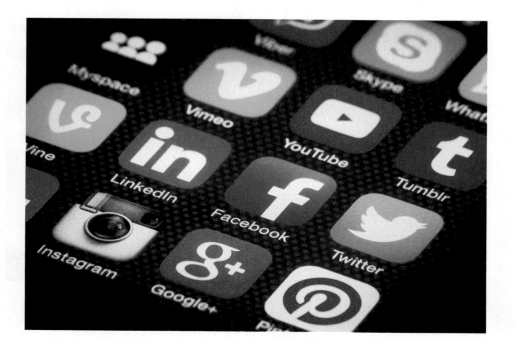

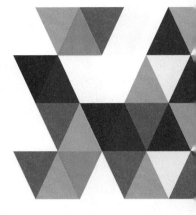

social media platforms, an instructor can better target their demographic by using the appropriate social media platform for their demographic.

Group Trainer
@Group_Trainer

How was your weekend? Join me at Cycle 101 Monday at 4:30PM, and let's get this week started!

↩ 127   ⇄ 85   ♥ 245

As powerful as social media can be in sharing positive, meaningful messages about fitness, a single post in poor taste shows a lack of etiquette and can turn off a new or existing follower—potentially for life. Before embarking on a social media campaign, instructors should know and understand a few simple standards. Instructors should:

▾ Make posts that support their fitness message, mission, and vision statements.

▾ Try to post original quotes and images as much as possible to let people know about personal mottos and spread *their* message.

▾ Give credit to original writers, artists, or owners when posting content from inspiring people or organizations and resonate with the brand. It also helps to explain why this content resonates.

▾ Post open-ended questions to engage the greatest number of participants and encourage them to create likes/reactions, comments, and shares.

▾ Include something visual; add a photograph or short video to the post to engage more participation.

CAUTION ⚠

It is important to consider club or fitness center policies before creating and adding participants to your social media network. Additionally, refer to any copyright or licensing guidelines before sharing proprietary materials.

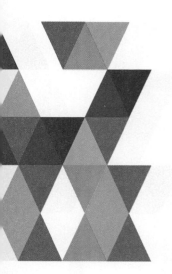

- ▼ Shoot any video clips with a smartphone in horizontal mode to capture a full image.
- ▼ Obtain permission from any individual before tagging them or publicly discussing anything about them.
- ▼ Make sure any content posted to public pages supports the brand. Delete spam or offensive material immediately, such as profanity, insults, hate speech, malicious links, fraudulent reviews, fake friends, and personally identifiable information.
- ▼ Avoid impolite topics such as politics and religion.
- ▼ Avoid aggressively requesting likes, shares, or comments.
- ▼ Try to have a "brand" account and a "personal" account to protect privacy and safety.
- ▼ Delete or remove tags that others make using their name that don't resonate with their brand.

Summary

There are many methods and strategies an instructor can try in order to engage more participants. However, it is important to remember that a Group Fitness Instructor does not have to perform every single technique all the time. Engagement strategies are meant to be cycled, tested, tweaked, and updated regularly over time. For the participant, it is not "just a workout," it is an experience that will be mentally, physically, and emotionally demanding, driving future decisions and about fitness and health. Each class experience influences participant health, club and member retention, and class size and energy; therefore, an instructor's motivation must be to prepare and execute the best workout experience possible.

Chapter in Review

- ▼ Elements of engagement
  - ▪ Performance & presence: cues, movements, music, ambiance, attire, volume, attitude,
  - ▪ Music: use variety, popular hits, dramatic segments, lyrics, and beat for engagement
  - ▪ Edutainment: combination of education and entertainment
  - ▪ Variety: add new moves and new music or change order and variables

- ▼ Motivational cues:
  - ▪ Time or rep countdown
  - ▪ Performance
  - ▪ Physical/emotional benefit
  - ▪ Competition
- ▼ Extrinsic motivation: reward separate from activity
- ▼ Intrinsic motivation: reward inherent to activity
- ▼ Influences on behavior

- Cognitive: confidence and self-talk
- Interpersonal: social support
- Affective: positive or negative emotions
- Sensation: physical feelings
- Behavior: self-monitoring & positive reinforcement

▼ Transtheoretical Model (Stages of Change): cyclical series of change behavior

- Precontemplation
- Contemplation
- Preparation
- Action
- Maintenance

▼ SMART Goals (specific, measureable, attainable, realistic, and time-oriented)

▼ Building a fitness brand (message, mission, vision)

- Engaging participants and building a community
- Social media etiquette

References

1. Kravitz L. Qualities of top teachers. *IDEA Fitness J.* 2012;9(8):20–23.
2. DeVore K. *The Voice Book: Caring For, Protecting, and Improving Your Voice.* Chicago, IL: Review Press; 2009.
3. Deci E, Ryan R. *Intrinsic Motivation and Self-Determination in Human Behavior.* New York: Plenum Press; 1985.
4. Deci E, Ryan R. The "what" and "why" of goal pursuits: Human needs and self-determination of behavior. *Psychol Inquiry.* 2000;11:227–268.
5. Alan K, McNab D. Instructor motivation and adherence: Getting them & keeping them. In L.A. Gladwin (Ed.). *Fitness: Theory & Practice.* 5th ed. Sherman Oaks, CA: Aerobics and Fitness Association of America; 2005:229–252.
6. Seligman MEP. *Authentic Happiness.* New York, NY: Free Press; 2002.
7. Rovinak L, Sallis J, Saelems B, Frank L, Marshall S, Norman G, Hovell MF. Adults' physical activity patterns across the life domains: Cluster analysis with repetition. *Health Psychol.* 2010;29:496–505.
8. Bandura A. *Self-Efficacy: The Exercise of Control.* New York, NY: Freeman; 1997.
9. Thayer R, Newman R, McClain T. Self-regulation of mood: Strategies for changing a bad mood, raising energy, and reducing tension. *J Pers Soc Behav.* 1994; *67*: 910–925.
10. Kroening R, Kim K. Premack principle. In N. J. Salkind (Ed.), *Encyclopedia of educational psychology.* Thousand Oaks, CA: SAGE Publications Ltd. 2008; 2: 814-814. doi:10.4135/9781412963848.n219
11. Smith R. Positive reinforcement, performance feedback, and performance enhancement. In: Williams J. (Ed.). *Applied Sport Psychology: Personal Growth to Peak Performance.* 5th ed. Mountain View, CA: Mayfield; 2006.
12. Prochaska J, DiClemente C. Stages and processes of self-change of smoking: Toward an integrative model of change. *J Consult Clin. Psychol.* 1983;51:390–395.
13. Prochaska O, Velicer W. Misinterpretation and misapplication of the transtheoretical model. *Am J Health Prom.* 1997;12:11–12.
14. Kravitz L. What motivates people to exercise! *IDEA Fitness J.* 2011;8(1):25–27.
15. Castells M. *Communication Power.* New York, NY: Oxford University Press; 2009.

Chapter 12
Professional and Legal Responsibilities

Learning Objectives

12.1.   **Describe** options for continuing education and developing experience.

12.2.   **Define** the professional expectations of a Group Fitness Instructor.

12.3.   **Describe** the legal and ethical expectations for Group Fitness Instructors.

12.4.   **Identify** self-care methods for Group Fitness Instructors.

Rationale for Continued Development

Throughout the course of their careers, Group Fitness Instructors affect the lives of countless individuals. Participants trust instructors to have the knowledge, skills, and abilities to lead safe, effective workouts. Instructors must strive to provide the best possible information, methodology, and experience to their groups. Obtaining an AFAA certification is a critical first step, but ongoing professional development is equally important to keep pace with changes in the fitness industry as exercise science and technology advance. For career development, an instructor should explore options to gain experience, seek feedback and evaluation, stay current with research and trends, and investigate specializations.

Feedback

Feedback offers an opportunity for learning, growth, and improved performance to expand future opportunities.[1] Instructors should anticipate and solicit feedback from participants, peers, and supervisors, as each contributes unique value. Although not all feedback will—or should—result in change, instructors can benefit by taking all feedback graciously and evaluating how to use it for improvement.

Participant Feedback

Positive feedback from participants is encouraging and validating. Conversely, negative feedback can feel defeating. Many factors may be influencing participant comments, including personal preferences, age, fitness level, past experiences, relationships with other instructors, and changing

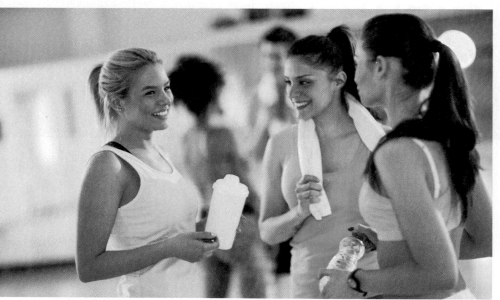

© Lucky Business/Shutterstock

moods. Even if it appears a participant may be reacting to elements beyond the control of the instructor, negative feedback should not be dismissed without considering its potential validity.

Peer Feedback

Feedback from fellow instructors is one of the most valuable types. Another instructor will typically have a better-informed perspective than a participant. When a peer comes to class, invite them to share specifically what worked, what did not, and how it could have been better; then, offer to do the same for them. When used for mutual benefit and improvement, peer-to-peer feedback is an excellent practice for instructors.

Supervisor Feedback

Regular feedback from a supervisor should also be expected and welcomed. Management's goal is to keep participants happy and classes well attended. Some facilities may also have specific standards, branded programs, or guidelines to which instructors must adhere. Supervisors also have a responsibility to uphold the standards specific to their respective programs and to meet the needs of participants.

Self-evaluation

Self-evaluation, or self-assessment, is a review of oneself or one's actions and attitudes, particularly with regard to one's performance at a job, viewed in relation to an objective standard. As it relates to the Group Fitness Instructor, self-evaluation is a vital and ongoing part of professional development.

Immediate Reflection

After every session, Group Fitness Instructors will typically have a sense of whether the class was good or bad. In either instance, an instructor can learn and grow from the experience. By identifying what factors contributed to the outcome, instructors can use the information to do more of what went right, and take action to avoid the elements that went wrong.

Long-term Evaluation

Unlike immediate reflection after a class, long-term evaluation refers to the practice of self-reflection over time. As an instructor gains more experience, it becomes possible to identify patterns or behaviors facilitating or impeding growth.

Long-term evaluation is also important for instructors deciding how to expand their education or career. After teaching for months or years, instructors might realize they are passionate about a specific format or population and less motivated to teach the format they started with. Based on that recognition, they may decide to pursue specialized education that enables them to work where they feel most satisfied.

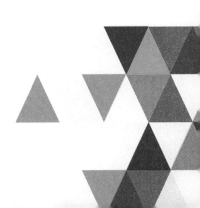

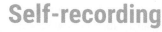
Self-recording

A video or voice recording of a live class can help an instructor identify opportunities for individual improvement. Voice recordings can help an instructor discover over-cueing, counting incessantly, speaking too fast, or engaging in unnecessary chatter that distracts from the primary objective.

When instructors watch themselves in action, they are able to look at their technique, movement quality, interactions with the group, and facial expressions in addition to hearing how they cue. They may discover their own movements do not accurately reflect what they are saying, or their own physical execution of an exercise does not match how they are cueing it.

Educational Development

Continued educational development is essential for instructors to provide up-to-date, accurate information and techniques. There are many resources and organizations dedicated to providing instructors with the best new research and methods available.

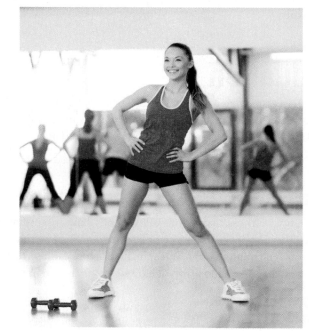

© Syda Productions/Shutterstock

Continuing Education

Continuing education refers to lectures, courses, webinars, and other programs designed to educate individuals and provide additional skills or knowledge. Continuing education may consist of workshops, trainings, assigned readings and quizzes, or online courses presented by an approved continuing education provider. It is important to verify the course has been pre-approved or is eligible to be petitioned for credit, as not all available continuing education options have been approved by AFAA.

Obtaining a specified number of approved continuing education units is required during each certification period to maintain active certification or as part of recurrent recertification.

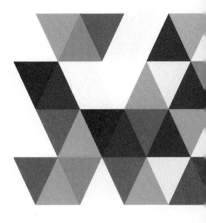

Recertification

Recertification ensures instructors stay current in information and approach as the industry evolves, preventing the instructor from stagnating. When instructors fail to seek new sources of continuing education, they limit their development and do a disservice to their participants, their fellow instructors, and the industry at large. It is important to visit and review the information at www.AFAA.com for the most up-to-date requirements and options for recertification.

Specialty Courses

Because of the intentionally broad focus of the AFAA Group Fitness Instructor certification program, additional, specific training is required to teach popular classes such as indoor cycling, mind-body, cardio-kickboxing, dance-based formats, water-based formats, and others specific to various populations like youth, older adult, or pre- and post-natal fitness. There are many different courses and format trainings that feature specialized equipment, pre-designed branded formats, or advanced instructor skills. Specialty courses enhance the skills, interests, and abilities of the instructor and also broaden his or her opportunities for employment.

Workshops and Live Events

Workshops delivered by a qualified provider can range from a few hours to a few days. Live, multi-day events and conferences offer the opportunity to attend various sessions on a wide

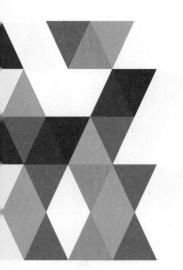

breadth of topics and formats from diverse educators. Each can be valuable to the instructor, not only to earn requisite credits to maintain certification status, but also for exposure to new areas of interest and specialization.

Credible Resources

Credible resources are supported by evidence-based, peer-reviewed research from respected organizations, groups, and individuals. When evaluating new information, instructors should consider the source and context before using it to influence their class design or cues. When in doubt, seek out established industry associations and businesses, and the works of the groups and individuals who contribute to them.

Experiential Development

There is no substitute for application and experience in the Group Fitness Instructor's development path. Being a successful instructor requires practice, observation, a commitment to grow, and patience. Experiential development can be acquired through a variety of resources:

▼ **Peer participation:** attending another instructor's class
▼ **Co-instruction**: instructing a class with a peer
▼ **Mentoring**: finding a mentor or serving as a mentor
▼ **Networking**: connecting with other professionals

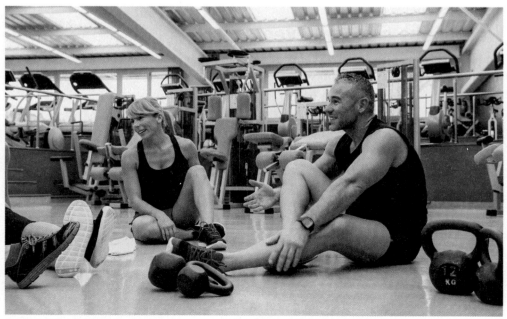

© David Pereiras/Shutterstock

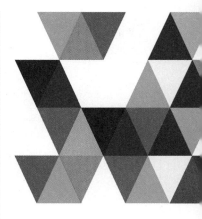

General Professionalism in Group Fitness

Professionalism starts with practicing basic principles of customer service, including arriving on time; communicating in a friendly, professional manner; and setting appropriate boundaries for contact with participants. As with any job that involves frequent and direct interaction with the public, instructors must be aware of the influence their attitudes, behaviors, and communication styles can have. To earn respect and trust, as well as to maintain the integrity of the profession, instructors should strive to act responsibly and professionally at all times. The following are some general professional guidelines for the Group Fitness Instructor:

▾ **Punctuality**: Every effort should be made to start and end class at the scheduled time.

▾ **Communication**: Instructors should communicate in a manner that is friendly, considerate, and inclusive. Vocal tone, choice of words, rate of speech, eye contact, and body language all contribute to professionalism or lack thereof.[2]

▾ **Physical Contact**: Due to the physical nature of teaching group fitness, it important for the instructor to maintain appropriate professional boundaries with regard to contact. If a participant agrees to physical contact, it should always be done with care and sensitivity for the individual. If a participant displays any sign of discomfort, contact should be immediately discontinued.[3]

▾ **Attire**: The instructor should dress in a manner that enables performance without creating discomfort or distraction for participants.[3]

▾ **Language**: In general, profanity or explicit language is best left out of the teaching environment.

▾ **Confidentiality**: The instructor should always maintain the confidentiality of the individual and avoid discussing a participant's personal information with others. In the case of health-related matters, sharing personal information could result in liability for both the instructor and the facility.

AFAA Group Fitness Instructors are also expected to adhere to *AFAA's Code of Professional Conduct*, conducting themselves in a manner that merits the respect of the public, other colleagues, and AFAA.

Legal and Ethical Considerations

Exercise programs, by nature, can result in injuries, from minor incidents to life-threatening events. The Group Fitness Instructor must not only have a working knowledge of legal and risk management concepts, but must also adhere to ethical practices to avoid legal consequences.[4]

Scope of Practice

When teaching, instructors must demonstrate sufficient knowledge of exercise science and an ability to provide safe and progressive exercise programming.[5] Participants expect their workouts will bring about positive change and their instructors have a sufficient grasp of anatomy, physiology, and exercise science to ensure safe and effective workouts.[5] Given that assumption, participants may also presume Group Fitness Instructors have more in-depth medical knowledge or credentials than they do, and thus may pose questions instructors are neither qualified nor licensed to answer.

Scope of practice refers to the limitations imposed by law on different vocational pursuits, pursuits which require specific education and experience or competency, as well as demonstrated competency. Scope of practice is used by national and state licensing boards, as well as various professions, to determine the procedures, actions, or processes permitted by a licensee or practitioner.[5] When an individual who is not licensed engages in the practices of a licensed profession, then he or she is violating scope of practice. Simply put, this means an instructor must understand what he or she is and is not qualified to do or say when working with participants; operating outside of those boundaries can constitute a violation of the law.

Common realms where instructors must be particularly cautious to not go beyond scope of practice include postural assessment, diagnosis or treatment of an injury, nutritional recommendations, and psychological advice.[5] The instructor should develop a network of trusted, qualified healthcare providers and refer clients to them accordingly.

Legal Practices

In addition to operating within scope of practice, instructors should also be aware of other legal liability exposures and risk management strategies. Incidents or injuries due to negligence (carelessness) can result in costly litigation for both the facility and the instructor.[4]

These claims may include:

- ▽ failing to provide a qualified instructor with sufficient knowledge, training, and experience to safely instruct the participant.
- ▽ failing to supervise or improperly instructing a participant.
- ▽ failing to have or to properly carry out a written emergency plan and procedure.

Risk management strategies for the Group Fitness Instructor include[4]:

- ▽ maintaining current Group Fitness Instructor and CPR/AED certification at all times.
- ▽ adhering to industry standards and guidelines for safety and efficacy when teaching group exercise.
- ▽ obtaining necessary training for all formats instructed and equipment used.
- ▽ operating within scope of practice.
- ▽ understanding and being able to execute emergency action plans.
- ▽ being familiar with and acting within all facility policies and procedures.
- ▽ completing incident reports properly and in a timely manner.

Group Fitness Instructors must be familiar with liability insurance and maintain those requirements, as well as participant liability waivers to minimize risk for themselves and the organization. There are two types of liability insurance: *general liability* and *professional liability*. General liability insurance protects the insured from ordinary negligence.[6] This refers to public liability and, in the case of a fitness facility, covers the premises and all equipment therein.[7] Professional liability insurance covers professional negligence which may be cited when a participant sustains a loss as a result of an instructor's negligent actions or behaviors (such as unsafe exercise or equipment misuse).[7] Professional liability insurance is recommended for all fitness professionals.[7]

The instructor can minimize risk by practicing common sense when dealing with participants, watching for potential problems, and making corrections before an accident happens. If an injury or incident should occur, the actions of the instructor immediately following can go a long way to mitigate the risk of negligence; it is important to promptly contact emergency or medical personnel and take detailed notes to provide to the insurer.[7]

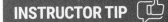

INSTRUCTOR TIP

Professional liability insurance can be obtained through a number of credible organizations. Instructors should carefully evaluate their coverage needs and liability risk when determining which type of professional liability insurance to purchase.

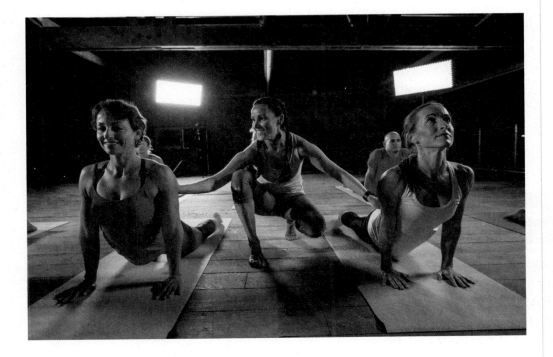

Ethics for Group Fitness Instructors

To be in alignment with ethical standards, Group Fitness Instructors commit to always act in the best interest of participants by maintaining the necessary education and knowledge, operating within their scope of practice, and behaving in a consistently positive, constructive, and professional manner.[3] The following are some of the most important ethical considerations for instructors[3]:

▼ Teach class with the best interests of the group in mind, while still acknowledging individual needs

▼ Prioritize safety

▼ Adhere to guidelines for proper music speed and volume

▼ Obtain and maintain necessary training and education for all formats instructed

▼ Work within scope of practice

▼ Be guided by truth, fairness, and integrity

▼ Respect professional boundaries

▼ Always uphold a professional image

Music Legalities

The act of teaching in a public place in front of groups of people and in a commercial setting requires a commercial music license. For music to be legal, two groups of contributors must be compensated:

▼ Publishers and songwriters

▼ Record labels and artists

Both parties contribute to a complete sound recording, but they are separate entities and each deserves fair compensation. According to the U.S. Copyright Office, publishers and songwriters create and manage the musical compositions; record labels and artists record and provide the sound equipment and vocal talent to make the recordings, and therefore own the actual recording. Legal music pays royalties to both parties. See Figure 12.1.

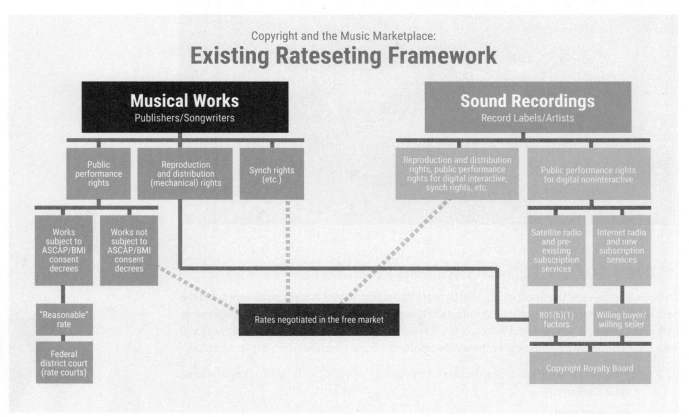

Figure 12.1
Existing Ratesetting Framework
"Copyright and the Music Marketplace" A Report of the Register of Copyrights, February 2015. United States Copyright Office.

Group Fitness Instructors who want an easy, legal music option should use music from a fitness music company, as these companies produce and own their own recordings and provide proper master recording licenses for commercial use.

Self-care

Due to the nature of the role, a fitness instructor can put tremendous stress on his or her body and their voice. To have a long and healthy career that sets an example, it is important to be mindful of some of the most common risks and how to avoid them.

Voice Care

As a result of long-term vocal strain, instructors can develop chronic laryngitis (i.e., long-term inflammation of the larynx and surrounding tissues), vocal nodules (i.e., benign growths on the vocal chords), and other symptoms of vocal damage.[8, 9] Like any other muscle in the body, the tissues involved in phonation (i.e, the production of vocal sounds) and speech can be damaged through overuse, misuse, and abuse.

In order to prevent such injuries, the Group Fitness instructor should be mindful of the following tactics to preserve his or her vocal health:

▼ **Project from the diaphragm.** Diaphragmatic or "belly" breathing is an important technique that supports the voice and enables the speaker to project with less strain on the vocal chords.

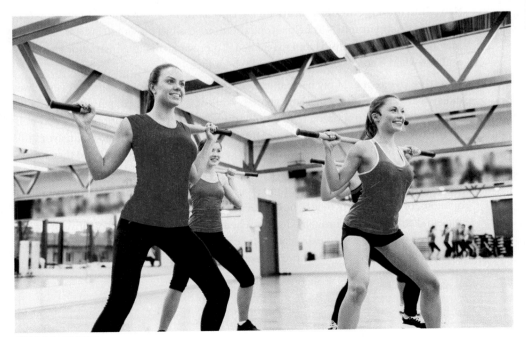

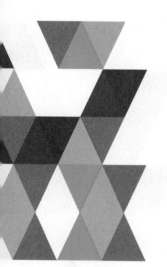

▼ **Avoid shouting and screaming.** Use vocal dynamics, body language, and visual cueing to engage participants, and use a microphone to be heard more easily.

▼ **Rest the voice.** Weekly or bi-weekly days of complete vocal rest (i.e., in which one avoids talking or making any vocal sounds) can be very beneficial in maintaining vocal health.

Overtraining

Because the Group Fitness Instructor's routine includes multiple classes each week—potentially hundreds each year—instructors must be careful to avoid overtraining.

In a healthy cycle of training and recovery, progressive overload combined with adequate recovery leads to performance improvements. However, when overload is uncontrolled without allowing for proper rest and rebuild, overtraining can result.[10, 11]

As instructors are a high-risk category for this condition, they should take immediate action, beginning with ample rest, if they develop symptoms of overtraining. The risk of overtraining may be reduced by diversifying the types of formats taught, managing personal intensity, coaching instead of demonstrating, and getting adequate rest and nutrition.

Stress Management

Teaching group fitness can be an exceptionally fun and rewarding occupation; flexible schedules, staying fit, constant interaction with like-minded individuals, and being compensated for helping others live a healthier life all contribute to the many benefits of being a Group Fitness Instructor. However, many of the same factors that make it attractive can become sources of stress when not properly managed. To reap the benefits of teaching without falling victim to some of the most commonly experienced causes of stress, instructors should be mindful of the following:

▼ **Schedule management.** In an attempt to earn more income or even simply to increase employment opportunities by helping out wherever possible, the Group Fitness Instructor may become overscheduled and exhausted. To prevent this, the instructor should be realistic when it comes to class load and scheduling.

▼ **Creative pressure.** Many instructors feel compelled to make changes to every class, due to fear participants will become bored. While it is important to periodically change class design or programming to maintain interest and create adaption to new stimuli, instructors often change more frequently than is necessary. Instructors can avoid this type of stress by planning how long they will keep a routine or sequence, and then inform participants so they can gauge progress.

▼ **Emotional considerations.** Although an instructor cannot control the perceptions, opinions, or comments of others, he or she can control how they affect his or her emotional state and stress levels. Through effective schedule planning, reducing creative pressure, and better managing emotionally loaded situations, the Group Fitness Instructor can spend less time feeling stressed and more time enjoying the many benefits of a fitness career.

Additional Opportunities in Fitness

In today's rapidly growing fitness industry, there are many options for the Group Fitness Instructor to extend his or her reach beyond teaching classes, from managing a group fitness staff, to personal training, to facilitating education for other instructors. By gaining experience and seeking additional opportunities, instructors can achieve a rewarding, full-time fitness career while maintaining their ability to teach a reasonable class load.

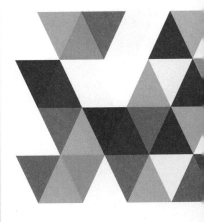

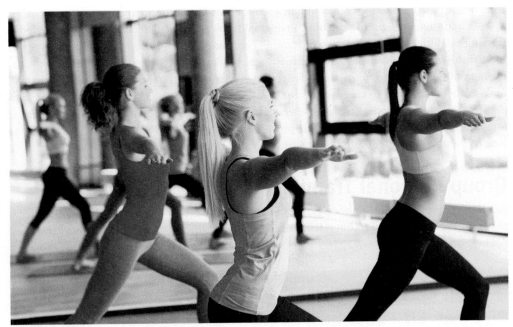

© Syda Productions/Shutterstock

Group Fitness Manager

The manager or coordinator of a group fitness program assumes responsibility not only for the delivery of his or her own classes, but also for the quality and variety of a well-balanced class schedule taught by other instructors. The responsibilities, time commitment, and compensation will vary with the type of facility. The aspiring group fitness manager should be prepared to manage and develop instructors, engage with members, track participation and payroll, and build an effective program that appeals to a wide variety of individuals.

Making the transition from instructor to manager can be both challenging and rewarding. Frequently, a popular and skilled instructor will be promoted into a management role based on his or her success in the fitness classroom. However, teaching skills and managerial skills are very different. To be a successful manager, the transitioning instructor should be committed

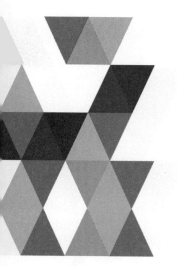

to professional development by seeking out leadership training, mentoring opportunities, and professional industry resources.

Some facilities will provide in-depth leadership training for management.

Personal Trainer

Personal training is a natural and complementary extension of the Group Fitness Instructor's career. Instead of interacting with a large group and creating programs designed to meet the needs of many, a personal trainer can specifically focus on the unique goals and needs of an individual. The dual role of Group Fitness Instructor and personal trainer is an excellent choice to maintain a great degree of autonomy while building a full- or part-time fitness career.

An additional benefit of becoming a personal trainer is the enhanced degree of knowledge it requires. With an additional personal training certification, the Group Fitness Instructor will increase his or her ability to design effective classes. Additionally, instructors who are also personal trainers often build a reputation for delivering classes that are particularly results-oriented, making them attractive to many participants.

If an instructor chooses to become a personal trainer, he or she should begin by obtaining an accredited certification. Through the process of certification, an individual will learn how to assess clients' goals and develop programs specific to their needs.

Group Personal Training

Another great option for the Group Fitness Instructor who is also a Certified Personal Trainer is to conduct group personal training sessions. Typically, group personal training refers to training

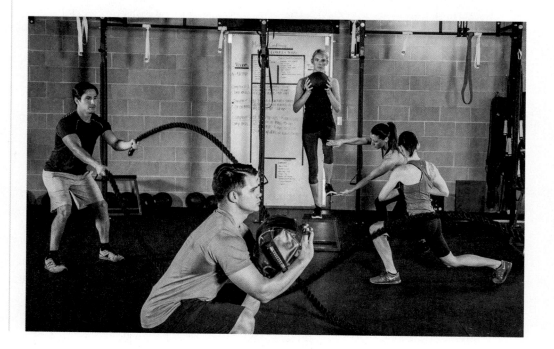

a small group of two or more (typically 3–5) clients at once. Like a group fitness class, group personal training provides individuals with the motivation and camaraderie of working out with others. However, because it enables instructors to provide more accountability, personalized attention, and individualized programming, it also allows clients to work toward more specific goals than group fitness classes can provide.

Conversely, by training a group, personal trainers can earn a higher per-session rate and serve more clients at once with creative program design that keeps sessions exciting and fun. Not only is it an excellent way to earn more income per session and provide additional revenue to facilities, it is also more affordable for clients than one-on-one training. All in all, group personal training is the perfect way to bridge the gap between teaching large group fitness classes and conducting one-on-one personal training.

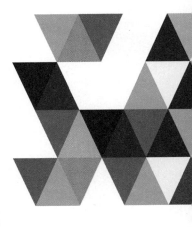

Workshop Facilitator

For the highly experienced instructor who desires to share knowledge with others, becoming a workshop facilitator can be an especially rewarding opportunity, both personally and financially. As an educator, one can contribute to the development of peers while expanding personal career opportunities and increasing income potential. In general, there are two types of workshop facilitators; one who presents original content, and one who presents the material of another individual or organization.

Regardless of whether the facilitator is presenting his or her own content, there are some basic prerequisites to be considered. These basic qualifications include dynamic public speaking skills, the ability to organize and present information clearly, and an in-depth knowledge of—and experience with—the topic being presented.

To get started, an aspiring facilitator may ask a group fitness manager or other supervisor for the opportunity to present a free workshop to fellow instructors. A low-pressure environment with support from others is an excellent first step to becoming a presenter. After gaining experience, the next step may be to apply to a local or regional conference. With time and the acquisition of skill, knowledge, and reputation, some exceptional presenters may find full-time employment as national and even international facilitators, considered by many to be the pinnacle of a fitness industry career.

Summary

In today's health and fitness industry, Group Fitness Instructors have a responsibility not only to themselves, but also to participants, peers, employers, and the industry at large, to pursue ongoing development, obtain continuing education, and adhere to ethical practices. With the influx of new information, trends, and social influences, instructors must constantly seek to learn, grow, and adapt in the dynamic fitness environment. To endure, he or she must also be open to feedback and be diligent about self-care. By being aware of and utilizing the many resources available for support and continued development, the Group Fitness instructor can look forward to a long, healthy, and rewarding career.

Chapter in Review

- ▼ Feedback resources: participants, peers, supervisors, self-evaluation
- ▼ Professional development
  - ▪ Recertification: maintaining certified status
  - ▪ Specialty courses: specific to modality, location, or groups of people
  - ▪ Workshops & live-events, conferences
- ▼ Credible resources: evidence-based, peer-reviewed
- ▼ Professional expectations
  - ▪ Punctuality
  - ▪ Friendly, considerate, inclusive communication
  - ▪ Physical contact by permission only
  - ▪ Appropriate attire
  - ▪ Appropriate language
  - ▪ Maintain participant confidentiality

- ▼ Legal and ethical expectations
  - ▪ Scope of practice: operating inside boundaries of profession
  - ▪ Liability (general and professional)
  - ▪ General ethics: prioritize safety and inclusivity, obtain appropriate education, general professionalism
  - ▪ Music licensing: purchase from fitness music companies
- ▼ Self-care
  - ▪ Voice care: use microphones and body language, avoid shouting
  - ▪ Overtraining: ensure proper rest and diversify formats
  - ▪ General stress management
- ▼ Related career opportunities (with training)
  - ▪ Group Fitness Management
  - ▪ Personal Training
  - ▪ Workshop Facilitation

References

1. The Ken Blanchard Companies. Take the fear out of feedback. *Perspectives*. (2016). http://www.kenblanchard.com/getattachment/Leading-Research/Research/Take-the-Fear-Out-of-Feedback/Blanchard-Take-the-Fear-out-of-Feedback.pdf. Accessed June 15, 2017.
2. Russell JEA. Career coach: The wrong tone can spoil the message. *The Washington Post*. February 7, 2011. http://www.washingtonpost.com/wp-dyn/content/article/2011/02/04/AR2011020406095.html. Accessed June 15, 2017.
3. International Dance Exercise Association (IDEA). *IDEA Codes of Ethics: Guidelines for Group Fitness Instructor, Personal Trainers, Owners and Managers*. Vol. 7 No. 7; June 2010. https://www.ideafit.com/fitness-library/idea-codes-of-ethics-for-fitness-professionals. Accessed June 15, 2017.
4. Eickhoff-Shemek JM. Minimizing legal liability for the exercise professional: strategies that work! *ACSM's Certified News* 2013;23(4). http://certification.acsm.org/files/file/ACSM%C2%B9sCertifiedNews_Q4_2013_web.pdf. Accessed June 15, 2017.
5. Abbott AA. The legal aspects: Scope of practice. *ACSM Health Fitness J.* 2012;16(1):31–34. http://journals.lww.com/acsmhealthfitness/Fulltext/2012/01000/The_Legal_Aspects__Scope_of_Practice.10.aspx. Accessed June 15, 2017.
6. Connaughton D, Eickhoff-Shemek J. Distinguishing "general" and "professional" liability insurance. *ACSM Health Fitness J.* 2003;7(1):28–30.

7. Riley S. Liability Insurance: Accidents Happen Regardless of How Diligent and Professional You Are. Protect Yourself. *IDEA Trainer Success* 2005;2(2). http://www.ideafit.com/fitness-library /liability-insuranceaccidents-happen-regardless-of-how-diligent-and-professional-you-are-protect -yourself. Accessed June 15, 2017.

8. Chinatti C. Sounding super: a guide to vocal health. *IDEA Fitness J.* 2010;7(11). http://www.ideafit.com /fitness-library/sounding-super-a-guide-to-vocal-health. Accessed June 15, 2017.

9. American Speech-Language, Hearing Association (ASHA). *Information for the Public/Speech, Language and Swallowing/Disorders and Diseases*. 2016. http://www.asha.org/public/speech/disorders/ NodulesPolyps/. Accessed June 15, 2017.

10. VanDusseldorp T, Kravitz L. All about overtraining. *IDEA Fitness J.* 2015;15(2). http://www.ideafit .com/fitness-library/all-about-overtraining. Accessed June 15, 2017.

11. VanDusseldorp T, Kravitz L. Heart rate variability and overtraining. *IDEA Fitness J.* 2015;12(1). http:// www.ideafit.com/fitness-library/heart-rate-variability-amp-overtraining. Accessed June 15, 2017.

Chapter 13
Nutrition

 Learning Objectives

13.1. **Explain** the structure and function of macronutrients.

13.2. **Explain** the role of water in the function of the body.

13.3. **Describe** effective pre-, peri-, and post-workout nutrition strategies.

Introduction to Basic Nutrition

Nutrition is founded in disciplines such as biochemistry, physiology, psychology, and food science. Research is sometimes misinterpreted, leading to confusion and misinformation. It is important to rely on licensed professionals, such as registered dietitians and nutritionists, to interpret the science. In most states, only licensed or registered dietitians can provide nutritional counseling and diet prescription.

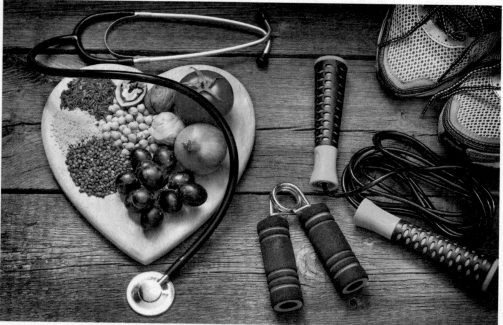

© udra11/Shutterstock

CAUTION ⚠

In most states only licensed professionals or registered dieticians can legally provide nutritional counseling and dietary recommendations to consumers.

Participants might ask questions about the latest nutritional trends, so it is critical for instructors to stay current. Additionally, networking and maintaining relationships with registered dietitians will ensure a go-to source when making referrals.

Dietary Guidelines

The Dietary Guidelines for Americans from the Department of Health and Human Services (HHS) and the U.S. Department of Agriculture (USDA) summarize science-based advice to promote health through diet and physical activity and reduce risk for major diseases such as heart disease and stroke. The recommendations reflect the knowledge that the major causes of death and disease in the United States are related to an unhealthy diet, a sedentary lifestyle, and obesity.

⊘ Check It Out

Visit www.health.gov/dietaryguidelines to access the latest Dietary Guidelines for Americans report.

Table 13.1

Dietary Reference Intake Terminology

Term	Definition
Estimated Average Requirement (EAR)	The average daily nutrient intake level estimated to meet the requirement of half the healthy individuals who are in a particular life stage and gender group.
Recommended Dietary Allowance (RDA)	The average daily nutrient intake sufficient to meet the nutrient requirements of nearly all (97-98%) healthy individuals who are in a particular life stage and gender group.
Adequate Intake (AI)	A recommended average daily nutrient intake level, based on observed (or experimentally determined) approximations or estimates of nutrient intake assumed to be adequate for a group (or groups) of healthy people. This measure is used when RDA cannot be determined.
Tolerable Upper Intake Level (UL)	The highest average daily nutrient intake level likely to pose no risk of adverse health effects to almost all individuals in a particular life stage and gender group. As intake increases above the UL, the potential risk of adverse health effects increases.

The overall purpose is to encourage most Americans to eat fewer calories, be more active, and make healthier food choices.

The nutrition label found on food can be used to implement these guidelines on a daily basis. The Dietary Guidelines are intended to be general, and do not provide information on the specific requirements of each nutrient. The requirements for essential nutrients are reported with Dietary Reference Intake (DRI) values. DRIs provide recommended intakes for specific nutrients, and can be used by registered dieticians to plan diets for individuals and groups. **Table 13.1** lists other dietary terminology.

Food Labels

Food labels are another tool for meal planning. They can help individuals make healthy food choices by listing information about the nutrient content of a food and how it fits into an overall healthy diet. The "overall diet" that the nutrient content of a specific food is compared to is called the *daily value*. It is like the DRI but is just one average value for each nutrient, because the label is not large enough to show values for different ages and genders and is based on a 2,000-calorie diet.

Macronutrients

The nutrients that provide the body's energy and mass are called macronutrients; they include the carbohydrates, fats, and proteins used by the body for energy metabolism, tissue growth and healing, and cellular function. Each macronutrient provides the body a different concentration of calories. A calorie is a scientific unit of energy, representing the amount of heat required to raise

Dietary Reference Intake (DRI)

Framework of dietary standards used to plan and evaluate diets.

Macronutrients

Nutrients that provide calories.

Calorie

A scientific unit of heat energy.

Table 13.2

Macronutrient Intake Recommendations	
Macronutrient	**Recommended Intake**
Carbohydrates	
General population	45–65% total daily calories OR 3 g/kg body weight
Those exercising more than 1 hour per day	4–5 g/kg body weight
Athletes or high-intensity exercisers training more than 4 hours per day	8–12 g/kg body weight
Proteins	
General population	0.8 g/kg OR 10–35% total daily calories
Endurance athletes	1.2–1.4 g/kg body weight
Strength athletes	1.6–1.7 g/kg body weight
Fats	
Total consumption	20–35% total daily calories
Saturated fat	Less than 10% total daily calories

Kilocalorie

A unit of energy equal to 1,000 calories.

Complex carbohydrate

A carbohydrate with more than 10 carbon-water units.

Glycogen

Complex carbohydrate stored in the liver and muscle cells.

Blood glucose

Sugar transported in the body to supply energy to the body's cells, including fueling the brain and other cells in the body that cannot use fat as a fuel (e.g., blood sugar).

the temperature of one kilogram of water 1°C. The *calories* used to measure food energy are called kilocalories—or, kcals—but are shortened to *calories* for use in food labeling. **Table 13.2** provides a summary of the recommended intakes of the three macronutrients for differing activity levels.[1, 2]

Carbohydrates

Carbohydrates supply energy (4 calories per gram), they spare protein for more efficient uses in the body, and they help to maintain blood sugar. Carbohydrates are a diverse class of nutrients, and the type of carbohydrate one consumes is important.

Carbohydrates are made of carbon and water and are categorized as *simple* or *complex* based on the carbon-water units they contain. A carbohydrate with more than 10 carbon-water units is a complex carbohydrate. Complex carbohydrates include the fiber and starch found in whole grains and vegetables. See **Table 13.3** for a summary of some food sources of simple and complex carbohydrates.

Function of Carbohydrates

The human body stores a limited amount of carbohydrates in the liver and the skeletal muscle in the form of glycogen. Liver glycogen helps to maintain blood glucose—the sugar transported in the blood to supply energy to the body, including fueling the brain and other cells in the body that cannot use fat as a fuel.

Table 13.3

Sources of Complex and Simple Carbohydrates	
Carbohydrate Type	**Food Sources**
Complex	
Starches	Grains, wheat, rice, corn, oats, potatoes, pasta, peas
Fiber	*Soluble:* Nuts, apples, blueberries, oatmeal, beans *Insoluble:* Bran, brown rice, fruit skins
Simple	
Disaccharides	Table sugar (sucrose), milk (lactose), ice cream (lactose), beer (maltose), sweet potatoes (maltose), molasses (maltose)
Monosaccharaides	Glucose, fructose, galactose

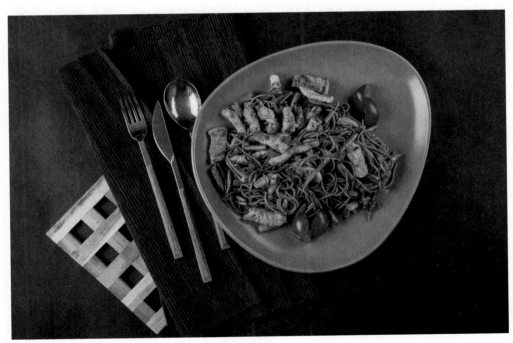

© Medolka/Shutterstock

Carbohydrates are an important source of fuel before, during, and after exercise. They are the predominant fuel source during high-intensity activities. The availability of carbohydrates as a fuel for both muscle contraction and the central nervous system—especially the brain—makes them critical to consume for optimal exercise performance.[3]

Nutrient density

Nutrient content of a food relative to its calories.

Recommended Intake of Carbohydrates

When expressed as a percentage of total calories, government recommendations direct adults to consume 45–65% of their total calories from carbohydrates, primarily in the form of complex carbohydrates and whole grains.[1] Individuals exercising more than 60–90 minutes a day or athletes training twice per day need more carbohydrates than an individual sitting at a desk all day with minimal activity.

Importance of Carbohydrate Type

Carbohydrates are naturally present in milk and in almost all plant foods—fruits, vegetables, grains, and legumes—primarily as complex carbohydrates; it is advised that most daily carbohydrate intake comes from these sources. The concept of consuming more nutrients per calorie is called nutrient density, and individuals are advised to center their meals around nutrient-dense foods, especially when trying to lose weight. See **Table 13.4** for information on the nutrient density of different foods.

Table 13.4

Nutrient Density	
High Nutrient Density (ideal)	Nonstarchy vegetables (raw leafy green veggies > solid green veggies > all other nonstarchy veggies)
	Beans
	Fresh fruit
	Starchy vegetables
	Whole grains
	Raw nuts and seeds
	Fish
	Fat-free dairy
	Poultry
	Eggs
Low Nutrient Density (less ideal)	Red meat
	Full-fat dairy
	Cheese
	Refined grains—crackers, chips, white pasta, etc.
	Oils
	Refined sweets—sugar, baked goods, candy, soda

Fats

Fats function as another primary source of energy for the body. Fats are also called lipids and are defined as substances that are insoluble in water. Lipids include fatty acids, triglycerides, phospholipids, and sterols (e.g., cholesterol). The fat stored in the human body is mostly in the form of triglycerides. While fats are typically the long-term storage mechanism for energy in the body, they also serve additional functions.

Lipids provide over twice as much energy as carbohydrates—9 calories per gram.[4] One pound of body fat constitutes about 3,500 calories. Fatty acids are chains of carbon linked together. Fats are classified based on their *saturation*—that is, the extent to which all possible carbon-hydrogen bonds are filled. A saturated fat consists of a chain of carbons bonded to all of the hydrogen atoms it can hold. Unsaturated fatty acids are those that have areas not completely saturated with hydrogen atoms. A fatty acid with just one missing hydrogen is a *monounsaturated fatty acid*. If several spots have hydrogen is missing, it is referred to as a polyunsaturated fatty acid. The level of saturation has important health implications.

There are two types of polyunsaturated fatty acids in the human diet: omega-3 and omega-6. Omega-3 fatty acids have anti-inflammatory effects and help to decrease blood clotting. Omega-6 fatty acids promote blood clotting and cell membrane formation.

Functions of Fat

Lipids serve many functions in the body, including:

- energy storage.
- providing essential fatty acids.
- absorption and transportation of fat-soluble vitamins.
- protection and insulation of vital organs.
- satiety and flavor in food.
- cell membrane structure.
- serving as a precursor for steroid hormones.

Recommended Intake of Fat

According to government recommendations, adults should consume 20–35% of their total calories from fats.[1] The types of fats consumed, rather than amount, have an important influence on the risk of cardiovascular and other diseases.

Animal fats tend to have a higher proportion of saturated fatty acids than plant-based foods.[4] A strong body of evidence indicates a higher intake of saturated fats is associated with increased levels of total blood cholesterol and low-density lipoprotein (LDL) cholesterol. Higher total and LDL cholesterol are risk factors for heart disease. Therefore, it is recommended adults consume fewer than 10% of their total calories from saturated fats, replacing them with polyunsaturated and monounsaturated fats.

Lipids

Group of compounds that includes triglycerides (fats and oils), phospholipids, and sterols.

Triglyceride

Chemical or substrate form in which most fat exists in food as well as in the body.

Saturated fat

Chain of carbons saturated with all of the hydrogens it can hold; there are no double bonds.

Low-density lipoprotein (LDL)

The molecule that carries lipids throughout the body and delivers cholesterol that can accumulate on artery walls.

Food Sources of Fats

Meat, cheese, butter, egg yolks, whole milk, and creamy sauces are all sources of *saturated fat*. Vegetable oils such as soybean, corn, and sunflower oils; fish (especially salmon and coldwater fish); and flaxseed and walnuts are all good sources of *polyunsaturated fats*. Olive, canola, peanut, safflower, and sesame oils, as well as nuts and avocados, are all good sources of *monounsaturated fats*.

Table 13.5 lists common food sources for the various types of dietary fats.

Table 13.5

Food Sources and Types of Fats			
Monounsaturated	**Polyunsaturated**	**Saturated**	***Trans*-fats**
Olive oil	*Vegetable oils:*	*Tropical oils:*	Stick margarine
Canola oil	Soy oil	Coconut oil	Shortening
Peanut oil	Corn oil	Palm oil	Some fried foods,
Sesame oil	Sunflower oils	Palm kernel oil	baked goods, and
Safflower oil	*Omega-3 fatty acids:*	Meat	pastries; many
Avocados	Herring	Poultry	restaurants and
Peanuts	Mackerel	Lard	food processors no
Almonds	Salmon	Butter	longer use *trans*-fat
Pistachios	Sardines	Cheese	lipid sources for fry-
	Flaxseeds	Cream	ing and baking
	Walnuts	Eggs	
		Whole milk	
		Many baked goods	

Table 13.6

Amino Acids	
Essential	**Nonessential**
Histidine	Alanine
Isoleucine	Arginine
Leucine	Asparagine
Lysine	Aspartic acid
Methionine	Cysteine
Phenylalanine	Glutamic acid
Threonine	Glutamine
Tryptophan	Glycine
Valine	Proline
	Serine
	Tyrosine

Protein

Long chains of amino acids that serve many essential functional roles in the body.

Proteins

Proteins are long chains of amino acids with nitrogen attached. Protein is an important part of a balanced diet and a vital macronutrient.

Like carbohydrates and fats, proteins contain carbon, hydrogen, and oxygen, but they also contain nitrogen. Proteins are made of amino acids linked together (**Table 13.6**). Essential amino acids cannot be made by the body and must be acquired in food. If essential amino acids are not consumed in adequate amounts, the body cannot make the proteins it needs for growth, maintenance, repair, or other functions without breaking down skeletal muscle. Nonessential amino acids can be made by the body, so they do not have to be consumed.

Functions of Proteins

Protein is known for its role in muscle growth and repair as well as its a vital role in the development, maintenance, and repair of all tissues in the body. It is involved in the following functions:

- fluid balance
- blood clotting
- enzyme production
- acid–base balance
- immune function
- hormone regulation
- carrier for several nutrients

Protein supplies energy (4 calories per gram), but providing energy is not its primary function.

Recommended Protein Intake

When expressed as a percentage of total calories, the recommendation is 10–35% of an individual's daily calories should come from protein.[1] Individuals regularly participating in endurance or resistance exercise require more protein than sedentary individuals.[5] By this rationale, recommendations are 1.2–1.4 grams per kilogram body weight for endurance athletes and 1.6–1.7 grams per kilogram body weight for strength athletes. Most athletes naturally consume adequate amounts of protein regardless of recommendations.[2]

Food Sources of Protein

A *high-quality protein*, also called a complete protein, provides all of the essential amino acids and is easy to digest and absorb (**Table 13.7**). Typically, animal proteins (those found in meats, eggs, and dairy products) are all considered highly digestible complete proteins.

Foods that do not contain all of the essential amino acids are called incomplete proteins, and include beans, legumes, grains, and vegetables. People who do not eat meat and dairy products can still consume an adequate intake of essential amino acids by combining incomplete proteins called complementary proteins (e.g., combining beans and rice).[4]

Amino acids

Building blocks of proteins; composed of a central carbon atom, a hydrogen atom, an amino group, a carboxyl group, and an R-group.

Essential amino acids

Amino acids that cannot be produced by the body and must be acquired by food.

Nonessential amino acids

Amino acids produced by the body that do not need to be consumed in dietary sources.

Complete protein

Protein that provides all of the essential amino acids in the amount the body needs and is also easy to digest and absorb (e.g., a *high-quality protein*).

Incomplete protein

Food that does not contain all of the essential amino acids in the amount needed by the body.

Complementary proteins

Two or more incomplete proteins that combined together provide all essential amino acids.

Table 13.7

Complete and Complementary Protein Food Sources	
Complete	**Complementary**
Eggs	Beans and rice
Milk and milk products	Beans and tortillas
Meats and poultry	Rice and lentils
Fish	Rice and black-eyed peas
Soy beans	Hummus (chickpeas and sesame paste) with whole grain pita

Hydration

While balance among all nutrients is important, water is essential to life and is required in the greatest amount. Water is important for controlling body temperature, maintaining the body's acid–base ratio, and regulating blood pressure.[4, 6] Water consists of two hydrogen atoms and one oxygen atom bonded together. This bond is unique, and allows other substances to dissolve in water.

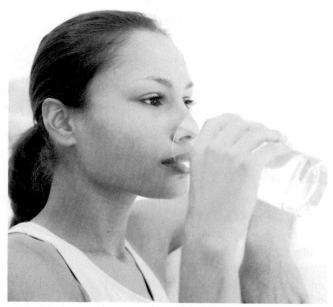

Table 13.8

Recommended Water Intake	
Sex or Exercise Status	**Recommended Intake**
Women	2.7 L (91 oz.) per day
Men	3.7 L (125 oz.) per day
2 hours pre-exercise	14–20 oz.
15 minutes pre-exercise	16 oz., if tolerated
During exercise	4–8 oz. every 15–20 minutes or 16–32 ounces every hour depending on rate of sweat
Post-exercise	16 ounces for every pound of body weight lost

Function of Water

Water serves a number of critical functions in the body as the medium by which the body transports nutrients, diffuses gases, and rids the body of waste as well as lubricating joints, cushioning vital organs, and providing structure to the skin and body tissue. Water also helps to stabilize body temperature by absorbing heat generated by exercise and environmental conditions[6] and releasing it via evaporation. As the body sweats and releases water through the skin, evaporation of the water helps cool the body.

General Guidelines for Water Intake

The Dietary Reference Intake (DRI) for water is a general recommendation. For women, the recommendation is approximately 2.7 liters (91 ounces) of total water from all beverages and foods each day; for men the recommendation is approximately 3.7 liters (125 ounces) per day.[7] Water needs can be met by drinking water and by consuming foods containing water. **Table 13.8** provides recommended water intake.[7]

Electrolytes

Electrolytes are minerals that include potassium, sodium, calcium, chloride, magnesium, and phosphate. The body needs and uses electrolytes for their electrical properties and to control fluid balance between the various systems of the body. Sodium and potassium are the most important electrolytes depleted in sweat. They must be replaced when significant amounts are lost or the condition of hyponatremia (low sodium) and/or hypokalemia (low potassium) may result.

Electrolyte replacement is most important during prolonged physical activity, and severe depletion is unlikely to occur during activities lasting under 2 hours unless an individual begins in a dehydrated or depleted state. Temperature and humidity also affect the rate of electrolyte loss; therefore, participants who have just started exercising or are new to being in a hot environment may be more at risk than those who are already acclimated.

Electrolytes

Minerals in blood and other body fluids that carry an electrical charge.

Water Balance

Hydration status depends on the balance between water loss and water intake. The following factors can influence how much water is lost per day:

- ▼ Temperature
- ▼ Humidity
- ▼ Age
- ▼ Intensity and duration of the activity
- ▼ Fitness level

To avoid dehydration, it is vital to balance water intake with water loss.

Water Loss

Overall water balance from input to output is summarized in **Table 13.9**.[4] During exercise, the body produces a large amount of heat, which must be released (typically through sweat) in order to keep body temperature in an acceptable range.

Dehydration

Dehydration can affect performance and threaten health, and even life. A loss of only 2–3% of body weight as water—roughly 3.0–4.5 pounds for a 150-pound person—can decrease exercise capacity and increase the risk of death. Even a small level of dehydration can cause fatigue and make it difficult to put forth the effort to get the most out of a workout.

Dehydration is often compounded with a severe loss of electrolytes. This can result in heat stroke. Confusion typically results from dehydration and heat stroke, causing poor decision-making, further worsening conditions. **Table 13.10** lists signs of dehydration to look out for.

Table 13.11 offers some general guidelines for fluid replacement in relation to exercise status.

Table 13.9

Water Balance from Intake and Output

Water Intake		Water Output	
Source	Intake	Source	Loss
Food	600–800 mL	Urine	900–1,200 mL
Beverages	1,000 mL	Mild sweating	400 mL
Metabolic water (from digestion)	200–300 mL	Lungs	300 mL
		Feces	200 mL
Total	1,800–2,100 mL	Total	1,800–2,100 mL

Table 13.10

Signs of Dehydration

Dry mouth	Sunken eyes	Headache
Sleepiness or tiredness	Low blood pressure	Constipation
Thirst	Rapid heartbeat	Dizziness
Decreased urine output	Rapid breathing	Delirium
Dry skin	Fever	Unconsciousness

Table 13.11

Guidelines for Fluid Replacement and Exercise[8]

Before Exercise

- Ensure high fluid intake for several days (urine should be pale in color).
- Consume 14–20 ounces (1.75–2.5 cups) of fluid 2 hours before exercise.
- Consume 16 ounces about 15 minutes before exercise, if tolerated.
- Consume water or sports drinks rather than soda or juice.
- Accelerate fluid absorption with a 6% carbohydrate drink (any popular sports drink).

During Exercise

- Drink 4–8 ounces (0.5–1.0 cup) every 15–20 minutes or 16–32 ounces of fluid every hour.
- Drink more fluids if the weather is very hot.
- Consume fluids with 500–700 milligrams of sodium per 33 ounces of water to enhance fluid replacement.
- Drink sports drinks containing 6–8% glucose (e.g., Gatorade, Powerade) for exercise lasting longer than 60 minutes.
- Avoid sodas, teas, and juices as they can upset the stomach.

After Exercise

- Consume 36 ounces of fluid for every kilogram (2.2 pounds) of body weight lost.
- Consume a drink that contains sodium and glucose to promote rapid rehydration for exercise longer than 1 hour in duration.

Monitoring Hydration Status

An objective way to check hydration status is assessing urine color and volume. If urine is light in color when the volume and frequency are near normal, then the individual is probably getting enough water; darker urine indicates a need to drink more water.

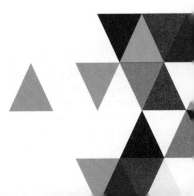

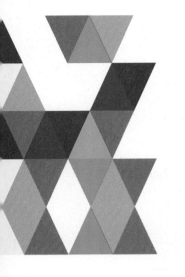

Nutrition Recommendations

Proper nutrition is directly related to exercise performance; what and when an individual eats can have a drastic influence on workout performance. It is important to maintain proper nutrition during and after exercise to help maximize the workout, as well as ensure optimal recovery.

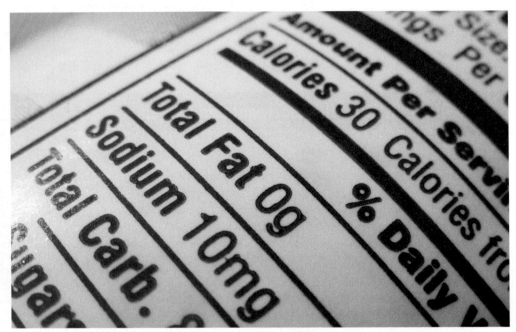

© Shutterstock

Pre-exercise

Eating before exercise has been shown to improve performance over exercising in a fasted state. The ideal situation for anyone is to arrive at the gym in a fed state (i.e., no hunger), yet without undigested food remaining in the stomach. The best way to accomplish this is to consume a larger, balanced meal roughly 3–4 hours before activity.

To boost available energy, enhance muscle synthesis, and promote gastric emptying for a speedy digestive process, the pre-exercise meal should be high in carbohydrates to optimize glycogen stores. The recommended amount will vary depending on individual appetite, metabolism, height and weight, and the intensity of the activity to be performed.

It is important to ensure the pre-workout meal is low in both fat and dietary fiber. The best options are healthy whole grains and starches, such as oatmeal, brown rice, or sweet potatoes. For protein, the source should be complete, meaning it provides all essential amino acids. Grilled chicken, lean red meat, pork, and low-fat dairy all accomplish this well when consumed according to dietary reference intake guidelines.

Another option is a meal replacement shake. These are engineered to have an optimal macronutrient balance, and tend to be much easier on the stomach. An ideal pre-workout liquid meal replacement should be high-carb, moderate protein, and low in fat.

During Exercise

Considerations for nutrition during exercise depend on the intensity and duration of the workout, as well as the environment in which it is being performed. Typically, activities lasting less than one hour do not warrant the need to eat during the activity. However, early-morning workouts may require nutrition, as glycogen stores can still be low from the overnight fast.

When activity is planned to last longer than one hour, additional macronutrient consumption may be necessary. The addition of 30–60 grams of carbohydrates per hour has been shown to boost performance in endurance athletes, allowing them to continue activity longer.[9]

Post-exercise

Post-exercise nutrition is also commonly related to the recovery period where the muscular and cardiovascular systems have been pushed and need to relax and rebuild. The key to maximizing recovery for both energy stores (glycogen) and muscle rebuild is to consume a meal with a carb-to-protein ratio of 4:1, roughly 30–45 minutes after exercise.[10] There is a narrow window of time after exercise where muscle cells are insulin-receptive; insulin is responsible for transporting glucose and amino acids into cells and initiating glycogen and protein synthesis, as well as reducing muscle protein breakdown.[11]

Consuming protein with carbohydrates immediately after exercise has also been shown to reduce muscle soreness. While adding protein beyond the 4:1 ratio does not improve glycogen repletion, it may be beneficial for muscle repair and synthesis by providing additional available amino acids for a more enhanced anabolic environment.[9]

 # Summary

To get the most out of a workout, it is essential to nourish the body, as well as maintain fluid and electrolyte balances. Insufficient nutrition, and particularly dehydration, can diminish performance and provoke medical emergency or even death. While it is out of the scope of practice for a Group Fitness Instructor to diagnose nutritional needs or prescribe diet plans for individuals, an understanding of how the human body obtains the fuel needed to function serves to benefit the overall health and well-being of instructors and participants alike.

Chapter in Review

- ▼ Carbohydrates (4 calories/gram): made of carbon and water
  - ▪ Simple: disaccharides, monosaccharaides
  - ▪ Complex: starches, fiber
  - ▪ Function: maintains blood glucose, supplies energy to the body, fuels the brain
  - ▪ Recommended intake: 45–65% of total calories

- ▼ Fats (9 calories/gram): made of chains of carbon
  - ▪ Types: saturated, unsaturated, polyunsaturated, trans-fats
  - ▪ Function: stores energy, supplies fatty acids, transport vitamins, protects organs, provides cell structure
  - ▪ Recommended intake: 20–30% of total calories

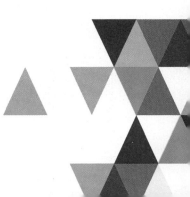

- ▼ Proteins (4 calories/gram): amino acids attached to nitrogen
  - ▪ Types: essential and nonessential
  - ▪ Function: growth and repair of muscle and tissues, balances fluids, clots blood, produces enzymes, balances acids, promotes immune function, regulates hormones
  - ▪ Recommended intake: 10–35% of total calories
- ▼ Hydration
  - ▪ Structure of water: two hydrogen atoms and one oxygen atom (H_2O)
  - ▪ Function: lubricates joints, cushions organs, provides tissue structure
  - ▪ Recommended intake: 2.7 liters/day for women; 3.7 liters/day for men
- ▼ Nutrition recommendations
  - ▪ pre-exercise: balanced meal 3-4 hours before activity
  - ▪ during exercise: for activity > 1 hour, add 30–60 grams of carbs per hour
  - ▪ post-exercise: 4:1 carb to protein ratio meal 30–45 minutes after exercise

References

1. Institute of Medicine, Food and Nutrition Board. *Dietary Reference Intakes for Energy, Carbohydrate, Fiber, Fat, Fatty Acids, Cholesterol, Protein, and Amino Acids.* Washington, DC: National Academies Press; 2005.
2. Jeukendrup A, Gleeson M. *Sports Nutrition: An Introduction to Energy Production and Performance.* Champaign, IL: Human Kinetics; 2010.
3. Burke LM, Hawley JA, Wonge SHS, Jeukendrup AE. Carbohydrates for training and competition. *J Sports Sci.* 2011;29(S1):S17–S27.
4. Hewlings SH, Medeiros DM. *Nutrition: Real People, Real Choices.* Dubuque, IA: Kendall Hunt; 2011.
5. Phillips SM, Van Loon LJC. Dietary protein for athletes: From requirements to optimum adaptation. *J Sports Sci.* 2011;29(Suppl. 1):S29–S38.
6. McArdle WD, Katch FI, Katch VL. *Exercise Physiology: Nutrition, Energy, and Human Performance* 8th ed. Baltimore, MD: Wolters Kluwer Health; 2015.
7. Institute of Medicine, Food and Nutrition Board. *Dietary Reference Intakes: Water, Potassium, Sodium, Chloride, and Sulfate.* Washington, DC: National Academies Press; 2004.
8. American College of Sports Medicine (ACSM). ACSM position stand: Exercise and fluid replacement. *Med Sci Sports Exerc.* 2009;39(2):377–390.
9. Dietitians of Canada/American Dietetic Association/American College of Sports Medicine. *Nutrition and Athletic Performance Position Statement, 2016.* https://www.dietitians.ca/Downloads/Public /noap-position-paper.aspx. Accessed June 16, 2017.
10. Ivy J, Portman R. *Nutrient Timing.* New York: Basic Health; 2004.
11. Houston ME. Gaining weight: The scientific basis of increasing skeletal muscle mass. *Can J Appl Physiol.* 1999;24(4):305–316.

Appendix A
The Kinetic Chain

The Nervous System
The Neuron

The functional unit of the nervous system is the neuron (**Figure A.1**). Billions of neurons make up the complex structure of the nervous system and provide it with the ability to communicate internally with itself, as well as externally with the outside environment. A neuron is a specialized cell that processes and transmits information through both electrical and chemical signals. Neurons form the core of the nervous system, which includes the brain, spinal cord, and peripheral ganglia.

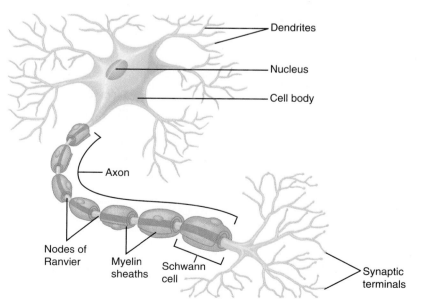

Dendrites

Nucleus

Cell body

Axon

Nodes of Ranvier

Myelin sheaths

Schwann cell

Synaptic terminals

Figure A.1
The neuron

Collectively, the merging of many neurons together forms the nerves of the body. Neurons are composed of three main parts: the cell body, axon, and dendrites.[1-4]

The cell body (or soma) of a neuron contains a nucleus and other organelles, including lysosomes, mitochondria, and a Golgi complex. The axon is a cylindrical projection from the cell body that transmits nervous impulses to other neurons or effector sites (i.e., muscles, organs, other neurons). The axon is the part of the neuron that provides communication from the brain and spinal cord to other parts of the body. The dendrites gather information from other structures and transmit it back into the neuron.[1-4]

The Central Nervous System

The nervous system is composed of two interdependent divisions: the central nervous system (CNS) and the peripheral nervous system (PNS). The CNS consists of the brain and the spinal cord; its primary function is to coordinate the activity of all parts of the body (**Figure A.2**).[1-5]

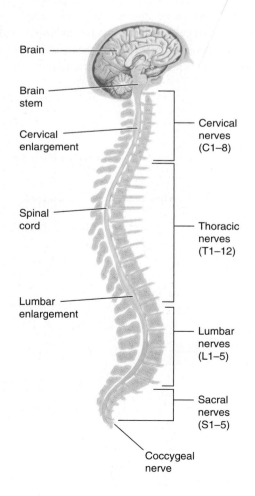

Figure A.2
The central nervous system

Brain

Brain stem

Cervical enlargement

Spinal cord

Lumbar enlargement

Cervical nerves (C1–8)

Thoracic nerves (T1–12)

Lumbar nerves (L1–5)

Sacral nerves (S1–5)

Coccygeal nerve

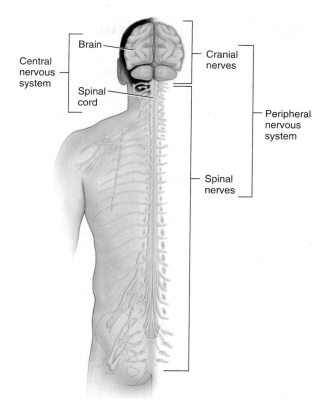

Central
nervous
system

Brain

Spinal
cord

Cranial
nerves

Peripheral
nervous
system

Spinal
nerves

The Peripheral Nervous System

The PNS consists of nerves that connect the CNS to the rest of the body and the external environment as well as 12 cranial nerves, 31 pairs of spinal nerves (which branch out from the brain and spinal cord), peripheral nerves, and sensory receptors (**Figure A.3**). The peripheral nerves serve two main functions. First, they provide a connection for the nervous system to activate different effector sites, such as muscles (motor function). Second, peripheral nerves relay information from the effector sites back to the brain via sensory receptors (sensory function), thus providing a constant update on the relation between the body and the environment.[1-4]

Two further subdivisions of the PNS include the somatic and autonomic nervous systems (**Figure A.4**). The somatic nervous system consists of nerves that serve the outer areas of the body and skeletal muscle, and they are largely responsible for the voluntary control of movement. The autonomic nervous system supplies neural input to the involuntary systems of the body (e.g., heart, digestive systems, and endocrine glands).[3,4]

The Muscular System

This section describes the isolated (concentric) and integrated (isometric, eccentric) actions of the major muscles of the human movement system.

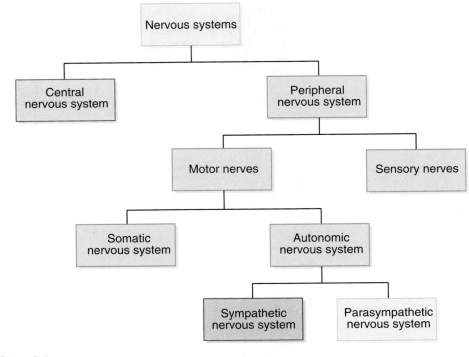

Figure A.4
Nervous system structure

This section also describes the origin, insertion, and function of each muscle. The origin and insertion refer to the anatomic locations of where a muscle attaches (usually a bone). The origin refers to the proximal attachment site that remains relatively flexed during contraction. The insertion refers to the muscle's distal attachment site to a moveable bone.

Lower Leg Musculature

Anterior tibialis

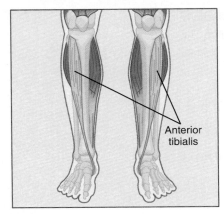

Anterior tibialis

Origin

▼   Lateral condyle and proximal two-thirds of the lateral surface of the tibia.

Insertion

▼   Medial and plantar aspects of the medial cuneiform and the base of the first metatarsal.

Isolated Function

▼   Concentrically accelerates dorsiflexion and inversion.

Integrated Function

▼   Eccentrically decelerates plantarflexion and eversion.

▼   Isometrically stabilizes the arch of the foot.

Posterior tibialis

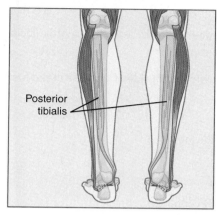

Origin

▼ Proximal two-thirds of posterior surface of the tibia and fibula.

Insertion

▼ Every tarsal bone (naviular, cuneiform, cuboid) but the talus plus the bases of the second through the fourth metatarsal bones.

▼ The main insertion is on the navicular tuberosity and the medial cuneiform bone.

Isolated Function

▼ Concentrically accelerates plantarflexion and inversion of the foot.

Integrated Function

▼ Eccentrically decelerates dorsiflexion and eversion of the foot.

▼ Isometrically stabilizes the arch of the foot.

Soleus

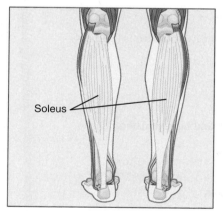

Origin

▼ Posterior surface of the fibular head and proximal one-third of its shaft and from the posterior side of the tibia.

Insertion

▼ Calcaneus via the Achilles tendon.

Isolated Function

▼ Concentrically accelerates plantarflexion.

Integrated Function

▼ Decelerates ankle dorsiflexion.

▼ Isometrically stabilizes the foot and ankle complex.

Gastrocnemius

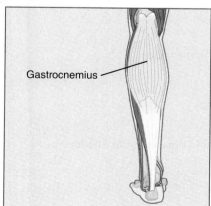

Origin

▼ Posterior aspect of the lateral and medial femoral condyles.

Insertion

▼ Calcaneus via the Achilles tendon.

Isolated Function

▼ Concentrically accelerates plantarflexion.

Integrated Function

▼ Decelerates ankle dorsiflexion.

▼ Isometrically stabilizes the foot and ankle complex.

Peroneus longus

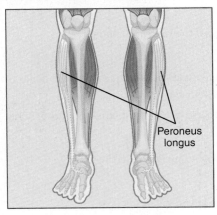

Peroneus longus

Origin

▼ Lateral condyle of tibia, head, and proximal two-thirds of the lateral surface of the fibula.

Insertion

▼ Lateral surface of the medial cuneiform and lateral side of the base of the first metatarsal.

Isolated Function

▼ Concentrically plantarflexes and everts the foot.

Integrated Function

▼ Decelerates ankle dorsiflexion.

▼ Isometrically stabilizes the foot and ankle complex.

Hamstring Complex

Biceps femoris: Long Head

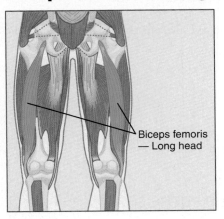

Biceps femoris — Long head

Origin

▼ Ischial tuberosity of the pelvis, part of the sacrotuberous ligament.

Insertion

▼ Head of the fibula.

Isolated Function

▼ Concentrically accelerates knee flexion and hip extension.

▼ Tibial external rotation.

Integrated Function

▼ Eccentrically decelerates knee extension.

▼ Eccentrically decelerates hip flexion.

▼ Eccentrically decelerates tibial internal rotation at midstance of the gait cycle.

▼ Isometrically stabilizes the lumbo-pelvic-hip complex (LPHC) and knee.

Biceps femoris: Short Head

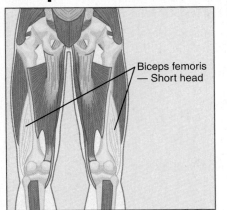

Biceps femoris — Short head

Origin

▼ Lower one-third of the posterior aspect of the femur.

Insertion

▼ Head of the fibula.

Isolated Function

▼ Concentrically accelerates knee flexion and tibial external rotation.

Integrated Function

▼ Eccentrically decelerates knee extension.

▼ Eccentrically decelerates tibial internal rotation.

▼ Isometrically stabilizes the knee.

Semimembranosus

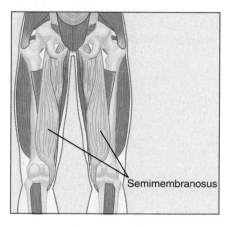

Origin

▼   Ischial tuberosity of the pelvis.

Insertion

▼   Posterior aspect of the medial tibial condyle of the tibia.

Isolated Function

▼   Concentrically accelerates knee flexion, hip extension, and tibial internal rotation.

Integrated Function

▼   Eccentrically decelerates knee extension.

▼   Eccentrically decelerates hip flexion.

▼   Eccentrically decelerates tibial external rotation.

▼   Isometrically stabilizes the LPHC and knee.

Semitendinosus

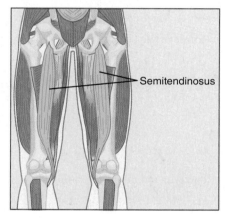

Origin

▼   Ischial tuberosity of the pelvis and part of the sacrotuberous ligament.

Insertion

▼   Proximal aspect of the medial tibial condyle of the tibia (pes anserine).

Isolated Function

▼   Concentrically accelerates knee flexion, hip extension, and tibial internal rotation.

Integrated Function

▼   Eccentrically decelerates knee extension.

▼   Eccentrically decelerates hip flexion.

▼   Eccentrically decelerates tibial external rotation.

▼   Isometrically stabilizes the LPHC and knee.

Quadriceps

Vastus lateralis

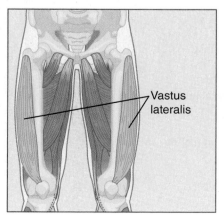

Origin

▼   Anterior and inferior border of the greater trochanter, lateral region of the gluteal tuberosity, lateral lip of the linea aspera of the femur.

Insertion

▼   Base of patella and tibial tuberosity of the tibia.

Isolated Function

▼   Concentrically accelerates knee extension.

Integrated Function

▼   Eccentrically decelerates knee flexion, adduction, and internal rotation.

▼   Isometrically stabilizes the knee.

Vastus medialis

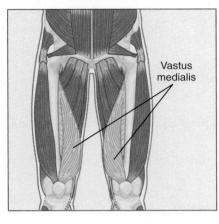

Origin

▼   Lower region of intertrochanteric line, medial lip of linea aspera, proximal medial supracondylar line of the femur.

Insertion

▼   Base of patella, tibial tuberosity of the tibia.

Isolated Function

▼   Concentrically accelerates knee extension.

Integrated Function

▼   Eccentrically decelerates knee flexion, adduction, and internal rotation.

▼   Isometrically stabilizes the knee.

Vastus intermedius

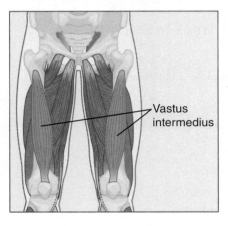

Origin

▼   Anterior-lateral regions of the upper two-thirds of the femur.

Insertion

▼   Base of patella, tibial tuberosity of the tibia.

Isolated Function

▼   Concentrically accelerates knee extension.

Integrated Function

▼   Eccentrically decelerates knee flexion, adduction, and internal rotation.

▼   Isometrically stabilizes the knee.

Rectus femoris

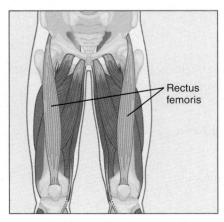

Origin

▼   Anterior-inferior iliac spine of the pelvis.

Insertion

▼   Base of patella, tibial tuberosity of the tibia.

Isolated Function

▼   Concentrically accelerates knee extension and hip flexion.

Integrated Function

▼   Eccentrically decelerates knee flexion, adduction, and internal rotation.

▼   Decelerates hip extension.

▼   Isometrically stabilizes the LPHC and knee.

Hip Musculature

Adductor longus

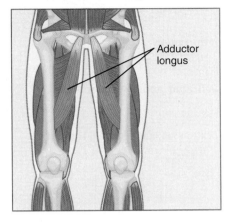

Origin

▼ Anterior surface of the inferior pubic ramus of the pelvis.

Insertion

▼ Proximal one-third of the linea aspera of the femur.

Isolated Function

▼ Concentrically accelerates hip adduction, flexion, and internal rotation.

Integrated Function

▼ Eccentrically decelerates hip abduction, extension, and external rotation.

▼ Isometrically stabilizes the LPHC.

Adductor magnus: Anterior Fibers

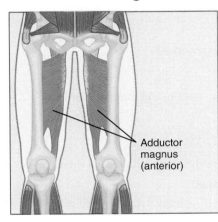

Origin

▼ Ischial ramus of the pelvis.

Insertion

▼ Linea aspera of the femur.

Isolated Function

▼ Concentrically accelerates hip adduction, flexion, and internal rotation.

Integrated Function

▼ Eccentrically decelerates hip abduction, extension, and external rotation.

▼ Dynamically stabilizes the LPHC.

Adductor magnus: Posterior Fibers

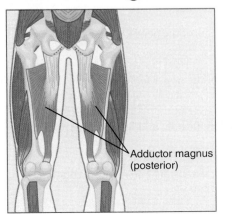

Origin

▼ Ischial tuberosity of the pelvis.

Insertion

▼ Adductor tubercle on femur.

Isolated Function

▼ Concentrically accelerates hip adduction, extension, and external rotation.

Integrated Function

▼ Eccentrically decelerates hip abduction, flexion, and internal rotation.

▼ Isometrically stabilizes the LPHC.

Adductor brevis

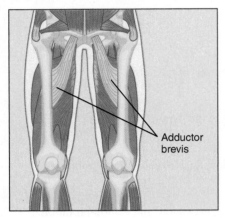

Origin

▼   Anterior surface of the inferior pubic ramus of the pelvis.

Insertion

▼   Proximal one-third of the linea aspera of the femur.

Isolated Function

▼   Concentrically accelerates hip adduction, flexion, and internal rotation.

Integrated Function

▼   Eccentrically decelerates hip abduction, extension, and external rotation.

▼   Isometrically stabilizes the LPHC.

Gracilis

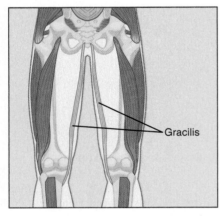

Origin

▼   Anterior aspect of lower body of pubis.

Insertion

▼   Proximal medial surface of the tibia (pes anserine).

Isolated Function

▼   Concentrically accelerates hip adduction, flexion, and internal rotation.

▼   Assists in tibial internal rotation.

Integrated Function

▼   Eccentrically decelerates hip abduction, extension, and external rotation.

▼   Isometrically stabilizes the LPHC and knee.

Pectineus

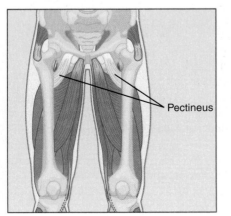

Origin

▼   Pectineal line on the superior pubic ramus of the pelvis.

Insertion

▼   Pectineal line on the posterior surface of the upper femur.

Isolated Function

▼   Concentrically accelerates hip adduction, flexion, and internal rotation.

Integrated Function

▼   Eccentrically decelerates hip abduction, extension, and external rotation.

▼   Isometrically stabilizes the LPHC.

Gluteus medius

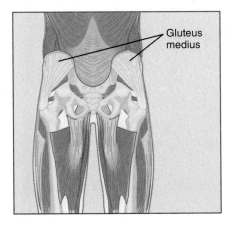

Origin

▼ Outer surface of the ilium of the pelvis.

Insertion

▼ Lateral surface of the greater trochanter on the femur.

Isolated Function

▼ Concentrically accelerates hip abduction and internal rotation (anterior fibers).

▼ Concentrically accelerates hip abduction and external rotation (posterior fibers).

Integrated Function

▼ Eccentrically decelerates hip adduction and external rotation (anterior fibers).

▼ Eccentrically decelerates hip adduction and internal rotation (posterior fibers).

▼ Isometrically stabilizes the LPHC.

Gluteus minimus

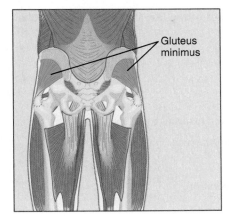

Origin

▼ Ilium of the pelvis between the anterior and inferior gluteal line.

Insertion

▼ Greater trochanter of the femur.

Isolated Function

▼ Concentrically accelerates hip abduction and internal rotation.

Integrated Function

▼ Eccentrically decelerates hip adduction and external rotation.

▼ Isometrically stabilizes the LPHC.

Gluteus maximus

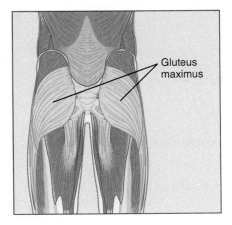

Origin

▼ Outer ilium of the pelvis, posterior side of sacrum and coccyx, and part of the sacrotuberous and posterior sacroiliac ligament.

Insertion

▼ Gluteal tuberosity of the femur and iliotibial tract.

Isolated Function

▼ Concentrically accelerates hip extension and external rotation.

Integrated Function

▼ Eccentrically decelerates hip flexion and internal rotation.

▼ Decelerates tibial internal rotation via the iliotibial band.

▼ Isometrically stabilizes the LPHC.

Tensor fascia latae (Including the Iliotibial Band)

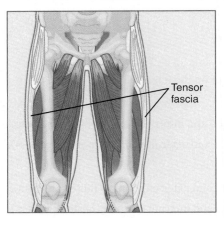

Origin

▼   Outer surface of the iliac crest just posterior to the anterior-superior iliac spine of the pelvis.

Insertion

▼   Proximal one-third of the iliotibial band.

Isolated Function

▼   Concentrically accelerates hip flexion, abduction, and internal rotation.

Integrated Function

▼   Eccentrically decelerates hip extension, adduction, and external rotation.

▼   Isometrically stabilizes the LPHC.

Psoas

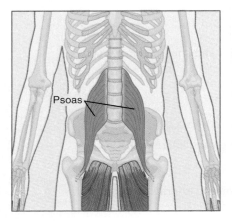

Origin

▼   Transverse processes and lateral bodies of the last thoracic and all lumbar vertebrae including intervertebral disks.

Insertion

▼   Lesser trochanter of the femur.

Isolated Function

▼   Concentrically accelerates hip flexion and external rotation.

▼   Concentrically extends and rotates lumbar spine.

Integrated Function

▼   Eccentrically decelerates hip internal rotation.

▼   Eccentrically decelerates hip extension.

▼   Isometrically stabilizes the LPHC.

Iliacus

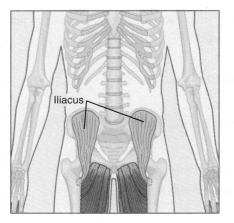

Origin

▼   Superior two-thirds of iliac fossa, inner lip of the iliac crest.

Insertion

▼   Lesser trochanter of femur.

Isolated Function

▼   Concentrically accelerates hip flexion and external rotation.

Integrated Function

▼   Eccentrically decelerates hip extension and internal rotation.

▼   Isometrically stabilizes the LPHC.

Sartorius

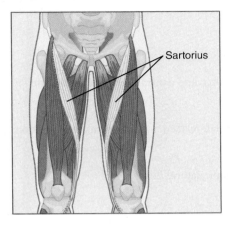

Origin

▼ Anterior-superior iliac spine of the pelvis.

Insertion

▼ Proximal medial surface of the tibia.

Isolated Function

▼ Concentrically accelerates hip flexion, external rotation, and abduction.

▼ Concentrically accelerates knee flexion and internal rotation.

Integrated Function

▼ Eccentrically decelerates hip extension and internal rotation.

▼ Eccentrically decelerates knee extension and external rotation.

▼ Isometrically stabilizes the LPHC and knee.

Piriformis

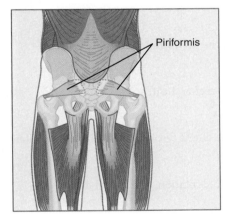

Origin

▼ Anterior side of the sacrum.

Insertion

▼ The greater trochanter of the femur.

Isolated Function

▼ Concentrically accelerates hip external rotation, abduction, and extension.

Integrated Function

▼ Eccentrically decelerates hip internal rotation, adduction, and flexion.

▼ Isometrically stabilizes the hip and sacroiliac joints.

Abdominal Musculature

Rectus abdominis

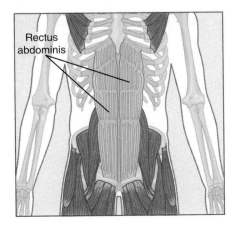

Origin

▼ Pubic symphysis of the pelvis.

Insertion

▼ Ribs 5–7.

▼ Xiphoid process of the sternum.

Isolated Function

▼ Concentrically accelerates spinal flexion, lateral flexion, and rotation.

Integrated Function

▼ Eccentrically decelerates spinal extension, lateral flexion, and rotation.

▼ Isometrically stabilizes the LPHC.

External oblique

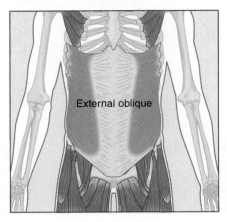

Origin

▼   External surface of ribs 4–12.

Insertion

▼   Anterior iliac crest of the pelvis, linea alba, and contralateral rectus sheaths.

Isolated Function

▼   Concentrically accelerates spinal flexion, lateral flexion, and contralateral rotation.

Integrated Function

▼   Eccentrically decelerates spinal extension, lateral flexion, and rotation.

▼   Isometrically stabilizes the LPHC.

Internal oblique

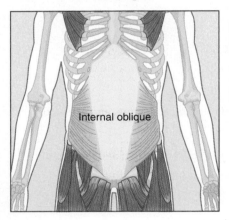

Origin

▼   Anterior two-thirds of the iliac crest of the pelvis and thoracolumbar fascia.

Insertion

▼   Ribs 9–12, linea alba, and contralateral rectus sheaths.

Isolated Function

▼   Concentrically accelerates spinal flexion, lateral flexion, and ipsilateral rotation.

Integrated Function

▼   Eccentrically decelerates spinal extension, rotation, and lateral flexion.

▼   Isometrically stabilizes the LPHC.

Transverse abdominis

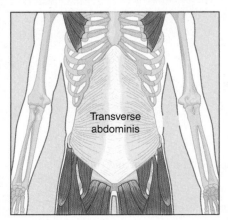

Origin

▼   Ribs 7–12, anterior two-thirds of the iliac crest of the pelvis, and thoracolumbar fascia.

Insertion

▼   Linea alba and contralateral rectus sheaths.

Isolated Function

▼   Increases intra-abdominal pressure.

▼   Supports the abdominal viscera.

Integrated Function

▼   Isometrically stabilizes the LPHC.

Diaphragm

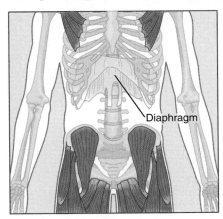

Origin

▼ Costal part: Inner surfaces of the cartilages and adjacent bony regions of ribs 6–12.

▼ Sternal part: Posterior side of the xiphoid process.

▼ Crural (lumbar) part: (1) Two aponeurotic arches covering the external surfaces of the quadratus lumborum and psoas major; (2) right and left crus, originating from the bodies of L1–L3 and their intervertebral disks.

Insertion

▼ Central tendon.

Isolated Function

▼ Concentrically pulls the central tendon inferiorly, increasing the volume in the thoracic cavity.

Integrated Function

▼ Stabilizes the LPHC.

Back Musculature

Superficial erector spinae: Iliocostalis, Longissimus, and Spinalis

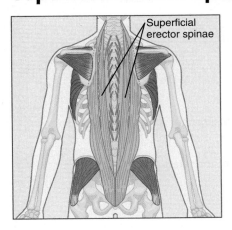

Division in the Group

▼ Lumborum (lumbar).

▼ Thoracis (thoracic).

▼ Cervicis (cervical).

Common Origin

▼ Iliac crest of the pelvis.

▼ Sacrum.

▼ Spinous and transverse process of T11–L5.

Insertion

Iliocostalis

▼ Lumborum: Inferior border of ribs 7–12.

▼ Thoracis: Superior border of ribs 1–6.

▼ Cervicis: Transverse process of C4–C6.

Longissimus

▼ Thoracis: Transverse process T1–T12; ribs 2–12.

▼ Cervicis: Transverse process of C6–C2.

▼ Capitis: Mastoid process of the skull.

Spinalis

▼ Thoracis: Spinous process of T7–T4.

▼ Cervicis: Spinous process of C3–C2.

▼ Capitis: Between the superior and inferior nuchal lines on occipital bone of the skull.

Isolated Function

▼ Concentrically accelerates spinal extension, rotation, and lateral flexion.

Integrated Function

▼ Eccentrically decelerates spinal flexion, rotation, and lateral flexion.

▼ Dynamically stabilizes the spine during functional movements.

Quadratus lumborum

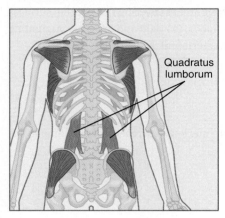

Origin

▼ Iliac crest of the pelvis.

Insertion

▼ 12th rib.

▼ Transverse process L2–L5.

Isolated Function

▼ Spinal lateral flexion.

Integrated Function

▼ Eccentrically decelerates contralateral lateral spinal flexion.

▼ Isometrically stabilizes the LPHC.

Multifidus

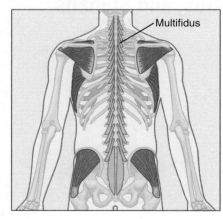

Origin

▼ Posterior aspect of the sacrum.

▼ Processes of the lumbar, thoracic, and cervical spine.

Insertion

▼ Spinous processes one to four segments above the origin.

Isolated Function

▼ Concentrically accelerates spinal extension and contralateral rotation.

Integrated Function

▼ Eccentrically decelerates spinal flexion and rotation.

▼ Isometrically stabilizes the spine.

Latissimus dorsi

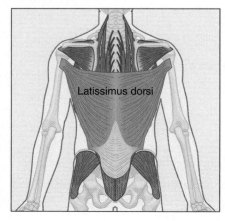

Origin

▼ Spinous processes of T7–T12.

▼ Iliac crest of the pelvis.

▼ Thoracolumbar fascia.

▼ Ribs 9–12.

Insertion

▼ Inferior angle of the scapula.

▼ Intertubercular groove of the humerus.

Isolated Function

▼ Concentrically accelerates shoulder extension, adduction, and internal rotation.

Integrated Function

▼ Eccentrically decelerates shoulder flexion, abduction, and external rotation.

▼   Eccentrically decelerates spinal flexion.

▼   Isometrically stabilizes the LPHC and shoulder.

Shoulder Musculature

Serratus anterior

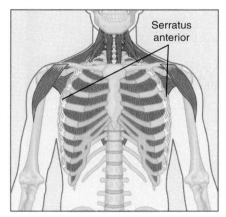

Origin

▼   Ribs 4–12.

Insertion

▼   Medial border of the scapula.

Isolated Function

▼   Concentrically accelerates scapular protraction.

Integrated Function

▼   Eccentrically decelerates dynamic scapular retraction.

▼   Isometrically stabilizes the scapula.

Rhomboid major

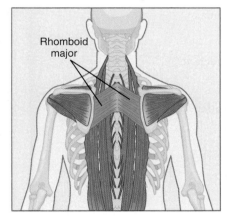

Origin

▼   Spinous processes C7–T5.

Insertion

▼   Medial border of the scapula.

Isolated Function

▼   Concentrically produces scapular retraction and downward rotation.

Integrated Function

▼   Eccentrically decelerates scapular protraction and upward rotation.

▼   Isometrically stabilizes the scapula.

Rhomboid minor

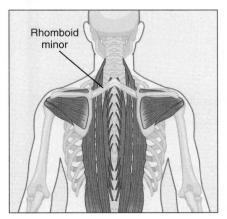

Origin

▼   Spinous processes C7–T1.

Insertion

▼   Medial border of the scapula superior to spine.

Isolated Function

▼   Concentrically produces scapular retraction and downward rotation.

Integrated Function

▼   Eccentrically decelerates scapular protraction and upward rotation.

▼   Isometrically stabilizes the scapula.

Lower trapezius

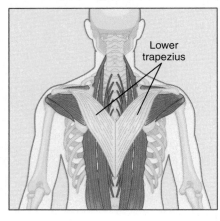

Origin

▼ Spinous processes of T6–T12.

Insertion

▼ Spine of the scapula.

Isolated Function

▼ Concentrically accelerates scapular depression.

Integrated Function

▼ Eccentrically decelerates scapular elevation.

▼ Isometrically stabilizes the scapula.

Middle trapezius

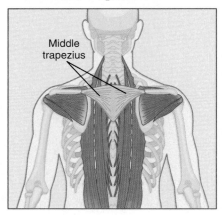

Origin

▼ Spinous processes of T1–T5.

Insertion

▼ Acromion process of the scapula.

▼ Superior aspect of the spine of the scapula.

Isolated Function

▼ Concentrically accelerates scapular retraction.

Integrated Function

▼ Eccentrically decelerates scapular elevation.

▼ Isometrically stabilizes the scapula.

Upper trapezius

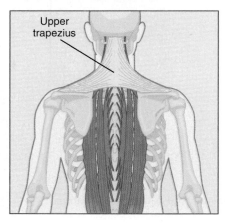

Origin

▼ External occipital protuberance of the skull.

▼ Spinous process of C7.

Insertion

▼ Lateral third of the clavicle.

▼ Acromion process of the scapula.

Isolated Function

▼ Concentrically accelerates cervical extension, lateral flexion, and rotation.

▼ Concentrically accelerates scapular elevation.

Integrated Function

▼ Eccentrically decelerates cervical flexion, lateral flexion, and rotation.

▼ Eccentrically decelerates scapular depression.

▼ Isometrically stabilizes the cervical spine and scapula.

Pectoralis major

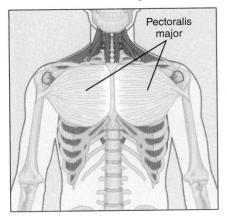

Origin

▼ Clavicular: Anterior surface of the clavicle.

▼ Sternocostal: Anterior surface of the sternum, cartilage of ribs 1–7.

Insertion

▼ Greater tubercle of the humerus.

Isolated Function

▼ Concentrically accelerates shoulder flexion (clavicular fibers), horizontal adduction, and internal rotation.

Integrated Function

▼ Eccentrically decelerates shoulder extension, horizontal abduction, and external rotation.

▼ Isometrically stabilizes the shoulder girdle.

Pectoralis minor

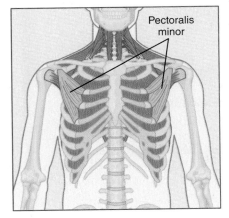

Origin

▼ Ribs 3–5.

Insertion

▼ Coracoid process of the scapula.

Isolated Function

▼ Concentrically protracts the scapula.

Integrated Function

▼ Eccentrically decelerates scapular retraction.

▼ Isometrically stabilizes the shoulder girdle.

Anterior deltoid

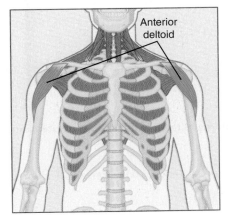

Origin

▼ Lateral third of the clavicle.

Insertion

▼ Deltoid tuberosity of the humerus.

Isolated Function

▼ Concentrically accelerates shoulder flexion and internal rotation.

Integrated Function

▼ Eccentrically decelerates shoulder extension and external rotation.

▼ Isometrically stabilizes the shoulder girdle.

Medial deltoid

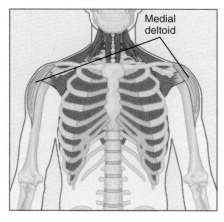

Origin

▼ Acromion process of the scapula.

Insertion

▼ Deltoid tuberosity of the humerus.

Isolated Function

▼ Concentrically accelerates shoulder abduction.

Integrated Function

▼ Eccentrically decelerates shoulder adduction.

▼ Isometrically stabilizes the shoulder girdle.

Posterior deltoid

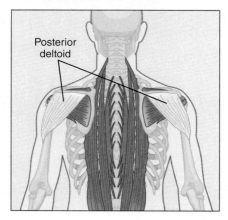

Origin

▼ Spine of the scapula.

Insertion

▼ Deltoid tuberosity of the humerus.

Isolated Function

▼ Concentrically accelerates shoulder extension and external rotation.

Integrated Function

▼ Eccentrically decelerates shoulder flexion and internal rotation.

▼ Isometrically stabilizes the shoulder girdle.

Teres major

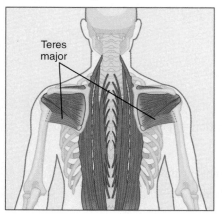

Origin

▼ Inferior angle of the scapula.

Insertion

▼ Lesser tubercle of the humerus.

Isolated Function

▼ Concentrically accelerates shoulder internal rotation, adduction, and extension.

Integrated Function

▼ Eccentrically decelerates shoulder external rotation, abduction, and flexion.

▼ Isometrically stabilizes the shoulder girdle.

Rotator Cuff

Teres minor

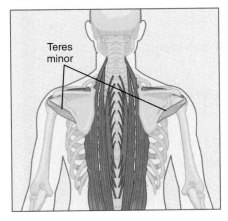

Origin

▼ Lateral border of the scapula.

Insertion

▼ Greater tubercle of the humerus.

Isolated Function

▼ Concentrically accelerates shoulder external rotation.

Integrated Function

▼ Eccentrically decelerates shoulder internal rotation.

▼ Isometrically stabilizes the shoulder girdle.

Infraspinatus

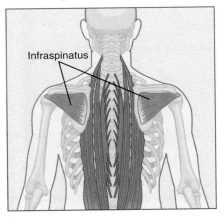

Origin

▼ Infraspinous fossa of the scapula.

Insertion

▼ Middle facet of the greater tubercle of the humerus.

Isolated Function

▼ Concentrically accelerates shoulder external rotation.

Integrated Function

▼ Eccentrically decelerates shoulder internal rotation.

▼ Isometrically stabilizes the shoulder girdle.

Subscapularis

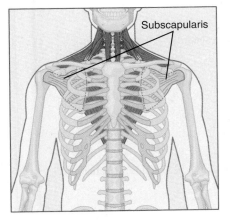

Origin

▼ Subscapular fossa of the scapula.

Insertion

▼ Lesser tubercle of the humerus.

Isolated Function

▼ Concentrically accelerates shoulder internal rotation.

Integrated Function

▼ Eccentrically decelerates shoulder external rotation.

▼ Isometrically stabilizes the shoulder girdle.

Supraspinatus

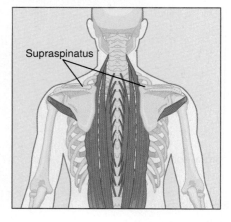

Origin

▼ Supraspinous fossa of the scapula.

Insertion

▼ Superior facet of the greater tubercle of the humerus.

Isolated Function

▼ Concentrically accelerates abduction of the arm.

Integrated Function

▼ Eccentrically decelerates adduction of the arm.

▼ Isometrically stabilizes the shoulder girdle.

Arm Musculature
Biceps brachii

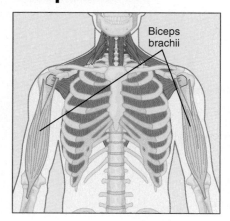

Origin

▼ Short head: Coracoid process of the scapula.

▼ Long head: Tubercle above glenoid cavity on the humerus.

Insertion

▼ Radial tuberosity of the radius.

Isolated Function

▼ Concentrically accelerates elbow flexion, supination of the radioulnar joint, and shoulder flexion.

Integrated Function

▼ Eccentrically decelerates elbow extension, pronation of the radioulnar joint, and shoulder extension.

▼ Isometrically stabilizes the elbow and shoulder girdle.

Triceps brachii

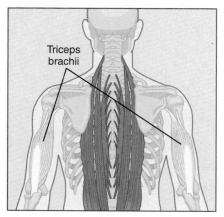

Origin

▼ Long head: Infraglenoid tubercle of the scapula.

▼ Short head: Posterior humerus.

▼ Medial head: Posterior humerus.

Insertion

▼ Olecranon process of the ulna.

Isolated Function

▼ Concentrically accelerates elbow extension and shoulder extension.

Integrated Function

▼ Eccentrically decelerates elbow flexion and shoulder flexion.

▼ Isometrically stabilizes the elbow and shoulder girdle.

Brachioradialis

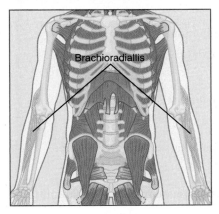

Origin

▼ Lateral supracondylar ridge of the humerus.

Insertion

▼ Lateral surface of distal radius, immediately above styloid process.

Isolated Function

▼ Concentrically accelerates elbow flexion.

Integrated Function

▼ Eccentrically decelerates elbow extension.

▼ Isometrically stabilizes the elbow.

Brachialis

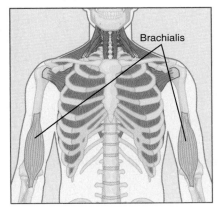

Origin

▼ Lower half of the anterior surface of the humerus.

Insertion

▼ Tuberosity and coronoid process of the ulna.

Isolated Function

▼ Concentrically accelerates elbow flexion.

Integrated Function

▼ Eccentrically decelerates elbow extension.

▼ Isometrically stabilizes the elbow.

Neck Musculature

Levator scapulae

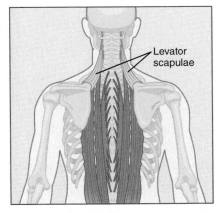

Origin

▼ Transverse processes of C1–C4.

Insertion

▼ Superior vertebral border of the scapulae.

Isolated Function

▼ Concentrically accelerates cervical extension, lateral flexion, and ipsilateral rotation when the scapulae is anchored.

▼ Assists in elevation and downward rotation of the scapulae.

Integrated Function

▼ Eccentrically decelerates cervical flexion and contralateral cervical rotation and lateral flexion.

▼ Eccentrically decelerates scapular depression and upward rotation when the neck is stabilized.

▼ Stabilizes the cervical spine and scapulae.

Sternocleidomastoid

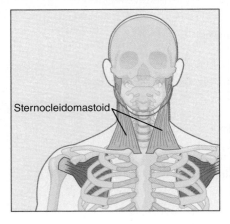

Origin

▼ Sternal head: Top of manubrium of the sternum.

▼ Clavicular head: Medial one-third of the clavicle.

Insertion

▼ Mastoid process, lateral superior nuchal line of the occiput of the skull.

Isolated Function

▼ Concentrically accelerates cervical flexion, rotation, and lateral flexion.

Integrated Function

▼ Eccentrically decelerates cervical extension, rotation, and lateral flexion.

▼ Isometrically stabilizes the cervical spine and acromioclavicular joint.

Scalenes

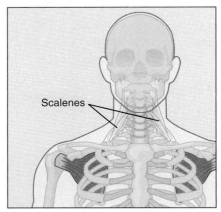

Origin

▼ Transverse processes of C3–C7.

Insertion

▼ First and second ribs.

Isolated Function

▼ Concentrically accelerates cervical flexion, rotation, and lateral flexion.

▼ Assists rib elevation during inhalation.

Integrated Function

▼ Eccentrically decelerates cervical extension, rotation, and lateral flexion.

▼ Isometrically stabilizes the cervical spine.

Longus coli

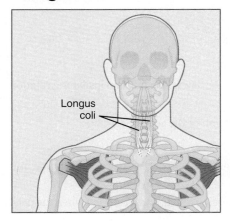

Origin

▼ Anterior portion of T1–T3.

Insertion

▼ Anterior and lateral C1.

Isolated Function

▼ Concentrically accelerates cervical flexion, lateral flexion, and ipsilateral rotation.

Integrated Function

▼ Eccentrically decelerates cervical extension, lateral flexion, and contralateral rotation.

▼ Isometrically stabilizes the cervical spine.

Longus capitis

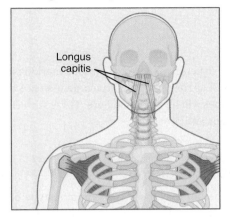

Longus capitis

Origin

▼ Transverse processes of C3–C6.

Insertion

▼ Inferior occipital bone.

Isolated Function

▼ Concentrically accelerates cervical flexion and lateral flexion.

Integrated Function

▼ Eccentrically decelerates cervical extension.

▼ Isometrically stabilizes the cervical spine.

The Skeletal System

Bone Growth

Throughout life, bone is constantly renewed through a process called remodeling. This process consists of resorption and formation. During resorption, old bone tissue is broken down and removed by special cells called osteoclasts. During bone formation, new bone tissue is laid down to replace the old. This task is performed by special cells called osteoblasts.

During childhood and through adolescence, new bone is added to the skeleton faster than old bone is removed. As a result, bones become larger, heavier, and denser. For most people,

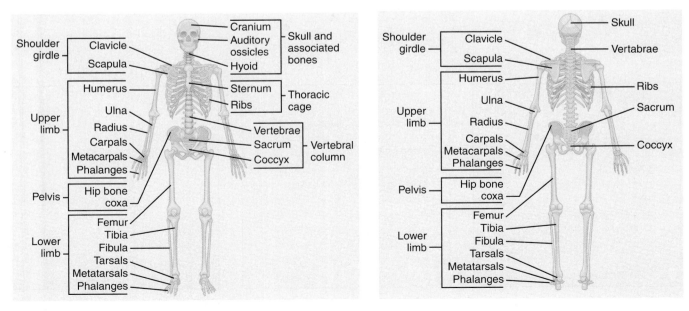

Figure A.5
The skeletal system

bone formation continues at a faster pace than removal until bone mass peaks, usually by the time individuals reach their 30s.[6]

Bone Markings

The majority of all bones have specific distinguishing structures known as surface markings. These structures are necessary for joint stability as well as for providing attachment sites for muscles. Some of the more prominent and important ones will be discussed here. These surface markings can be divided into two categories: depressions and processes.[3]

Depressions

Depressions are flattened or indented portions of the bone. A fossa is a common type of depression. An example is the supraspinous or infraspinous fossa located on the scapulae (**Figure A.6**). These are attachment sites for the supraspinatus and infraspinatus muscles, respectively.[3]

A sulcus is another type of depression. A sulcus is a groove in a bone that allows soft tissue (i.e., tendons) to pass through. An example is the intertubercular sulcus located between the greater and lesser tubercles of the humerus (**Figure A.7**). This is commonly known as the groove for the biceps tendon.[3]

Processes

Processes are projections that protrude from the bone to which muscles, tendons, and ligaments can attach (**Figure A.8**). Processes include condyles, epicondyles, tubercles, and trochanters. Examples of processes include the spinous processes found on the vertebrae and the acromion and coracoid processes found on the scapulae.[3]

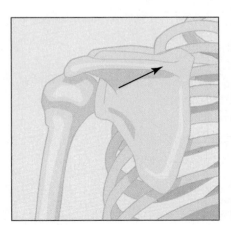

Figure A.6
Fossa

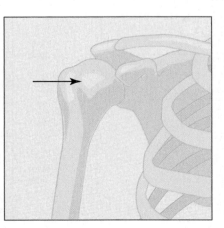

Figure A.7
Sulcus

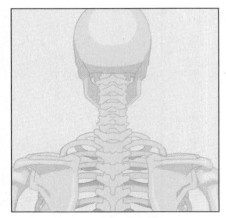

Figure A.8
Process

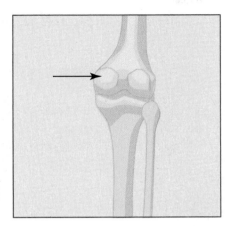

Figure A.9
Condyle

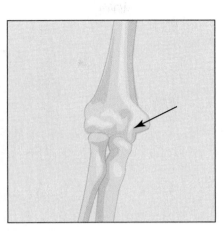

Figure A.10
Epicondyle

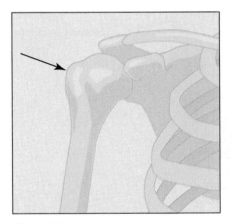

Figure A.11
Tubercle

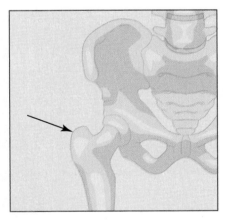

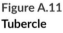

Figure A.12
Trochanter

Condyles are located on the inner and outer portions at the bottom of the femur and top of the tibia to form the knee joint (**Figure A.9**). Epicondyles are located on the inner and outer portions of the humerus to help form the elbow joint (**Figure A.10**).

The tubercles are located at the top of the humerus at the glenohumeral joint (**Figure A.11**). There are the greater and lesser tubercles, which are attachment sites for shoulder musculature.

Finally, the trochanters are located at the top of the femur and are attachment sites for the hip musculature (**Figure A.12**). The greater trochanter is commonly called the hipbone.[3]

Vertebral Column

The first seven vertebrae starting at the top of the spinal column (**Figure A.13**) are called the cervical vertebrae (cervical spine, C1–C7). These bones form a flexible framework and provide support and motion for the head.

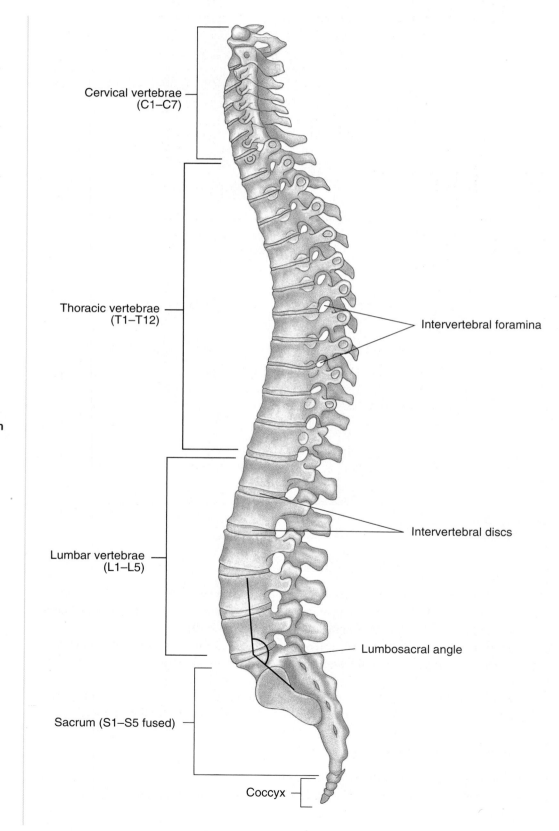

Cervical vertebrae
(C1–C7)

Thoracic vertebrae
(T1–T12)

Intervertebral foramina

Figure A.13
The vertebral column

Intervertebral discs

Lumbar vertebrae
(L1–L5)

Lumbosacral angle

Sacrum (S1–S5 fused)

Coccyx

The next 12 vertebrae located in the upper and middle back are called the thoracic vertebrae (thoracic spine, T1–T12). These bones articulate with the ribs to form the rear anchor of the rib cage. Thoracic vertebrae are larger than cervical vertebrae and increase in size from top to bottom.

Below the thoracic spine are the five vertebrae comprising the lumbar vertebrae (lumbar spine, L1–L5). These bones are the largest in the spinal column. These vertebrae support most of the body's weight and are attached to many of the back muscles.

The sacrum is a triangular bone located just below the lumbar vertebrae. It consists of four or five sacral vertebrae in a child, which become fused into a single bone during adulthood.

The bottom of the spinal column is called the coccyx or tailbone. It consists of three to five bones fused together in an adult. Many muscles connect to the coccyx.

In between the vertebrae are intervertebral discs made of fibrous cartilage that act as shock absorbers and allow the spine to move. In addition to allowing humans to stand upright and maintain their balance, the vertebral column serves several other important functions. It helps to support the head and arms, while permitting freedom of movement. It also provides attachment for many muscles, the ribs, and some of the organs, and it protects the spinal cord, which controls most bodily functions (National Institute of Neurological Disorders and Stroke, 2010).

The optimal arrangement of curves is referred to as a neutral spine and represents a position in which the vertebrae and associated structures are under the least amount of load. The adult human spine has three major curvatures:

▼ *Posterior cervical curvature*: The posterior concavity of the cervical spine.

▼ *Anterior thoracic curvature*: The posterior convexity of the thoracic spine.

▼ *Posterior lumbar curvature*: The posterior concavity of the lumbar spine.

References

1. Fox SI. *Human physiology*. (9th ed.). New York, NY: McGraw-Hill; 2006.
2. Milner-Brown A. *Neuromuscular physiology*. Thousand Oaks, CA: National Academy of Sports Medicine; 2001.
3. Tortora GJ. *Principles of human anatomy*. (9th ed.). New York, NY: John Wiley & Sons; 2001.
4. Vander A, Sherman L, Luciano D. *Human physiology: The mechanisms of body function*. (8th ed.). New York, NY: McGraw-Hill; 2001.
5. Cohen H. *Neuroscience for rehabilitation*. (2nd ed.). Philadelphia, PA: Lippincott Williams & Wilkins; 1999.
6. National Institute of Arthritis and Musculoskeletal and Skin Diseases. What is bone? 2015. Retrieved from at: www.niams.nih.gov/Health_Info/bone/Bone_Health/default.asp
7. Watkins J. *Structure and function of the musculoskeletal system*. Champaign, IL: Human Kinetics; 1999.
8. National Institute of Neurological Disorders and Stroke. Low back pain fact sheet. Retrieved from at: www.ninds.nih.gov/disorders/backpain/detail_backpain.htm#102183102

Appendix B
Expanded Human Movement Science

Nervous System

The nervous system handles thousands of signals per second. When outcomes do not turn out favorably, like when a class participant struggles through their first yoga pose or boot camp exercise, the nervous system can influence future outcomes through repetition. The nervous system, through practice, can be trained to achieve a specified outcome, like a lunge performed with proper form in a full range of motion. It is the physical application of the adage "practice makes perfect."

Participants often only hear about the muscular system and don't understand the role of the nervous system when learning and performing exercises. Take, for example, a balance exercise: New participants often struggle when being asked to balance on one foot. But as they learn to mentally focus or think about the musculature needed to stabilize for this movement, the nervous system can recruit the necessary muscles to be successful.

The Central Nervous System

The brain is where **motor control**, **motor learning**, and **motor development** are honed in order to produce skilled movement over time. The spinal cord serves as the gathering point for all nerve pathways and builds the connection between the peripheral nervous system (PNS) and the brain.

Group Fitness Instructors need to recognize training the nervous system happens over time. In a class setting, motor patterns vary from individual exercises (e.g., squats, burpees) to complex choreography sequences (e.g., an hour-long dance-oriented routine).

Afferent and Efferent Neurons and Interneurons

The consecutive linking of neurons conducts electrochemical signals called **nerve impulses** that travel throughout the nerve fiber. Nerve impulses that move *toward* the spinal cord and brain from the periphery of the body are sensory in nature and are known as **afferent neurons**. Afferent neurons rely on sensory receptors to recognize environmental stimuli.

Nerve impulses that move from the brain and spinal cord are termed *efferent*. **Efferent neurons** stimulate muscle contraction, which is why they are also referred to as *motor neurons* since they create movement. **Interneurons** are only located within the spinal cord and brain; they receive impulses from afferent (sensory) neurons and conduct signals back out to provide an efferent (motor) response.

Creation of Efficient Movement (Motor Behavior)

The creation of efficient movement is made possible by the repetition of sensory inputs and the refinement of **motor outputs**. Group Fitness Instructors should know what an exercise should look like and provide cues necessary to elicit a change in a participant's form. The change in form is a change in motor recruitment patterns to allow for safer, more efficient, and more effective motor behavior.

Motor behavior is the response of the Human Movement System to internal and external environmental stimuli. The study of motor behavior examines the manner by which the nervous, muscular, and skeletal systems interact to produce skilled movement, using sensory information from internal and external environments. Motor behavior is the combination of three distinct concepts:

▼ Motor control: how the CNS integrates internal and external sensory information with previous experiences to produce a motor response.

▼ Motor learning: the capacity to produce skilled movements through practice and experience.

▼ Motor development: the change in motor behavior over time throughout the lifespan.

Muscular System

The muscular system is part of the kinetic chain and is composed of three different types of muscles: smooth, cardiac, and skeletal. Smooth muscles are involuntary muscles, meaning they are not consciously controlled. They are found in the walls of blood vessels and hollow organs. Cardiac muscles are the involuntary muscles that exclusively make up the heart. There are approximately 640 skeletal muscles in the body. These muscles are voluntary—or consciously controlled—muscles that provide both movement and stability to the skeletal system.

Behavioral Properties of Muscle

Muscle is the only tissue in the human body to allow movement at a joint and to exert a force on the bone it is trying to move.[1-4] Skeletal muscle allows the body to remain upright, to move its limbs, and to absorb shock from external forces. The nervous system controls the timing and rate of a muscle action. The nervous system must work together with the muscular system in order for these movements to occur efficiently. Having a general understanding of how muscle behaves can help Group Fitness Instructors conceptualize how muscles respond during various types of movements in a class setting. Muscle has four behavioral properties:

▼ Extensibility

▼ Elasticity

▼ Irritability

▼ Ability to develop tension

The first behavioral property is extensibility. **Extensibility** refers to the ability to be stretched or lengthened, which is commonly referred to as "flexibility." A participant lacking extensibility of a muscle will be limited in his or her ability to lengthen that muscle. **Elasticity** refers to a muscle's ability to return to normal or resting length after it has been stretched. Muscle is elastic, much like a rubber band that can be elongated with stretching and can resume its original position after being released. In addition, skeletal muscle has a viscoelastic property that allows it to extend and recoil with time. This is also the property that explains why muscles are more responsive to extension at a slower speed. Viscous materials are thick and sticky. If you push too fast and too hard, a viscous material will push back.

Another behavioral property is irritability. **Irritability** means a muscle is able to respond to a stimulus from internal nerve impulses and external forces. Finally, a muscle has the **ability to develop tension**. Traditionally, the development of tension in a muscle has been called a "contraction"; however, a muscle only contracts during the concentric phase of the muscle action spectrum. In reality, all phases of the muscle action spectrum (i.e., concentric shortening, eccentric lengthening, and isometric stabilization) develop tension in the muscle to accomplish movement around the joints.[3,5,6]

Because of these behavioral properties, individuals can improve their mobility and have the potential to improve their performance of activities of daily living. Irritability of a muscle means it is sensitive to neural stimulation so an individual can move a limb at any time. Lastly, the ability to develop tension in a muscle is what allows it to produce the force that moves a joint, which in turn moves a limb.

Skeletal System

The skeletal system is made up of 206 bones. The axial skeleton has 80 bones, including the skull, rib cage, and spinal column, and creates the protective structure for vital organs and nervous system. The axial skeleton can be further broken down to its individual segments:

▼ Skull: 28 bones

▼ Hyoid bone: 1 bone (U-shaped bone in the neck that supports the tongue)

▼ Sternum and ribs: 25 bones

▼ Spinal column: 26 bones (including sacrum and coccyx)

Though instructors do not deal with pain management, they are often presented with participant questions during or after classes regarding back issues, so it is helpful to be informed

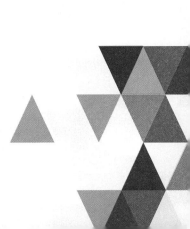

on the subject. The bones of the spinal column are divided into five major categories. From the top down, they are as follows:

- ▼ Cervical vertebrae (C1–C7)
- ▼ Thoracic vertebrae (T1–T12)
- ▼ Lumbar vertebrae (L1–L5)
- ▼ Sacrum
- ▼ Coccyx

The appendicular skeleton is composed of 126 bones and is divided into the upper and lower extremities. The upper extremity is made up of 64 bones, including the shoulder girdle:

- ▼ Clavicle: 2 bones
- ▼ Scapula: 2 bones
- ▼ Humerus: 2 bones
- ▼ Radius: 2 bones
- ▼ Ulna: 2 bones
- ▼ Carpals: 16 bones
- ▼ Metacarpals: 10 bones
- ▼ Phalanges: 28 bones

The lower extremity is made up of 62 bones, including the pelvic girdle:

- ▼ Innominate (os coxa, hemi-pelvis): 2 bones
- ▼ Femur: 2 bones
- ▼ Patella: 2 bones
- ▼ Tibia: 2 bones
- ▼ Fibula: 2 bones
- ▼ Tarsals: 14 bones
- ▼ Metatarsals: 10 bones
- ▼ Phalanges: 28 bones

Types of Bones

The bones of the skeletal system are primarily categorized into major categories based on their shape. The five types of bones in the human body are long, short, flat, irregular, and sesamoid.

Long Bones

Long bones have a cylindrical body called a shaft; they are longer than they are wide and enlarge and widen at each end. They can vary in size; in fact, some can be quite short. Long bones are made up of compact and spongy bone tissue. This enables them to tolerate considerable leverage forces, support a large amount of weight, and absorb shock. They often have a slight curve, both

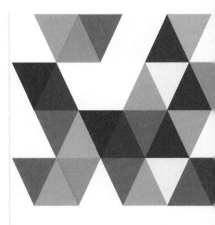

for efficiency and for better force distribution. The following are the long bones of the upper body (**Figure B.1**):

- ▼ Clavicle
- ▼ Humerus
- ▼ Radius
- ▼ Ulna
- ▼ Metacarpals
- ▼ Phalanges

The following are the long bones of the lower body (**Figure B.2**):

- ▼ Femur
- ▼ Tibia
- ▼ Fibula
- ▼ Metatarsals
- ▼ Phalanges

Short Bones

Short bones are cube- or box-shaped bones nearly as wide as they are long (**Figure B.3**). They are made up of mostly spongy bone tissue to maximize shock absorption. The tarsals of the foot and carpals of the hand are examples of short bones.

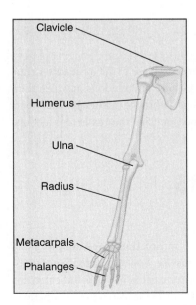

Figure B.1
Long Bones of the Upper Body

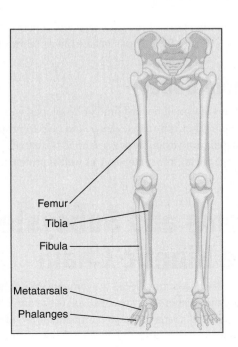

Figure B.2
Long Bones of the Lower Body

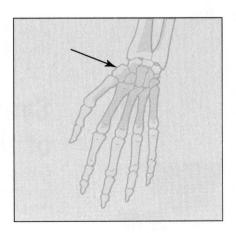

Figure B.3
Short Bones

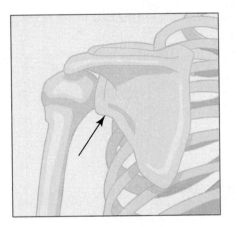

Figure B.4
Flat Bones

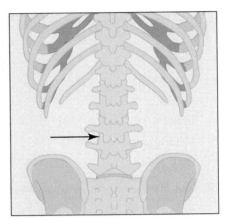

Figure B.5
Irregular Bones

Flat Bones

Flat bones are thin bones made up of two layers of compact bone tissue surrounding a layer of spongy bone tissue (**Figure B.4**).[7,8] These bones are involved in protection of internal structures and also provide broad attachment sites for muscles.[7] The flat bones include the sternum, scapulae, ribs, ilium, and cranial bones.[7-9]

Irregular Bones

Irregular bones are bones of unique shape and function that do not fit the characteristics of the other categories (**Figure B.5**). These include the vertebrae, pelvic bones, and certain facial bones.[7-9]

Sesamoid Bones

Sesamoid bones are small bones found or developed within tendons close to the joint and within the joint capsule. They improve leverage and help to protect the joint and tendons in which they reside. The patella is an example of a sesamoid bone that develops within the quadriceps tendon to provide leverage during knee extension, as well as protect the knee joint and the quadriceps tendon.

Systems and Subsystems of the Kinetic Chain

As previously discussed, functional movements do not happen in isolation. For example, side-lying leg abduction is commonly used to isolate the outer hip muscles; however, activities of daily living that require this type of isolated movement are rare, if they exist at all. This indicates the need for multiple muscles to work in tandem to allow multiple joints to move together to function. The complexities of functional movements require stabilization of the kinetic chain, as well as synchronized activation from the nervous system to create and refine global movement patterns. There are two main systems in the kinetic chain: the local muscular (stabilization system) and the global muscular (movement) system.

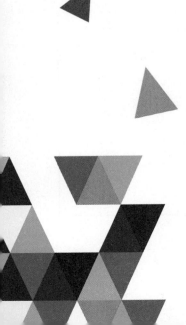

Local Muscular (Stabilization) System

The **local muscular system** is also called the stabilization system. It is composed of muscles that have the primary function of providing joint support and stabilization.[10-14] These muscles connect directly to the spine to provide support for the vertebrae during functional movement. They stabilize the spine so there is a central place from which to produce force, allowing for peripheral movement. In other words, the body is not able to properly move the extremities without a stable base of support. The following are the principal core stabilization muscles:[10,11,14,15]

- ▼   Transverse abdominis
- ▼   Multifidus
- ▼   Internal oblique
- ▼   Diaphragm
- ▼   Pelvic floor muscles

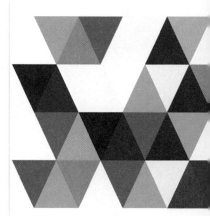

Global Muscular (Movement) System

The **global muscular system** consists of generally larger muscles that work synergistically to transfer and stabilize forces through the body to the ground. The global movement system has four subsystems: deep longitudinal, lateral, anterior oblique, and posterior oblique.

Details of the four global musculature subsystems include:

- ▼   **Deep longitudinal subsystem (DLS):** Consists of the peroneus longus, anterior tibialis, long head of the biceps femoris, sacrotuberous ligament, thoracolumbar fascia, and erector spinae (**Figure B.6**). A good exercise to train the DLS is a sagittal plane single-leg hop (front-to-back) with stabilization (hold).

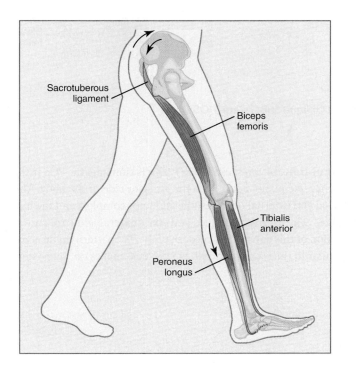

Figure B.6
Deep Longitudinal
Subsystem (DLS)

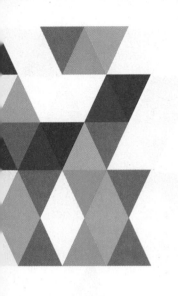

▼ **Posterior oblique subsystem (POS)**: Consists of the latissimus dorsi and the contralateral gluteus maximus, with the thoracolumbar fascia creating a fascial bridge for the cross-body connection (**Figure B.7**). Good exercises to train this subsystem include the squat-to-row and the lunge-to-row.

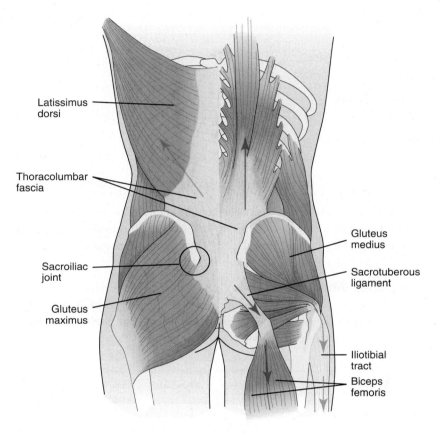

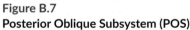

Figure B.7
Posterior Oblique Subsystem (POS)

▼ **Anterior oblique subsystem (AOS)**: This is similar to the POS in that it also functions in the transverse plane, but it is on the anterior side of the body. The muscles include the internal and external obliques, the adductor complex, and the hip external rotators (**Figure B.8**). The external obliques and contralateral adductors are the most common visualization of this subsystem because of the "X" pattern made across the front of the body, similar to the cross-body pattern the POS makes on the posterior.

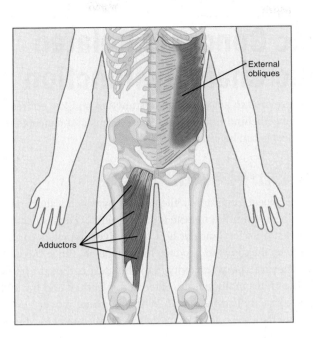

**Figure B.8
Anterior Oblique
Subsystem (AOS)**

▼ **Lateral subsystem (LS)**: Also called the frontal plane stabilization subsystem, it is made up of the gluteus medius, tensor fascia latae (TFL), the adductors on the same side (ipsilateral) of the body, and the quadratus lumborum (QL) on the opposite side (contralateral) (**Figure B.9**).

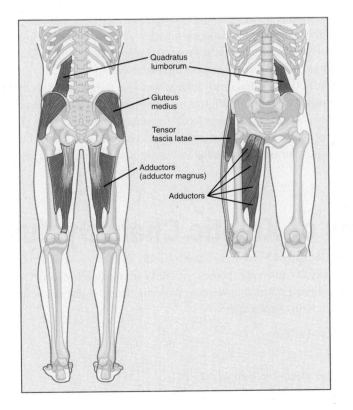

**Figure B.9
Lateral Subsystem
(LS)**

Scientific Concepts Related to Kinetic Chain Dysfunction

Various concepts are related to kinetic chain dysfunction and are addressed frequently when talking about the science behind imbalances. These terms and concepts build the foundation from which other concepts can be introduced.

Altered Reciprocal Inhibition

Recall that altered reciprocal inhibition is the process by which a short muscle, a tight muscle, and/or myofascial adhesions in the muscle (i.e., overactive) causes decreased neural drive of its functional antagonist muscle. Consider how overactive hip flexors could reciprocally inhibit the ability of the gluteus maximus to produce hip extension. Since the glutes are a functional antagonist to the hip flexors, the overactivity in the hip flexors thus prevents optimal activation of the glutes. With the glutes inhibited, hip extension is limited and the ability to jump, squat, or hold a yoga pose correctly is diminished. With the prime mover now inhibited, synergist muscles will work more than they should to assist the prime mover to complete the task, known as synergistic dominance.

Synergistic Dominance

Synergistic dominance occurs when synergists take over the function of a weak or inhibited prime mover. In the above example, it was demonstrated that tight hip flexors can inhibit the gluteus maximus, diminishing its ability to extend the hip. The inhibited gluteus maximus muscle now requires other synergist hip extensor muscles, such as the hamstrings, to assist more than it should to perform the joint action; the synergists of hip extension (i.e., hamstrings and posterior adductor magnus) become the dominant hip extensors.

Coincidentally, the most frequently injured muscle in the lower body is the hamstring, specifically the biceps femoris. This muscle performs as a synergist to the gluteus maximus for hip extension. When the biceps femoris is synergistically dominant, it will perform the job of hip extension that the gluteus maximus should be performing. This will lead to the biceps femoris becoming overwhelmed and overused, potentially leading to muscle strains as a repetitive stress injury.

Areas of Kinetic Chain Dysfunction

The Human Movement System, or kinetic chain, is composed of several major joints where various and excessive movements occur. As links in the kinetic chain, these joints are the areas of focus in identifying optimal movement patterns. These major segments are commonly called the *five kinetic chain checkpoints*:

- ▼ Foot and ankle
- ▼ Knee
- ▼ Lumbo-pelvic-hip complex (LPHC)
- ▼ Shoulder girdle
- ▼ Head (cervical spine)

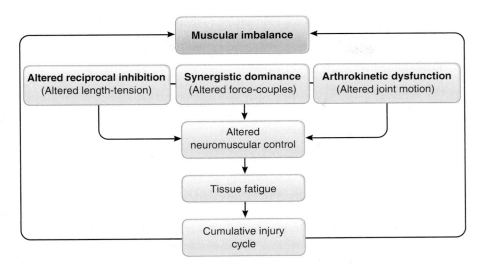

Figure B.10
Muscular Imbalance

These kinetic chain checkpoints can be used to recognize muscular imbalances. Imbalances create muscles or groups of muscles that are weak, short, lengthened and/or overactive. These imbalances may also contribute to a change/loss in **tensegrity**, leaving the body susceptible to injury or suboptimal movement patterns. Tensegrity refers to tensional integrity, and explains how the bones, which are surrounded by soft tissue, stay in place; the tension of the muscles is what keeps the bones in position.

Like a domino effect, a change in tensegrity causes other muscles to compensate or suffer a potential injury during movement patterns. Once injured, the body can heal itself to a degree to continue life and movement. The body can also actively, even subconsciously, compensate to avoid pain, or allow for particular desired outcomes. For example, an instructor with hip pain may subconsciously internally rotate the knee and pronate the foot to compensate for the pain.

Muscle imbalance may be caused by, or result in, altered reciprocal inhibition, synergistic dominance, arthrokinematic dysfunction, and overall decreased neuromuscular control (**Figure B.10**).

A variety of mechanisms can cause muscle imbalance,[16,17] including:

▼ Postural stress

▼ Emotional duress

▼ Repetitive movement

▼ Cumulative trauma

▼ Poor training technique

▼ Lack of core strength

▼ Lack of neuromuscular efficiency

Foot and Ankle

The foot and ankle complex has many bones and associated joints that support the body during various movements. When issues arise within the foot and ankle complex, it can lead to altered mechanics throughout the entire Human Movement System. Foot and ankle injuries are among the most common musculoskeletal injuries.[18] Common injuries include:

▼   Plantar fasciitis

▼   Achilles tendinopathy

▼   Medial tibial stress syndrome

▼   Ankle sprains and chronic ankle instability

The foot and ankle complex is a focus of warm-up, movement prep, and rehabilitation in many fitness and sporting events because so many activities take place with the foot and ankle complex supporting the weight of the entire body. Exercises where the foot and ankle play a dominant role are usually some variation of running, squatting, or jumping. Many issues develop as a result of deceleration forces, which include the lowering component of the squat and the impacting phases of running and jumping. Two common movement impairments of the foot and ankle are:

▼   **Lack of ankle dorsiflexion:** Excessive forward lean, knees do not bend properly during a squat.

▼   **Excessive foot pronation**: Feet visibly turn out; the sequential combination of dorsiflexion, eversion, and abduction.

Knee

The knee is a common site of injury in athletes and fitness enthusiasts alike. Anatomically, knee injuries are so common because the knee is a relatively stable joint stuck directly between two highly mobile joints (ankle and hip) with very long levers (tibia and femur). It only takes limited range of motion, poor neuromuscular recruitment, and altered arthrokinematics at one of these two joints to cause a potentially devastating injury at the knee. Common knee injuries include:

▼   Patellar tendonopathy (jumper's knee)

▼   Iliotibial band (IT-band) syndrome (runner's knee)

▼   Patellofemoral pain syndrome

▼   Anterior cruciate ligament (ACL) injury (along with injuries to the posterior cruciate [PCL], medial collateral [MCL], and lateral collateral [LCL] ligaments)

▼   Meniscus tears

By demonstrating and cueing proper posture and technique in classes, the Group Fitness Instructor may help alleviate pain while providing participants with exercise options they once deleted from their repertoire of possibilities. Common observable movement impairments are pronation distortion syndrome of the lower extremity:

▼   *Foot and ankle complex*: Dorsiflexion, eversion, and external rotation.

▼   *Knee*: Knee flexes and adducts; tibia and femur rotate toward midline.

▼   *Hips*: Flexion, adduction, internal rotation.

▼   *Hip and/or the foot and ankle*: Pronation of the knee; can appear as though the knee is caving in.

Lumbo-pelvic-hip Complex

The lumbo-pelvic-hip complex (LPHC) is commonly viewed as the core of the Human Movement System. It is the center of the human body and is directly connected to, influenced by, and has influence on both the upper and lower extremities. This is why LPHC stability is vitally important to injury prevention and sport performance. A properly stabilized core can be properly mobilized. Injuries associated with LPHC movement compensations are as follows:

- Local injuries:
  - Low back pain
  - Sacroiliac joint dysfunction
  - Hamstring, quadriceps, and groin strains
- Injuries above the LPHC:
  - Shoulder and upper extremity injuries
  - Cervical-thoracic spine
  - Rib cage dysfunction
- Injuries below the LPHC:
  - Patellar tendonitis
  - IT-band syndrome
  - Medial, lateral, or anterior knee pain
  - Chondromalacia patellae (knee inflammation and cartilage softening)
  - Plantar fasciitis
  - Achilles tendonitis
  - Posterior tibialis tendonitis (shin splints)

Common observable movement impairments of the LPHC are:

- **Excessive posterior tilt when seated**: Combine slouching and sitting, and a posterior pelvic tilt will present itself.
- **Excessive anterior tilt when standing**: Excessive curve seen in the lower back; tight hip flexors and low back extensors are contributors.

Shoulder

The shoulder joint, specifically the glenohumeral joint, is a mobile joint because of its unique anatomic features. It is a ball-and-socket joint that favors range of motion over stability. The shoulder joint is a part of the shoulder girdle, which is composed of the scapula, clavicle, and humerus. Much like the LPHC, the shoulder girdle moves in a particular rhythm to allow for increased range of motion. For example, as a participant raises his arms overhead, the scapula rotates upward. As the arms are brought down, the scapula rotates back downward. When these joints become locked down or limited in their ROM, the glenohumeral joint is often the point of pain. Common shoulder injuries include:

- Rotator cuff strains/tears
- Shoulder impingement
- Biceps tendinopathy
- Shoulder instability

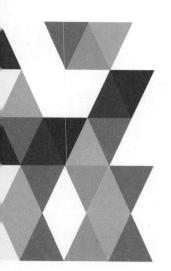

Shoulder impairment can also lead to cervical spine issues and headaches. Below the shoulder, the dysfunction can travel down and possibly lead to low back pain and dysfunction in the sacroiliac joint. Common observable movement impairments of the shoulder are:

▼ **Scapular winging**: Scapula protrudes excessively during prone exercises.

▼ **Overactive traps, rhomboids, and posterior deltoids; overactive anterior delts and pectorals**: Shoulder-forward posture; "slouching."

Cervical Spine

Neck pain is the fourth leading cause of disability, with over 30% of adults worldwide complaining of neck pain at some point in their lives.[19] As with other structures of the body, the cervical spine has an effect on the structures above and below it. Neck problems can lead to pain and dysfunction through headaches, back pain, and compensations to adjust for posture and balance control. Poor cervical spine mechanics can lead to neck injuries and other problems, such as:

▼ Neck stiffness

▼ Headaches

▼ Dizziness

▼ Temporomandibular joint-related (jaw-related) symptoms

▼ Cervical strains

▼ Cervical disk lesions

Many people will experience cervical spine dysfunction due to their lifestyle. Sitting at a desk, carrying heavy backpacks, purses, or children can strain the trapezius and levator scapulae muscles leading to dysfunction and pain that transfers to the cervical spine. Those with jobs that require a great deal of overhead work may show signs of cervical spine dysfunction for the same reason. Flexibility exercises for the sternocleidomastoid, levator scapulae, and upper trapezius musculature will become an important part of the workout for formats that include pushing and pulling movements. Strengthening the deep cervical flexors, lower trapezius, and cervical-thoracic extensors will also help to alleviate such dysfunction. Common observable movement impairments of the cervical spine are:

▼ **Forward head posture**: Commonly occurs from sitting at a desk and computer for long periods of time.

References

1. Hall S. *Basic Biomechanics*. (7th ed.). New York, NY: McGraw-Hill Education, 2017.
2. Hamill J, Knutzen K, Derrick T. *Biomechanical Basis of Human Movement*. (4th ed.). Philadelphia, PA: Lippincott Williams & Wilkins, 2015.
3. Knudson D. *Fundamentals of Biomechanics*. (2nd ed.). New York, NY: Springer, 2007.
4. Levangie P, Norkin C. Basic concepts in biomechanics. In *Joint Structure and Function: A Comprehensive Analysis*. (3rd ed.). Philadelphia, PA: F.A. Davis, 2001.
5. Brooks G, Fahey T, Baldwin K. *Exercise Physiology: Human Bioenergetics and Its Applications* (4th ed.). New York, NY: McGraw-Hill, 2005.

6. Neumann D. *Kinesiology of the Musculoskeletal System: Foundations for Rehabilitation.* (2nd ed.). St. Louis, MO: Mosby/Elsevier, 2010.

7. Hamill J, Knutzen JM. *Biomechanical Basis of Human Movement.* (2nd ed.). Baltimore, MD: Lippincott Williams & Wilkins, 2003.

8. Tortora GJ. *Principles of Human Anatomy.* (9th ed.). New York, NY: John Wiley & Sons, 2001.

9. Luttgens K, Hamilton N. *Kinesiology: Scientific Basis of Human Motion* (11th ed.). New York, NY: McGraw-Hill, 2007.

10. Bergmark A. Stability of the lumbar spine. A study in mechanical engineering. *Acta Ortho Scand.* 1989; *230*(suppl): 20–24.

11. Crisco JJ, Panjabi MM. The intersegmental and multisegmental muscles of the spine: A biomechanical model comparing lateral stabilizing potential. *Spine.* 1991;7:793–799.

12. Mooney V. Sacroiliac joint dysfunction. In A. Vleeming, V. Mooney, T. Dorman, C. Snijders, R. Stoeckhart (Eds.), *Movement, Stability, and Low Back Pain.* London, UK: Churchill Livingstone, 1997:37–52.

13. Panjabi MM. The stabilizing system of the spine. Part I. Function, dysfunction, adaptation, and enhancement. *J Spinal Disord Techn.* 1992;5:383–389; discussion 397.

14. Richardson C, Jull G, Hodges P, Hides J. *Therapeutic Exercise for Spinal Segmental Stabilization in Low Back Pain.* London, UK: Churchill Livingstone, 1999.

15. Schmidt RA, Lee TD. *Motor Control and Learning: A Behavioral Emphasis.* (3rd ed.). Champaign, IL: Human Kinetics, 1999.

16. Alter MJ. *Science of Flexibility.* (2nd ed.). Champaign, IL: Human Kinetics, 1996.

17. Gossman MR, Sahrman SA, Rose SJ. Review of length-associated changes in muscle: Experimental evidence and clinical implications. *Phys Ther.* 1982;62:1799–1808.

18. Doherty C, Delahunt E, Caulfield B, Hertel J, Ryan J, Bleakley C. The incidence and prevalence of ankle sprain injury: A systematic review and meta-analysis of prospective epidemiological studies. *Sports Med.* 2014;44(1):123–140.

19. Goode AP, Freburger J, Carey T. Prevalence, practice patterns, and evidence for chronic neck pain. *Arthritis Care Res.* 2010;62(11):1594–1601. doi:10.1002/acr.20270

20. Cohen SP. Epidemiology, diagnosis, and treatment of neck pain. *Mayo Clinic Proc.* 2015;90(2):284–299. doi:http://dx.doi.org/10.1016/j.mayocp.2014.09.008

Appendix C
Other Systems Related to Human Movement

Endocrine System

The endocrine system is a system of organs known as glands that secrete hormones into the bloodstream to regulate a variety of bodily functions, such as mood, growth and development, tissue function, and metabolism (**Figure C.1**). Hormones are the chemical messengers that enter the bloodstream and attach to target tissues and target organs. The target cells have hormone-specific receptors, ensuring each hormone will communicate only with specific target cells.

The endocrine system is responsible for regulating multiple bodily functions to stabilize the body's internal environment. Hormones produced by the endocrine system affect virtually all of the body's functions (e.g., triggering muscle contraction, stimulating protein and fat synthesis, activating enzyme systems, regulating growth and metabolism, and determining how the body will physically and emotionally respond to stress).[1]

Endocrine Glands

The primary endocrine glands are the hypothalamus, pituitary, thyroid, and adrenal glands. The pituitary gland is often referred to as the "master gland" of the endocrine system because it controls the function of the other endocrine glands. The pituitary gland and hypothalamus, which are both located in the brain, ultimately control much of the hormonal activity in the body. Together they represent an important link between the nervous and endocrine systems.[2]

Catecholamines

The two catecholamines—epinephrine (or adrenaline) and norepinephrine (noradrenaline)—are hormones produced by the adrenal glands situated on top of the kidneys. These hormones help prepare the body for activity; they are part of the stress response known as the *fight-or-flight response*. In preparation for activity, the hypothalamus triggers the adrenal glands to secrete more epinephrine. The increase in epinephrine results in specific physiological effects that help to sustain exercise activity:[2,3]

▼ Increases heart rate and stroke volume
▼ Redistributes blood to working tissues
▼ Elevates blood glucose (for energy)
▼ Mobilizes fats (for energy)

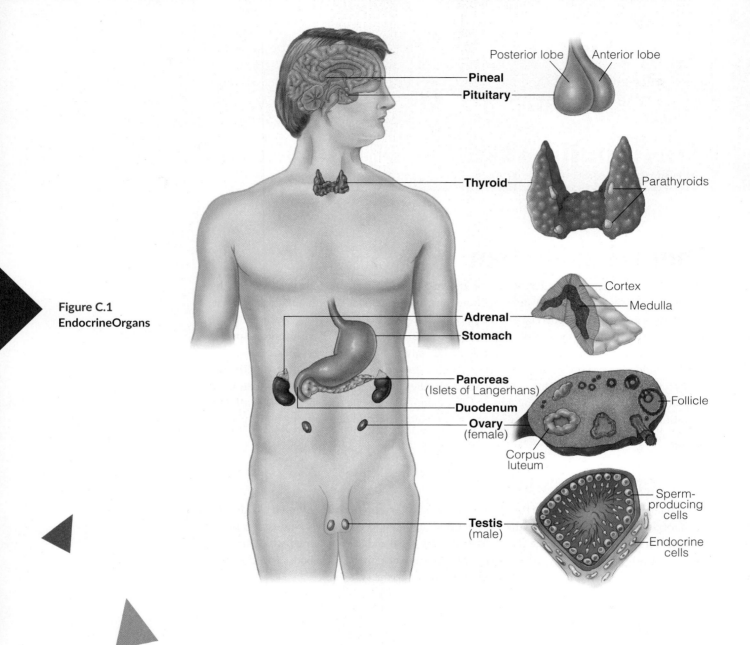

Figure C.1
EndocrineOrgans

- ▼ Stimulates sweating
- ▼ Promotes vasodilation (dilation of blood vessels) in needed areas versus vasoconstriction (constriction of blood vessels) in non-needed areas
- ▼ Norepinephrine rise >50% $\dot{V}O_2$max
- ▼ Epinephrine rises >70% $\dot{V}O_2$max

Testosterone and Estrogen

Testosterone is produced in the testes of the male and in small amounts in the ovaries and adrenal glands of the female. Males produce up to 10 times more testosterone than females.[1] Testosterone is primarily responsible for the development of male secondary sexual characteristics, such as facial and body hair and greater muscle mass. Estrogen is produced primarily in the ovaries in the female, with small amounts produced in the adrenal glands in males. For both males and females, however, testosterone plays a fundamental role in the growth and repair of tissue. Increased levels of testosterone are indicative of anabolic (tissue-building) training status.

Cortisol

Cortisol is referred to as a catabolic hormone, which means it is associated with the breaking down of tissue. Chronic stress from overtraining, excessive stress, poor sleep, and inadequate nutrition can elevate cortisol levels, leading to unwanted and potentially harmful side effects,[1] such as:

- ▼ Breakdown of muscle tissue
- ▼ Decreased fat utilization
- ▼ Increased body fat composition (specifically abdominal fat)
- ▼ Decreased metabolism

Growth Hormone

Growth hormone is an anabolic hormone responsible for most of the growth and development that occurs during childhood up until puberty, when the primary sex hormones take over. Growth hormone increases the development of bone and muscle and promotes protein synthesis and fat burning; it also strengthens the immune system. Growth hormone is stimulated by:

- ▼ Estrogen
- ▼ Testosterone
- ▼ Deep sleep
- ▼ Hypertrophy training
- ▼ Maximal strength training

Thyroid Hormones

The thyroid gland releases vital hormones primarily responsible for human metabolism, namely triiodothyronine (T3) and thyroxine (T4). Thyroid hormones have been shown to be responsible for:

- ▼ Carbohydrate, protein, and fat metabolism
- ▼ Basal metabolic rate
- ▼ Protein synthesis
- ▼ Sensitivity to epinephrine
- ▼ Heart rate
- ▼ Breathing rate
- ▼ Body temperature

Effects of Exercise on the Endocrine System

The general effects of exercise on the endocrine system are as follows:

▼ A person's activity level has an effect on hormone levels.

▼ Hormone levels can affect exercise performance.

▼ When participants are stressed, tired, actively overtraining, or only training in one format, hormones may become imbalanced.

▼ Lack of physical activity and obesity may alter normal hormone levels.

▼ When a person becomes active or maintains a healthy weight, hormone levels are more likely to be balanced (with the exception of medical conditions).

Digestive System

The digestive system performs the vital function of getting nutrients to cells and removing food waste; it includes everything from the mouth to the anus. The term *gastrointestinal (GI) tract* refers specifically to the stomach and intestines.[4]

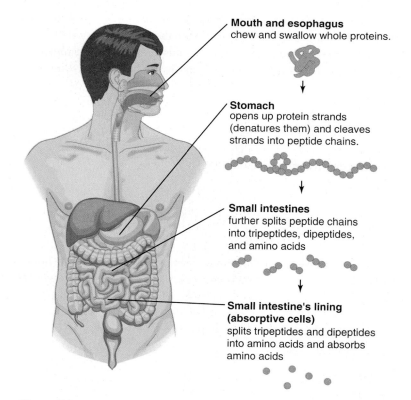

Mouth and esophagus
chew and swallow whole proteins.

Stomach
opens up protein strands (denatures them) and cleaves strands into peptide chains.

Small intestines
further splits peptide chains into tripeptides, dipeptides, and amino acids

Small intestine's lining (absorptive cells)
splits tripeptides and dipeptides into amino acids and absorbs amino acids

Figure C.2
The Digestive System

The process of getting food into the digestive system starts at the mouth with eating, or *ingestion*, and begins the digestion process by mechanically breaking down food through chewing. Accessory organs of the digestive system help begin the process:

- ▼ The salivary glands produce saliva to assist with the chemical breakdown of food.
- ▼ The tongue has taste receptors and helps with food manipulation.
- ▼ Teeth provide the initial and greatest amount of mechanical breakdown of food.
- ▼ As food is swallowed, it leaves the mouth and enters the pharynx.

Pharynx and Esophagus

The pharynx is the space between the mouth and both the trachea and esophagus. With swallowing, the opening to the trachea (airway) closes so food can enter the esophagus. The esophagus is about 10 inches long and provides passage of food to the stomach. The muscular mechanism that causes food to travel down the esophagus is called *peristalsis*.

Stomach

The stomach is a C-shaped muscular pouch where the second phase of digestion takes place by both chemical and physical breakdown. Gastric enzymes and hydrochloric acid are secreted to assist in the chemical breakdown of food, while (involuntary) smooth muscular contractions work to physically break down food. This second phase of digestion usually lasts between 40 minutes and a few hours.

Small Intestine

The small intestine is the longest section of the alimentary tube (about 23 feet, average) that serves as a passage from the stomach to the large intestine. It is a twisted, coiled, and muscular tube. It is where the majority of digestion actually takes place. It has three main areas:

- ▼ Duodenum (Latin for "12 finger widths")
- ▼ Jejunum (Latin for "empty")
- ▼ Ileum (Latin for "twisted intestine")

Because the small intestine can only process food in small amounts, the pyloric sphincter serves as the "gatekeeper" between the stomach and small intestine. As food travels through the small intestine and digestion occurs, it allows desired nutrients to get into the bloodstream.

Large Intestine

The large intestine starts where the small intestine ends (ileocecal valve) and ends at the anus. The large intestine has several jobs, but ultimately its role is to absorb water and electrolytes (sodium and potassium) and dry out undigested "leftover" food in the intestines and to eliminate it as feces.

Digestion of Nutrients

Because food is the fuel that drives movement, it is important to understand the basic digestive anatomy and how food is broken down and enters the bloodstream to feed the cells, tissues, and organs of the body through the circulatory system.

Protein Digestion, Absorption, and Utilization

Proteins must be broken down into their constituent amino acids before the body can use them. The fate of the amino acids after digestion and absorption by the intestines depends on the body's needs, which can range from tissue replacement or addition to a source of energy.

As ingested proteins enter the stomach, they encounter hydrochloric acid, which denatures (i.e., uncoils) the protein so digestive enzymes can begin dismantling the peptide bonds. In addition, the enzyme pepsin begins to cleave the protein strand into smaller polypeptides (i.e., strands of several amino acids) and single amino acids. As these protein fragments leave the stomach and enter the small intestine, pancreatic and intestinal proteases (i.e., enzymes that aid in protein digestion) continue to dismantle the protein fragments.

The resulting dipeptides, tripeptides, and single amino acids are absorbed through the intestinal wall into the enterocytes and released into the blood supply to the liver. Once in the bloodstream, the free-form amino acids have several possible fates: they can be used for protein synthesis (i.e., building and repairing tissues or structures), immediate energy, or potential energy (i.e., fat storage).

Amino Acids for Immediate Energy

The body has a constant need for energy; the brain and nervous system, in particular, have a constant need for glucose. If carbohydrate or total energy intake is too low, the body has the ability to use amino acids (from dietary or body proteins) to provide energy.[5,6] This process is typically known as *gluconeogenesis*. The amino acids are first deaminated (i.e., stripped of their amine group), allowing the remaining carbon skeleton to be used for the production of glucose or ketones to be used for energy. The removed amine group produces ammonia, a toxic compound, which is converted to urea in the liver and excreted as urine by the kidneys.

Amino Acids for Potential Energy (Fat)

If protein intake exceeds the amount needed for tissue synthesis, and the body's energy needs have been met, then amino acids from dietary protein are de-aminated, and their carbon fragments may be stored as fat. Among Americans, protein and caloric intakes are typically well above the body's requirements, allowing protein to contribute significantly to individuals' fat stores.[7]

Carbohydrate Digestion, Absorption, and Utilization

The principal carbohydrates present in food are in the form of simple sugars, starches, and cellulose. Simple sugars are very easily digested. Double sugars require some digestive action, but are not nearly as complex as starches. Starches require prolonged enzymatic action to be broken down into simple sugars (i.e., glucose) for use. Cellulose is largely indigestible by humans and contributes little energy value to the diet. It provides the bulk necessary for intestinal motility and aids in elimination.[8,9]

The rate at which ingested carbohydrates raise blood sugar, and its accompanying effect on insulin release, is referred to as the glycemic index (GI; **Table C.1**). The GI for a food is determined when the particular food is consumed by itself on an empty stomach. Mixed meals of protein, other carbohydrates, and fat can alter the glycemic effect of single foods.[10] One can see in **Table C.2** that foods lower on the glycemic index are good sources of complex carbohydrates, as well as being high in fiber and overall nutritional value.

Table C.1

Glycemic Index	
High	>70
Moderate	56–69
Low	<55

Table C.2

Glycemic Index for Assorted Foods					
Low		**Moderate**		**High**	
Food	**GI**	**Food**	**GI**	**Food**	**GI**
Peanuts	14	Apple juice	40	LifeSavers (hard candy)	70
Plain yogurt	14	Snickers	41	White bread	70
Soybeans	18	Peach	42	Bagel	72
Peas	22	Carrots	47	Watermelon	72
Cherries	22	Brown rice	50	Popcorn	72
Barley	25	Strawberry jam	51	Graham crackers	74
Grapefruit	25	PowerBar	53	French fries	75
Link sausage	28	Orange juice	53	Grape-Nuts cereal	75
Black beans	30	Honey	55	Shredded wheat	75
Lentils	30	Pita bread	57	Gatorade	78
Skim milk	32	Plain oatmeal	58	Corn flakes	81
Fettuccine	32	Pineapple	59	Rice cakes	72
Chickpeas	33	Sweet potato	61	Pretzels	83
Chocolate milk	32	Coca Cola	63	Baked white potato	85
Whole-wheat spaghetti	37	Raisins	64	Instant rice	87
Apple	38	Cantaloupe	65	Gluten-free bread	90
Pinto beans	39	Whole-wheat bread	67	Dates	103

Through the processes of digestion and absorption, all disaccharides and polysaccharides are ultimately converted into simple sugars such as glucose or fructose. However, fructose must be converted to glucose in the liver before it can be used for energy. Some of the glucose (i.e., blood sugar) is used as fuel by tissues of the brain, nervous system, and muscles. Because humans are periodic eaters, a small portion of the glucose is converted to glycogen after a meal and stored within the liver and muscles. Any excess is converted to fat and stored throughout the body as a reserve source of energy. When total caloric intake exceeds output, any excess carbohydrate, dietary fat, or protein may be stored as body fat until energy expenditure once again exceeds energy input.

Role of Fiber in Health

One of the greatest contributions made by complex carbohydrates is fiber. Higher intakes of dietary fiber are associated with lower incidence of heart disease and certain types of cancer.[11,12] Fiber is an indigestible carbohydrate that is either soluble or insoluble. Soluble fiber is dissolved by water and forms a gel-like substance in the digestive tract. Soluble fiber has many benefits, including moderating blood glucose levels and lowering cholesterol. Good sources of soluble fiber include oats and oatmeal, legumes (e.g., peas, beans, lentils), barley, and many uncooked fruits and vegetables (especially oranges, apples, and carrots).

Insoluble fiber does not absorb or dissolve in water. It passes through the digestive tract close to its original form. Insoluble fiber offers many benefits to intestinal health, including a reduction in the risk of colorectal cancer and occurrence of hemorrhoids and constipation. Most insoluble fibers come from the bran layer of cereal grains. The recommended intake of fiber is set at 38 grams per day and 25 grams per day for young men and women respectively.[13] Additional benefits of fiber include the following: [11,14-16]

- ▼ Provides bulk in the diet, thus increasing the satiety value of foods.
- ▼ Delays emptying of the stomach, further increasing satiety.
- ▼ Prevents constipation and establishes regular bowel movements.
- ▼ May reduce the risks of heart and artery disease by lowering blood cholesterol.
- ▼ Regulates the body's absorption of glucose (diabetics included), perhaps because fiber is believed to be capable of controlling the rate of digestion and assimilation of carbohydrates.
- ▼ High-fiber meals have been shown to exert regulatory effects on blood glucose levels for up to 5 hours after eating.

Fat Digestion, Absorption, and Utilization

Digestion of dietary fat starts in the mouth, moves to the stomach, and is completed in the small intestine. In the intestine, the fat interacts with bile to become emulsified so pancreatic enzymes can break the triglycerides down into two fatty acids and a monoglyceride. Absorption of these constituents occurs through the intestinal wall into the blood. In the intestinal wall, they are reassembled into triglycerides that are then released into the lymph in the form of a lipoprotein called chylomicron. Chylomicrons from the lymph move to the blood. The triglyceride content of the chylomicron is removed by the action of the enzyme lipoprotein lipase (LPL), and the released fatty acids are taken up by the tissues. Throughout the day, triglycerides are constantly cycled in and out of tissues, including muscles, organs, and adipose tissue.

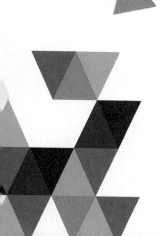

References

1. McArdle W, Katch F, Katch V. *Exercise Physiology: Nutrition, Energy, and Human Performance.* (7th ed.). Philadelphia, PA: Lippincott Williams Wilkins; 2010.

2. Tortora GJ, Grabowski SR. *Principles of Anatomy and Physiology.* (8th ed.). New York, NY: HarperCollins; 1996.

3. Wilmore JH, Costill DL. *Physiology of Sport and Exercise.* Champaign, IL: Human Kinetics; 2004.

4. Patton K, Thibodeau G. *The Human Body in Health and Disease* (6th ed.). New York, NY: Elsevier Science Health Science; 2015.

5. Berdanier CD. *Advanced nutrition: Macronutrients.* Boca Raton, FL: CRC Press; 1995.

6. Martineau A, Lecavalier L, Falardeau P, Chiasson JL. Simultaneous determination of glucose turnover, alanine turnover, and gluconeogenesis in human using a double stable-isotope-labeled tracer infusion and gas chromatography-mass spectrometry analysis. *Anal Biochem.* 1985;151(2):495–503.

7. Seagle HM, Strain GW, Makris A, Reeves RS, American Dietetic Association. Position of the American Dietetic Association: Weight management. *J Am Diet Assoc.* 2009;109:330–346.

8. Jenkins DJ, Vuksan V, Kendall CW, Würsch P, Jeffcoat R, Waring S, Wong E. Physiological effects of resistant starches on fecal bulk, short chain fatty acids, blood lipids and glycemic index. *J Am Coll Nutr.* 1998;17(6):609–616.

9. Lewis SJ, Heaton KW. Increasing butyrate concentration in the distal colon by accelerating intestinal transit. *Gut.* 1997;41(2):245–251.

10. Järvi AE, Karlström BE, Granfeldt YE, Björck IM, Vessby BO, Asp NG. The influence of food structure on postprandial metabolism in patients with non-insulin-dependent diabetes mellitus. *Am J Clin Nutr.* 1995;61(4):837–842.

11. Anderson JW, Smith BM, Gustafson NJ. Health benefits and practical aspects of high-fiber diets. *Am J Clin Nutr.* 1994;59(5 Suppl):1242S–1247S.

12. Wolk A, Manson JE, Stampfer MJ, Colditz GA, Speizer FE, Hennekens CH, Willett WC. Long-term intake of dietary fiber and decreased risk of coronary heart disease among women. *JAMA.* 1999;281(21):1998–2004.

13. Aldoori WH, Giovanucci EL, Rockett HR, Sampson L, Rimm EB, Willett WC. A prospective study of dietary fiber types and symptomatic diverticular disease in men. *J Nutr.* 1998;128(4):714–719.

14. Fernstrom JD, Miller GD. *Appetite and Body Weight Regulation.* Boca Raton, FL: CRC Press; 1994.

15. Howe GR, Benito E, Castelleto R, Cornée J, Estève J, Gallagher RP, et al. Dietary intake of fiber and decreased risk of cancers of the colon and rectum: Evidence from the combined analysis of 13 case-control studies. *J Natl Cancer Inst.* 1992;84(24):1887–1896.

16. Rimm EB, Ascherio A, Giovanucci E, Spiegelman D, Stampfer MJ, Willett WC. Vegetable, fruit, and cereal fiber intake and risk of coronary heart disease among men. *JAMA.* 1995;275(6):447–451.

Appendix D
Chronic Conditions and Expanded Emergencies in the Fitness Environment

Expanded Chronic Conditions
Diabetes

Diabetes is a metabolic disorder in which the body does not produce enough insulin (type 1) or the body cannot respond normally to the insulin made (type 2). An estimated 23.6 million children and adults in the United States (7.8% of the population) have diabetes, and 1.6 million new cases are diagnosed each year.[1] Diabetes is the seventh leading cause of death in the United States and is associated with a greater risk for heart disease, hypertension, and adult-onset blindness.[1] It has been shown that people who develop diabetes before the age of 30 are 20 times more likely to die by age 40 than those who do not have diabetes.[2]

There are two primary forms of diabetes: type 1 (insulin-dependent diabetes) and type 2 (non–insulin-dependent diabetes). Although type 2 is referred to as non–insulin-dependent diabetes, some individuals with type 2 diabetes cannot manage their blood glucose levels and do require additional insulin. Type 2 diabetes is strongly associated with an increase in childhood and adult-onset obesity.

Type 1 diabetes is typically diagnosed in children, teenagers, or young adults. With type 1 diabetes, specialized cells in the pancreas called beta cells stop producing insulin, causing blood sugar levels to rise, resulting in hyperglycemia (high levels of blood sugar). To control this high level of blood sugar, the individual with type 1 diabetes must inject insulin to compensate for what the pancreas cannot produce. Exercise increases the rate at which cells use glucose, which may mean that insulin levels may need to be adjusted with exercise. If the individual with type 1 diabetes does not control his or her blood glucose levels (via insulin injections and dietary carbohydrates) before, during, and after exercise, blood sugar levels can drop rapidly and cause a condition called hypoglycemia (low blood sugar), leading to weakness, dizziness, and fainting. Although insulin, proper diet, and exercise are the primary components prescribed for individuals with type 1 diabetes, these individuals must still be monitored throughout exercise to ensure safety.

Individuals with type 2 diabetes usually produce adequate amounts of insulin; however, their cells are resistant to the insulin (the insulin present cannot transfer adequate amounts of blood sugar into the cell). This condition can lead to hyperglycemia (high blood sugar). Chronic hyperglycemia is associated with a number of diseases associated with damage to the

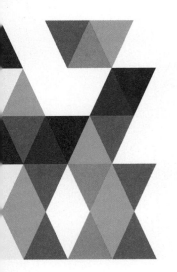

kidneys, heart, nerves, eyes, and circulatory system. Although individuals with type 2 diabetes do not experience the same fluctuations in blood sugar as those with type 1, it is still important to be aware of the symptoms, particularly for individuals with type 2 diabetes who use insulin medications.

Exercise and Diabetes

The most important goals of exercise for individuals with either type of diabetes are glucose control and, for those with type 2 diabetes, weight loss. Exercise is effective with both goals because it has a similar action to insulin by enhancing the uptake of circulating glucose by exercising skeletal muscle. Research has shown that exercise improves a variety of glucose measures, including tissue sensitivity, improved glucose tolerance, and even a decrease in insulin requirements.[3,4] Thus, exercise has been shown to have a substantial positive effect on the prevention of type 2 diabetes.

There are specific exercise guidelines and recommendations to follow when working with a diabetic population, including strategies to prevent hypoglycemic and hyperglycemic events during or after exercise as well as when to defer exercise based on resting blood glucose levels or symptoms. In most cases, excluding other health-related problems, the exercise management goals for individuals with diabetes are similar to those for physical inactivity and excess body weight. In contrast to walking being a highly preferred form of exercise for obese participants, care must be taken when recommending walking to participants with diabetes to prevent blisters and foot microtrauma that could result in foot infection. Special care should also be taken with respect to giving advice to participants with diabetes regarding carbohydrate intake and insulin use, not only before exercise but afterward, to reduce the risk of a hypoglycemic or hyperglycemic event.

Exercise guidelines for participants with diabetes (**Table D.1**) are similar to those advised for obese adults, as many participants with type 2 diabetes are obese.

Table D.1

Basic Exercise Guidelines for Individuals with Diabetes	
Mode	Low-impact activities (such as cycling and low-impact or step aerobics)
Frequency	4–7 days per week
Intensity	50–90% of maximum heart rate Stage I cardiorespiratory training (may be adjusted to 40–70% of maximal heart rate if needed) progressing to stages II and III based on a physician's approval.
Duration	20–60 minutes
Special Considerations	Make sure participant has appropriate footwear and have participant or physician check feet for blisters or abnormal wear patterns. Advise participant to keep a snack (quick source of carbohydrate) available during exercise, to avoid sudden hypoglycemia. Avoid excessive plyometric training, and higher-intensity training is not recommended for typical participant.

Arthritis

Arthritis is an inflammatory condition that mainly affects the joints of the body. Arthritis is the leading cause of disability among U.S. adults and is also associated with significant activity limitation, work disability, reduced quality of life, and high healthcare costs. Currently an estimated 21.6% of the adult U.S. population (46.4 million individuals) have arthritis.[5] Two of the most common types of arthritis are osteoarthritis and rheumatoid arthritis.

Osteoarthritis is caused by degeneration of cartilage within joints. This lack of cartilage creates a wearing on the surfaces of articulating bones, causing inflammation and pain at the joint. Some of the most commonly affected joints are in the hands, knees, hips, and spine.

Rheumatoid arthritis is a degenerative joint disease in which the body's immune system mistakenly attacks its own tissue (in this case, tissue in the joints or organs). This can cause an inflammatory response in multiple joints, leading to pain and stiffness. The condition is systemic and may affect both a variety of joints and organ systems. Joints most commonly affected by this condition include the hands, feet, wrists, and knees. It is usually characterized by morning stiffness, lasting more than a half hour, which can be both acute and chronic, with eventual loss of joint integrity.

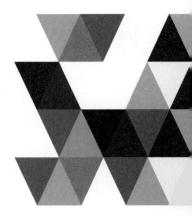

Exercise and Arthritis

Improving muscle strength and enhancing flexibility through exercise can assist in decreasing symptoms associated with arthritis. Static and active forms of stretching can be used and may be better tolerated from a seated or standing position. The use of self-myofascial release can be used if tolerated.

Table D.2 provides exercise guidelines for participants with arthritis. Cardiorespiratory training should begin in stage I and may progress to stage II or stage III, depending on the participant's

Table D.2

Basic Exercise Guidelines for Individuals with Arthritis	
Mode	Cycle and low-impact or step aerobics
Frequency	3–5 days per week
Intensity	60–80% of maximal heart rate Stage I cardiorespiratory training progressing to stage II (may be reduced to 40–70% of maximal heart rate if needed)
Duration	30 minutes
Special Considerations	Avoid heavy lifting and high repetitions. Stay in pain-free ranges of motion. There may be a need to start out with only 5 minutes of exercise and progressively increase, depending on the severity of conditions.

capabilities and a physician's advice. Core and balance exercises will be very important for this population to increase levels of joint stability and balance. Plyometric training is not recommended for arthritic participants.

Musculoskeletal Injuries

Musculoskeletal injuries are often painful, but they are rarely life-threatening. However, they can have serious consequences and even result in permanent disability if ignored or not cared for properly. It is important to understand the differences between various types of musculoskeletal injuries, both acute and chronic. When assessing a group fitness class, instructors should look out for the following signs of musculoskeletal injury:

▼   Abnormal lumps or deformities (usually only with fracture and/or dislocation)

▼   Discolored skin (will look red at first, then will look bruised)

▼   Inability to use or move the affected part (loss of motion, or inability to support weight)

▼   Numbness

▼   Pain, swelling (can appear rapidly or gradually)

When it is unknown how severe an injury is, always treat it as if it were serious. Some signs of serious injuries include popping or snapping of the bone, numbness, tingling, or change of color in the extremities. The cause of a musculoskeletal injury may also suggest its severity. Emergency services should be called whenever:

▼   A fracture, dislocation, deformity, or point of tenderness over bone is suspected.

▼   An individual is unable to move or use the injured body part.

▼   The injury involves the head, neck, or back.

Acute Injury

All injuries, at some point, are considered acute. Acute injuries occur as trauma to the body. Some examples of acute injuries are fractures, dislocations, subluxations, sprains, contusions, and strains. Additionally, acute injuries may present as cramps or soreness but can also include injuries to the nerves.[6] **Table D.3** provides descriptions for some of the most commonly seen acute musculoskeletal injuries in the group fitness setting.

Chronic Conditions

Chronic conditions are ongoing, persistent medical conditions often unrelated to physical injury. Sometimes, however, they can be the result of continued use of a body segment that had a previous acute injury. The term *inflammation* tends to carry a negative connotation in today's popular culture; however, it is an essential process to initiate healing after injury.[6] The inflammatory response should last around 4 days from the time of injury.[6] It is when other factors exist to extend this period of inflammation that chronic conditions arise from acute

Table D.3

Acute Musculoskeletal Injury Response

Injury or Condition	Description	Common Signs or Symptoms
Sprain	Damage to a ligament or joint capsule.	• Pain • Swelling • Stiffness
Strain	A result of a muscle being overstretched or force to contract against too much resistance, sometimes resulting in separation or tearing of the muscle fibers.	• Tenderness • Depression in muscle • Impairment or loss of movement
Dislocation	At least one bone in a joint is forced completely out of its normal and proper alignment. Dislocations require the bone to be manually or surgically put back into place, which always demands medical intervention. Dislocations that are inadequately or inappropriately tended can exacerbate the issue, creating further injury. Subluxation is similar to a dislocation except that the displaced bone goes right back into place.[6]	• Deformity • Pain or tenderness
Fracture	Broken bones are a result of extreme stresses to the skeletal system. If not managed properly, fractures can be very serious and create long-term issues for the injured individual. Fractures can only be diagnosed by a medical professional with an x-ray. There are many different types of fractures, each with different treatments and healing times.[6]	• Deformity • Tenderness • Swelling • Pain during active and passive movement • Popping or grating sound
Contusion	Contusions are commonly known as bruises and are not typically serious. They can be created from impact to the soft tissues of the body, causing the capillaries to tear and bleed into the tissues. Often, this creates a bluish-purple discoloration of the skin and some tenderness at the area of impact. Typically, the pain will dissipate within a few days and the discoloration will disappear within a few weeks.	• Tenderness • Discoloration

injury causes. Chronic conditions of this nature are most often attributed to overuse, postural and movement dysfunction, or not allowing a previous acute injury to heal correctly. While all chronic conditions should be diagnosed and treated under the care of a licensed medical professional, **Table D.4** provides a basic outline of some of the most common chronic conditions seen in participants.

Table D.4

Chronic Musculoskeletal Injury Response

Injury or Condition	Description	Common Signs or Symptoms
Tendinitis	Inflammation of a tendon often resulting from overuse.	• Pain • Swelling • Crepitus (crackling sound when moving)
Plantar fasciitis	Irritation and swelling of the thick tissue on the bottom of the foot associated with a difficulty in performing ankle dorsiflexion.	• Medial heel pain • Pain during dorsiflexion
Medial tibial stress syndrome (shin splints)	Pain in the front of the tibia caused typically by a strain of the posterior tibialis muscle. Can also be caused by stress fractures, compartment syndromes, or tendinitis in the lower leg.	• Anterior pain in the lower leg
Iliotibial (IT) Band syndrome (runner's knee)	Overuse running and cycling injury; the result of inflammation and irritation of the distal portion of iliotibial tendon as it rubs against the lateral femoral condyle. Often the result of musculoskeletal malalignments in the feet and legs.	• Mild swelling • Increased warmth and redness • Tenderness • Pain increases with activity
Patellofemoral pain syndrome	Discomfort of the inner knee area and may be caused by the abnormal tracking of the patella within the femoral trochlea.	• Anterior knee pain during flexion • Grating sensation during flexion • Recurrent swelling
Low back pain	Most common human ailment, usually resulting from suboptimal movement patterns, faulty posture, congenital anomalies, or trauma to the lumbar region.	• Pain in the posterior lumbar area • Muscular weakness

Metabolic Emergencies

Metabolic emergencies include acute exacerbations of chronic medical conditions, such as hypoglycemia in diabetes, and are associated with extreme or rapid changes in blood glucose levels. Typically, participants diagnosed with metabolic conditions will be familiar with the signs and symptoms of their ailment; however, given the nature of these particular conditions, affected individuals may not be able to respond appropriately to their symptoms, as they often cause weakness and disrupt mental capabilities. **Table D.5** outlines metabolic conditions that would constitute an emergency during a group fitness class.

Table D.5

Metabolic Emergency Response			
Injury or Condition	**Description**	**Common Signs or Symptoms**	**Response Protocols**
Hypoglycemia	Hypoglycemia is associated with diabetes, and is related to a rapid drop in blood glucose levels. This drop can be associated with exercise, so individuals with diabetes, especially those taking insulin, should be careful in timing their workouts to prevent hypoglycemia both during and after exercise.	• Weakness • Shaking • Sweating • Anxiety • Tingling of the extremities • Headache • Confusion • Seizures	• Call 9-1-1 for emergency services right away. • If the individual can drink and swallow, offer fruit juices or non-diet soda that are high in sugar and can be absorbed quickly. • Continue to monitor for changes in respiration and heart rate while waiting for EMS to arrive.
Hyperglycemia	Diabetes is a disease by which the pancreas in unable to secrete sufficient insulin levels to support the uptake and utilization of glucose in the body, resulting in high blood sugar levels. For non–insulin-dependent (type 2) diabetics, drinking water and exercising will help reduce blood glucose levels. In type 1 diabetics, injecting insulin is the only appropriate therapy, and *must* be done by the participant, as insulin dosing is outside scope of practice. In type 1 diabetics and (very rarely) type 2 diabetics, diabetic ketoacidosis (DKA) may develop. DKA is a medical emergency.	• Increased thirst • Headache • Increased need to urinate • Dehydration With severely high blood glucose levels (>300 mg/dL), additional symptoms indicative of DKA include: • Confusion • Shortness of breath • Breath that smells fruity • Nausea and vomiting • Very dry mouth	• Encourage participant to drink water and test blood sugar. • Encourage participant to take an insulin dose if he or she is insulin-dependent. • After insulin administration, discourage exercise participation until blood glucose test shows reduced blood sugar levels. For severely high blood glucose (>300 mg/dL), if participant is unable to inject insulin and/or symptoms of DKA are present, • Call 9-1-1 for emergency services right away. • Continue to monitor for changes in respiration and heart rate while waiting for EMS to arrive.

Cardiorespiratory Emergencies

Cardiorespiratory emergencies can occur anytime in the fitness setting, and even affect those who are in peak physical condition. For this reason, all Group Fitness Instructors are required to be certified in the life-saving techniques of CPR and AED operation. **Table D.6** lists what to watch for and how to react when presented with a cardiorespiratory emergency during a group fitness class.

Table D.6

Cardiorespiratory Emergency Response

Injury or Condition	Description	Common Signs or Symptoms	Response Protocols
Heart Attack	A heart attack is the result of a blockage of one of the arteries that supply blood to the heart muscles, preventing the delivery of an adequate oxygen supply. Decreased oxygen supply can create changes to a portion of the cardiac muscle. Such changes can prevent the heart from pumping adequate amounts of blood to the rest of the system. The most serious complication of a heart attack can be arrhythmias, cardiogenic shock (total heart failure), or cardiac arrest.	• Dizziness • Nausea • Pain or squeezing in the middle of the chest • Pain radiating in the arm (usually the left), jaw, or back • Pain in the sternum area (often mistaken for indigestion) • Profuse sweating • Shortness of breath • Weakness	• Direct the individual to stop activity and lie down, and call 9-1-1 immediately. • If the individual becomes unconscious and/or has no pulse and respiration, begin performing CPR protocols while waiting for emergency services to arrive.
Asthma Attack	In the asthmatic patient, bronchiolar spasms are responsible for decreasing air flow. High levels of activity can precipitate an asthma attack. In fact, some individuals suffer from exercise-induced asthma.	• Bluish tint to the nails, lips, or skin • Shortness of breath and difficulty exhaling • Skin color may change to a dusky hue • Sweating and increase in heart rate • Wheezing or a "squeaking" or "whistling" sound when exhaling	• The first reaction to an individual with difficulty breathing is to stop the exercise, which will decrease the oxygen demand. Have the individual sit down or lie down with their shoulders and chest elevated. It may be helpful to have them lean against a wall when seated. • If they have constrictive clothing, loosen or remove the constrictive pieces. • Many asthmatics carry bronchodilator medications for inhalation during attacks—ask whether they have this medication and help them administer it. • Observe them frequently for improvement or deterioration. If their condition continues to worsen, call 9-1-1 for emergency services immediately.
Choking	Choking occurs any time the airway is blocked by an external object. Participants often chew gum while exercising, which presents a high risk for choking by having an object in the mouth while respiration is heavy.	• Participant visibly shows panic and difficulty breathing. • Face becomes flush, then pale as oxygen depletion takes hold.	• If the individual is conscious, perform back blows or abdominal thrusts to force the obstruction out of the airway. • If the individual is unconscious, perform techniques learned in CPR/AED training to clear the airway.

Cerebrovascular Emergencies

Cerebrovascular emergencies are made up of injuries or conditions that directly affect the brain. These include, but are not limited to, strokes, seizures, and traumatic brain injuries (TBI) such as concussions. These are some of the most serious medical emergencies that can occur to an exerciser, so if one of the conditions listed in **Table D.7** is identified, 9-1-1 should be dialed immediately to activate emergency services.

Table D.7

Cerebrovascular Emergency Response

Injury or Condition	Description	Common Signs or Symptoms	Response Protocols
Stroke	A stroke or Cerebral Vascular Accident (CVA) is a sudden, often severe impairment of body functions brought on by a disruption of blood flow to the brain. When blood flow fails to reach parts of the brain, the affected brain cells die and leave an infarcted area. The location and magnitude of the injury determines the residual damage to the individual.	• Change of mood • Confusion, disorientation to self, time, or place • Difficulty speaking • Difficulty swallowing • Dizziness, loss of balance, unexplained fall • Headache, usually sudden and severe • Numbness, paralysis, or weakness of face, neck, or limbs; occurring on one or both sides of the body • Persistent ringing in the ears • Sudden blurred vision or loss of vision in one or both eyes	• Call 9-1-1 immediately • Keep the individual lying down and protected. • Do not give them anything to eat or drink. • If the individual is semi-conscious or unconscious, turn them to their side to prevent secretion from falling back into their lungs (aspiration). Due to the potential pressure in the brain, stroke individuals may vomit. • Reassess the person's respiratory status in case their condition deteriorates and begin CPR if necessary. • In cases where the stroke passes and the individual seems to regain all faculties, do not allow him or her to resume activity, and direct them to seek medical attention as soon as possible.
Concussion	The immediate post-trauma impairment of neural functions due to a direct blow to the head that causes a shaking of the brain within the skull.[6]	• Alteration of consciousness (not necessarily fully knocked unconscious) • Blurred vision • Dizziness • Amnesia (in some cases) • Headache • Tinnitus (ringing of the ears) • Light sensitivity • Sleep disturbance • Difficulty concentrating	• If the individual is still conscious, have him or her cease activity and direct the individual to seek medical attention at once. • If the individual is knocked unconscious, or if symptoms do not subside quickly, call 9-1-1 right away for emergency medical attention. • If the individual remains unconscious and has no pulse and respiration, begin performing CPR protocols while waiting for emergency services to arrive.

(continues)

Table D.7

Cerebrovascular Emergency Response (*continued*)

Injury or Condition	Description	Common Signs or Symptoms	Response Protocols
Seizure	A seizure is a sudden brief attack of altered consciousness, motor activity, and sensory phenomena. Seizures can be brief episodes (petit mal) or major occurrences (grand mal). Anyone can experience a seizure; however, those with epilepsy are at constant risk and should only take part in athletic activity with the clearance and guidance of a physician.	• Uncontrollable shaking, jerking motions • Rigid, flexed muscles (tonic-clonic muscle contractions) • Drooling • Foaming at the mouth • Periods of unconsciousness	• Call 9-1-1 right away. • Do not restrain seizing individuals. Protect them from injury by moving objects away from them. Never attempt to put anything into their mouths or force anything between their teeth. Never attempt to insert fingers in their mouth. • When the jerking movements stop, position the individual on one side to allow for drainage from the mouth. Keep their airway open and reassess frequently to make sure they are breathing. • Seizure attacks are generally followed by periods of rest or sleep, and continued moving around can precipitate another attack. Allow the individual to comfortably rest while waiting for medical personal arrive.

Environmental Emergencies

All environmental emergencies are due to overexposure to heat or cold, and all are preventable. By wearing appropriate clothing for the external conditions, and maintaining a proper hydration and electrolyte balance, individuals can easily avoid environmentally induced injury or illness. The signs, symptoms, and response protocols for hot and cold weather injuries should be fully understood (**Table D.8**).

Table D.8

Environmental Emergency Response

Injury or Condition	Description	Common Signs or Symptoms	Response Protocols
Heat cramps	Heat cramps are muscle spasms that are painful. It could be a warning signal or sign of a heat-related emergency.	• Painful muscle spasms in the legs or abdominal region	• Rest the individual in a cool place. • Provide cool water. • Do not give salt tablets or salt water to drink.
Heat exhaustion	More severe than heat cramps and usually occurs after a long period of strenuous exercise or work in the heat and/or humidity.	• Cool, moist, pale, or red skin • Headache or dizziness • Nausea • Normal or below normal body temperature • Weakness and/or exhaustion	• Get the individual out of the heat. • Call 9-1-1 right away. • Cool the body with cool, wet cloths, such as towels. • Loosen all tight clothing. • If the individual is able to swallow, give cool water to drink (slowly). • Monitor vital signs and wait for EMS.
Heat stroke	The least common, but the most severe heat emergency. Usually occurs after the signals of heat exhaustion are ignored. In heat stroke, dangerously elevated internal temperatures cause vital body systems to fail.	• Change in consciousness • Rapid, shallow breathing • Rapid, weak pulse • Red, hot, dry skin	• Get the individual out of the heat. • Call 9-1-1 immediately. • Cool the body with cool, wet cloths, such as towels. • Loosen all tight clothing. • Do not give anything by mouth. • Monitor vital signs and wait for EMS.
Hypothermia	Hypothermia occurs when the body can no longer generate enough heat to maintain normal body temperature.	• Apathy and decreased levels of consciousness • Numbness or glassy stare • Shivering (could be absent in latter stages) • Slow, irregular pulse • Pale cool skin • Patches of cyanosis, or blue color to lips and skin	• Call 9-1-1 immediately. • Remove wet clothing and dry the individual (if applicable). • Gradually warm up the body with blankets and dry clothes. • Move to a dry, warmer environment. • Do not warm individual too quickly as this could lead shock. • Monitor vital signs and wait for EMS.

Table D.9

Response for Pregnancy-Related Emergencies	
Potential Complications from Pregnancy	**Response Protocols**
• Bloody show (spotting or frank bleeding) • Cramping (possibly severe) • Premature contractions or labor • Dyspnea before exertion • Dizziness • Headache • Chest pain • Muscle weakness • Calf pain or swelling • Decreased fetal movement • Amniotic fluid leakage • Pregnancy-related hypoglycemia	• Call 9-1-1 immediately. • Have the individual stop exercising and sit or lie down. • If cramping and contractions continue, make arrangements to transport the individual to the hospital. • If bloody show is severe, lie the person down with legs elevated. In advanced pregnancy, do not lie the individual flat since this will limit breathing and decrease blood flow to the fetus. • Re-evaluate the individual frequently for changes in breathing or cardiac status while waiting for medical personnel to arrive.

Pregnancy-Related Emergencies

Prior to beginning any exercise program, a pregnant participant needs medical clearance from her obstetrician. Generally, pregnancy is not a contraindication to exercise. In addition, any activity performed by a pregnant individual that results in one or more signs or symptoms (**Table D.9**) should be immediately ceased, and medical follow-up or emergency services should be pursued.[7]

Skin Wounds

A skin wound is defined as trauma to tissues that causes a break in the continuity of that tissue; skin is soft and pliable and easily traumatized.[6] There are four types of skin wounds overtly common in the sport and fitness realm: abrasions, lacerations, puncture wounds, and avulsion wounds. All skin wounds follow the same treatment protocol to be cleaned and dressed, but, depending on the severity of the wound, emergency services may need to be called so the injured individual can receive the appropriate medical care. Regardless, individuals experiencing any type of injury should always be referred to a medical professional for care beyond the initial first aid response.

A main concern when reacting to skin wounds is the biological hazard presented to the both the class and the instructor; specifically, blood-borne pathogens. If a participant experiences an injury of this nature, it is important to first clear other participants away from any areas contaminated with blood. If at all possible, it is imperative to wear medical gloves when coming into contact with another's blood. Then, depending on the type of skin wound, the correct application of cleaning and dressing should be performed. Furthermore, cleanup of the contaminated area should be reserved for janitorial staff trained in biohazard cleanup protocols. All fitness facilities should have an emergency response plan for biohazards, with which Group Fitness Instructors should be familiar before working.

Abrasions

Abrasions are when the skin is scraped away by a rough surface such as a playing field, floor, or exercise mat; the top layer of skin is removed, exposing numerous blood capillaries.[6] The nature of this type of wound creates large exposed areas, so it is essential to cleanse and dress it with clean water and a sterile gauze pad to stop the bleeding, then refer the participant to seek additional medical care if necessary.

Lacerations

Lacerations happen when a sharp object tears the skin tissue, giving the wound the look of a jagged edge cavity.[6] The main concern with lacerations is the quantity of bleeding. The first response should be for the injured participant to place direct pressure on the wound to slow or (hopefully) stop the bleeding. If direct pressure is not enough, a tourniquet should be applied and 9-1-1 should be called immediately, as the wound may require sutures to close.

Puncture Wounds

Puncture wounds occur when a sharp, pointed object penetrates the skin and typically intrudes through deeper layers of bodily soft tissues; due to the deep, penetrating nature of a puncture wound, there is a strong risk of tetanus being introduced into the bloodstream.[6] Procedures to stop the bleeding and clean and dress the wound follow the same protocols as lacerations; however, all puncture wounds should be treated immediately by a physician.

Avulsion Wounds

An avulsion wound is when the skin is torn from the body.[6] This is often seen in classes that utilize barbells or other handheld implements, as the skin of the palm can be ripped by the bar spinning in the hands during movement. Like abrasions, avulsion wounds expose large areas of capillaries and are often associated with heavy bleeding. As with all other wound types, contact with another's blood should be avoided, pressure should be applied to stop or at least slow the bleeding, the wound should be cleaned and dressed, and the individual should be directed to the appropriate medical care. In cases where bleeding is not easily controlled or stopped, 9-1-1 should always be contacted right away.

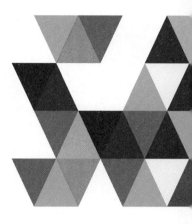

References

1. American Diabetes Association. *Diabetes statistics.* Available at: http://www.diabetes.org/diabetes-basics/diabetes-statistics. Accessed October 20, 2010.
2. Slemenda C, Heilman DK, Brandt KD, et al. Reduced quadriceps strength relative to body weight. A risk factor for knee osteoarthritis in women? *Arthritis Rheum.* 1998;41:1951-1959.
3. *ACSM's Exercise Management for Persons with Chronic Diseases and Disabilities.* (3rd ed.). Champaign, IL: Human Kinetics; 2009.
4. American Diabetes Association. Diabetes mellitus and exercise. *Diabetes Care.* 2002;25(Suppl 1):s64.
5. Centers for Disease Control and Prevention (CDC). Prevalence of doctor-diagnosed arthritis and arthritis-attributable activity limitation—United States, 2003-2005. *MMWR Morb Mortal Wkly Rep.* 2006;55(40):1089-1092.
6. Prentice WE. *Essentials of athletic injury management.* (10th ed.). New York: McGraw-Hill; 2016.
7. American College of Sports Medicine. *ACSM's Guidelines for Exercise Testing and Prescription* (9th ed.). Philadelphia: Wolters Kluwer/Lippincott Williams & Wilkins; 2014.

Appendix E
Expanded Nutritional Concepts

Nutrition Guidelines

A very basic definition of a healthy diet is a plan of eating that incorporates balance, variety, and moderation while meeting individual nutritional needs and goals and balancing energy intake to maintain a healthy weight. It is important to note that nutritional needs change over the life span differ for athletes and those who are sick, pregnant, or taking certain medications. Another factor to consider is the nutrient density of foods. Nutrient density refers to the nutrient content of a food relative to its calories.

These basic concepts can be incorporated into a healthy eating plan in a number of ways. As part of its role in improving the health of all Americans, the U.S. government has developed resources such as MyPlate and the Dietary Guidelines for Americans, as well as laws governing what must appear on food labels. Each provides general information to be individualized for variety of eating needs. Group Fitness Instructors should refer participants to these resources when they have questions about healthy eating.

MyPlate

MyPlate (choosemyplate.gov) is a planning and assessment tool that individuals can use to incorporate the recommendations into daily meal choices. It provides useful meal planning and healthy eating tools and promotes physical activity. If participants require detailed assistance with the information they receive, an instructor can refer them to a registered dietitian.

Dietary Reference Intakes

The Dietary Reference Intakes (DRI) are reference values used to plan and assess nutrient intakes of healthy individuals. The DRIs include four nutrient-based reference values: Recommended Dietary Allowance (RDA), Adequate Intake (AI), Estimated Average Requirement (EAR), and Tolerable Upper Intake Level (UL). The DRIs are established for healthy individuals and do not apply to those with chronic or acute disease (who may need extra nutrients) or those recovering from a diagnosed deficiency. DRIs can be used by registered dieticians to plan menus for individuals, as well as institutions, such as hospitals and school cafeterias, that use the DRIs to ensure they provide adequate nutrition.

Table E.1

Comparison of Dietary Reference Intake Values for Adult Men and Women and Daily Values for Micronutrients with the Tolerable Upper Intake Levels, Safe Upper Levels, and Guidance Levels.[a]

Nutrient	RDA/AI (Men/Women) ages 31–50	Daily Value (Food Labels)	UL	SUL or Guidance Level	Selected Potential Effects of Excess Intake
Vitamin A (µg)	900/700	1,500 (5,000 IU)	3,000	1,500[c] (5,000 IU)	Liver damage, bone and joint pain, dry skin, loss of hair, headache, vomiting
β-carotene (mg)	–	–	–	7 (11,655 IU)	Increased risk of lung cancer in smokers and those heavily exposed to asbestos
Vitamin D (µg)	5[b]	10 (400 IU)	50	25 (1,000 IU)	Calcification of brain and arteries, increased blood calcium, loss of appetite, nausea
Vitamin E (mg)	15	20 (30 IU)	1,000	540 (800 IU)	Deficient blood clotting
Vitamin K (µg)	120/90[b]	80	–	1,000[c]	Red blood cell damage or anemia, liver damage
Thiamin (B$_1$) (mg)	1.2/1.1	1.5	–	100[c]	Headache, nausea, irritability, insomnia, rapid pulse, weakness (7,000+ mg dose)
Riboflavin (B$_2$) (mg)	1.3/1.1	1.7	–	40[c]	Generally considered harmless; yellow discoloration of urine
Niacin (mg)	16/14	20	35	500[c]	Liver damage, flushing, nausea, gastrointestinal problems
Vitamin B$_6$ (mg)	1.3	2	100	10	Neurological problems, numbness and pain in limbs
Vitamin B$_{12}$ (µg)	2.4	6	–	2,000[c]	No reports of toxicity from oral ingestion
Folic acid (µg)	400	400	1,000	1,000[c]	Masks vitamin B$_{12}$ deficiency (which can cause neurological problems)

Nutrient	RDA/AI (Men/Women) ages 31–50	Daily Value (Food Labels)	UL	SUL or Guidance Level	Selected Potential Effects of Excess Intake
Pantothenic acid (mg)	5[b]	10	–	200[c]	Diarrhea and gastrointestinal disturbance
Biotin (µg)	30[b]	300	–	900[c]	No reports of toxicity from oral ingestion
Vitamin C (mg)	90/75[b]	60	2,000	1,000[c]	Nausea, diarrhea, kidney stones
Boron (mg)	–	–	20	9.6	Adverse effects on male and female reproductive systems
Calcium (mg)	1,000[b]	1,000	2,500	1,500[c]	Nausea, diarrhea, kidney stones
Chromium (µg)	35[b]	120	–	10,000[c]	Potential adverse effects on liver and kidneys; picolinate form possibly mutagenic
Cobalt (mg)	–	–	–	1.4[c]	Cardiotoxic effects; not appropriate in a dietary supplement except as vitamin B_{12}
Copper (µg)	900	2,000	10,000	10,000	Gastrointestinal distress, liver damage
Fluoride (mg)	4/3[b]	–	10	–	Bone, kidney, muscle, and nerve damage; supplement only with professional guidance
Germanium	–	–	–	zero[c]	Goutlike symptoms, joint pains, increased uric acid
Iodine (µg)	150	150	1,100	500[c]	Elevated thyroid hormone concentration
Iron (mg)	8/18	18	45	17[c]	Gastrointestinal distress, increased risk of heart disease, oxidative stress
Magnesium (mg)	420/320	400	350[d]	400[c]	Diarrhea
Manganese (mg)	2.3/1.8[b]	2	11	4[c]	Neurotoxicity

(*continues*)

Table E.1

Comparison of Dietary Reference Intake Values for Adult Men and Women and Daily Values for Micronutrients with the Tolerable Upper Intake Levels, Safe Upper Levels, and Guidance Levels.[a] (*continued*)

Nutrient	RDA/AI (Men/Women) ages 31–50	Daily Value (Food Labels)	UL	SUL or Guidance Level	Selected Potential Effects of Excess Intake
Molybdenum	45	75	2,000	zero[c]	Goutlike symptoms, joint pains, increased uric acid
Nickel (µg)	–	–	–	260[c]	Increased sensitivity of skin reaction to nickel in jewelry
Phosphorus (mg)	700	1,000	4,000	250[c]	Alteration of parathyroid hormone levels, reduced bone mineral density
Potassium (mg)	–	–	–	3,700[c]	Gastrointestinal damage
Selenium (µg)	55	70	400	450	Nausea, diarrhea, fatigue, hair and nail loss
Silicon (mg)	–	–	–	700	Low toxicity, possibility of kidney stones
Vanadium (mg)	–	–	1.8	Zero	Gastrointestinal irritation; fatigue
Zinc (mg)	11/8	15	40	25	Impaired immune function, low HDL-cholesterol

[a] Food and Nutrition Board, Institute of Medicine (U.S.). Dietary Reference Intake Tables. Available at http://nationalacademies.org/hmd/activities/nutrition/summarydris/dri-tables.aspx.

[b] Indicates adequate intake (AI).

[c] Indicates guidance levels, set by the Expert Group on Vitamins and Minerals of the Food Standards Agency (FSA), United Kingdom. These are intended to be levels of daily intake of nutrients in dietary supplements that potentially susceptible individuals could take daily on a lifelong basis without medical supervision in reasonable safety. When the evidence base was considered inadequate to set a safe upper level (SUL), guidance levels were set based on limited data. SULs and guidance levels tend to be conservative, and it is possible that for some vitamins and minerals, great amounts could be consumed for short periods without risk to health. The values presented are for a 60-kg (132-lb) adult. Consult the full publication for values expressed per kilogram of body weight. This FSA publication, *Safe Upper Levels for Vitamins and Minerals*, is available at: https://cot.food.gov.uk/cotreports/cotjointreps/evmreport.

[d] The UL for magnesium represents intake specifically from pharmacologic agents and dietary supplements in addition to dietary intake. *RDA*, recommended dietary allowance; *UL*, tolerable upper intake level; *AI*, adequate intake; *SUL*, safe upper level.

Energy and Macronutrient Requirements

A general recommendation for how many calories one should consume is the Estimated Energy Requirement (EER). It is based on formulas designed to include individual characteristics such as age, gender, height, weight, and level of physical activity. The tools used to assess DRIs will also calculate the user's calorie needs based on a set of formulas.

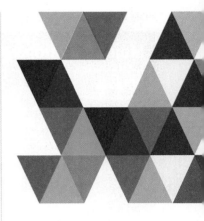

The recommendations for carbohydrates, fats, and proteins are provided under the Acceptable Macronutrient Distribution Range (AMDR). The AMDR is a recommended range of macronutrient requirements based on a person's total daily calorie needs and the balance of nutrients associated with a decreased risk of chronic disease:

▼ Protein: 10–35% of total daily calories

▼ Fat: 20–35% of total daily calories

▼ Carbohydrates: 45–65% of total daily calories

There is some debate surrounding these numbers; however, they provide a place to start that can be adjusted to meet individual goals and needs. For example, an endurance athlete would need to eat more carbohydrates than an inactive person.

Vitamins and Minerals

Vitamins and minerals are often referred to as *micronutrients* because they are required in smaller amounts than the macronutrients. These are essential to health and vitality because of the important roles they play in every function in the body and their role in the body's ability to obtain energy from carbohydrates, fats, and proteins.

The recommended amounts of essential vitamins and minerals can be obtained through a healthy diet with plenty of vegetables, fruits, whole grains, fat-free dairy, and lean meats.[1] However, many people feel they are unable to eat healthy every day, and therefore choose to take a multivitamin that will supply 100% of the recommended vitamins and minerals. Multivitamins are fine if taken as a supplement to a healthy diet, but they should not be considered a replacement for a healthy diet. Taking multivitamins containing more than 100% of what is recommended or using many additional individual vitamin and mineral supplements introduces the risk of toxicity. Having too much of one nutrient can also sometimes interfere with the absorption of another.

Tables E.2 and **E.3** provide a brief overview of some of the major functions of important vitamins and minerals, respectively, with good food sources for each. Instructors can use this information for encouraging participants to obtain the vitamins and minerals they need from a balanced diet. However, it is not within the Group Fitness Instructors' scope of practice to prescribe diets or supplements to their participants.

Table E.2

Major Functions of Vitamins in the Body and Good Food Sources[2]

Vitamin	Role in Body	Good Food Sources
Vitamin A	Essential for proper development and maintenance of eyes and vision. Needed to maintain integrity of skin, digestive tract, and other tissues. Required for proper immune system function. Support of cell differentiation.	Eggs Vitamin A–fortified dairy products Green, leafy vegetables
Beta-carotene (provitamin A)	Antioxidant role. Like other provitamin A carotenoids (alpha-carotene and beta-cryptoxanthin), can be converted to vitamin A in the body.	Sweet potatoes Carrots Pumpkin

(continues)

Table E.2

Major Functions of Vitamins in the Body and Good Food Sources[2] (*continued*)

Vitamin	Role in Body	Good Food Sources
Vitamin D	Helps maintain calcium in the blood by increasing calcium absorption in the digestive tract and decreasing calcium loss in urine.	Milk Salmon Tuna
Vitamin E	Antioxidant role. Protects red blood cells, muscles, and other tissues from free-radical damage.	Vegetable oil Wheat germ Nuts
Vitamin K	Necessary for normal blood clotting. Required for strong bones.	Collards and kale Spinach Brussel sprouts
Vitamin C (ascorbic acid)	Antioxidant role. Involved in collagen formation. Aids in iron absorption.	Oranges and other citrus fruits Green peppers Broccoli (cooked)
Thiamin (vitamin B_1)	Coenzyme for several reactions in energy metabolism. Necessary for muscle coordination and proper development and maintenance of central nervous system.	Cereal and grains Pork Nuts and seeds
Riboflavin (vitamin B_2)	Coenzyme for several reactions in energy metabolism.	Milk and yogurt Green, leafy vegetables Eggs
Niacin (vitamin B_3)	Coenzyme for several reactions in energy metabolism. In very large doses, lowers cholesterol. (Note: Large doses should only be taken under physician supervision.)	Peanuts, roasted Tuna Whole grains
Vitamin B_6 (pyridoxine)	Coenzyme for reactions involved in amino acid processing. Aids in breakdown of carbohydrate stores (glycogen) in muscles and liver.	Fish Beans and peas Spinach and greens Bananas
Folic acid (folacin)	Essential for manufacture of genetic material. Aids in red blood cell formation. Required for cell division.	Asparagus Brussel sprouts Spinach Cantaloupe Whole grains
Vitamin B_{12} (cobalamin)	Essential for proper DNA synthesis and regulation. Helps form red blood cells. Maintains myelin sheath of nerves.	Meat and seafood Milk products Eggs
Pantothenic acid	Coenzyme for reactions involved in energy metabolism.	Abundant in many foods
Biotin	Energy metabolism	Abundant in many foods

Table E.3

Major Functions of Minerals in the Body and Good Food Sources[2]

Mineral	Role in Body	Food Sources
Calcium	Component of mineral crystals in bone and teeth. Involved in muscle contraction, initiation of heartbeat, blood clotting, and release and function of several hormones and neurotransmitters.	Yogurt Milk Green, leafy vegetables Legumes
Phosphorus	As phosphate, a component of mineral crystals in bone and teeth. Component of high-energy molecules in cells (ATP, CP). Found in cell membranes.	Nuts and seeds Milk Meat
Magnesium	Involved in energy metabolism. Component of many different enzymes.	Nuts Grains Split peas
Iron	Component of heme structure found in hemoglobin, myoglobin, and cytochromes that transports oxygen in blood or stores and handles oxygen in cells. Found in molecules involved in collagen production and energy metabolism. Antioxidant properties.	Meat Prune juice Spinach Fortified cereals
Zinc	Component of numerous enzymes.	Raw oysters Meat Pecans Wheat germ
Copper	Component of several enzymes involved in energy metabolism. Antioxidant activity. Plays role in collagen production and hormone and neurotransmitter production.	Beef liver Oysters Clams (cooked)
Selenium	Component of antioxidant enzymes. Involved in thyroid hormone function.	Tuna Brown rice Eggs
Iodine	Component in thyroid hormone.	Codfish Iodized salt Shrimp
Fluoride	Involved in strengthening teeth and bones.	Shrimp (canned) Fluoridated water Carrots (cooked)
Chromium	Involved in glucose metabolism.	Broccoli Grape juice Potatoes (mashed)

(continues)

Table E.3

Major Functions of Minerals in the Body and Good Food Sources[2] (*continued*)

Mineral	Role in Body	Food Sources
Sodium	Promotes blood volume balance. Nerve impulse generation. Muscle contraction. Acid–base balance.	Processed foods Table salt Soy sauce Soups
Potassium	Cell membrane balance. Nervous impulse generation. Muscle contraction. Acid–base balance.	Potatoes Bananas Avocado Bran

The Science Behind Weight Loss and Weight Gain

Helping an individual lose weight can be a daunting task; although instructors may have control over participant's workouts, the influence is minimal when it comes to their eating habits. In addition, many approaches for weight loss have been developed and will have varying results from person to person; there is no such thing as a "one size fits all" diet. Creating a caloric deficit (by consuming less calories and burning more) is the most basic and successful method to lose weight, regardless of the specific approach taken.[3]

In order to lose weight, a calorie deficit must be created; an individual must burn more calories than are consumed. In turn, to maintain weight, a person must burn as many calories as are consumed; to gain weight, more calories must be consumed than are burned. Any successful weight loss strategy must create a caloric deficit either by decreasing caloric intake or increasing caloric expenditure through exercise and increasing lean body mass.[4] **Table E.4** lists the calories expended when engaging in various types of activities.

Foundations of Supplementation Concepts

The Dietary Supplement Health and Education Act of 1994 (DSHEA) was enacted by Congress following public debate concerning the importance of dietary supplements in promoting health, the need for consumers to have access to current and accurate information about supplements, and controversy over the FDA's regulatory approach to this product category. According to the DSHEA, a supplement is[6]:

▼   A product intended to supplement the diet that contains one or more of the following dietary ingredients: a vitamin, a mineral, an herb or other botanical, an amino acid, or any other dietary substance used to supplement the diet by increasing a total daily intake.

Table E.4

Calories Burned by Various Physical Activities[5]	Approximate Calories Used (Burned) by a 154-Pound Man	
MODERATE Physical Activities	**In 1 hour**	**In 30 minutes**
Hiking	370	185
Light gardening/yard work	330	165
Dancing	330	165
Golf (walking and carrying clubs)	330	165
Bicycling (less than 10 mph)	290	145
Walking (3.5 mph)	280	140
Weight training (general light workout)	220	110
Stretching	180	90
VIGOROUS Physical Activities	In 1 hour	In 30 minutes
Running/Jogging (5 mph)	590	295
Bicycling (more than 10 mph)	590	295
Swimming (slow freestyle laps)	510	255
Aerobics	480	240
Walking (4.5 mph)	460	230
Heavy yard work (splitting wood)	440	220
Weight lifting (vigorous effort)	440	220
Basketball (vigorous)	440	220

▼   Intended for ingestion in pill, capsule, tablet, or liquid form.

▼   Not represented for use as a conventional food or as the sole item of a meal or diet.

▼   Labeled as a dietary supplement.

In defining a supplement, it is also important to understand how the supplement industry is regulated. Since the passing of the DSHEA in 1994, the FDA regulates dietary supplements under a different set of regulations from those covering "conventional" foods and drugs (i.e., prescription and over the counter). Under the DSHEA, the supplement manufacturer, not the FDA, must ensure a dietary supplement is safe before it is marketed.

The important thing to remember is the FDA does not get involved until *after* the product has been on the market. In other words, the FDA does *post-marketing surveillance* of supplements, but it does not ensure their safety or effectiveness.

Many supplements can be safely consumed without adverse effects on health if consumed correctly. However, the instructor should not provide guidance or advice in regard to the consumption of supplements by participants. Instructors should direct participants to a medical professional or registered dietitian for discussions on supplement usage.

Supplement Types

There are various types of supplements with supporting rationales for their use.

Protein Supplements

Protein supplements are frequently consumed by athletes and active people to achieve greater increases in muscle mass and strength, and also improve overall physical performance. They are marketed as providing superior muscle-building properties to the protein provided in food. Although these supplements provide a convenient source of protein after a workout or when a protein-rich meal is needed on the run, they are not superior to protein-rich foods such as egg whites in stimulating muscle growth.[7]

A variety of protein supplements are available. Whey and casein constitute the two major protein groups of cow's milk; milk protein is 80% casein and 20% whey protein. Whey is a byproduct of cheese making. In its raw form, whey consists of fat, lactose, and other substances. Supplement manufacturers take this raw form and process it to produce whey protein concentrate and whey protein isolate. Whey is considered a fast protein because the body absorbs it quickly. Casein is a slow protein and takes longer to absorb. Because of this, most supplements contain whey protein. A few different types of whey proteins are marketed. Whey protein concentrates are rich in whey proteins and also contain fat and lactose. Whey protein isolates are low in fat and lactose. Although whey proteins are a good source of protein, they are not superior to other forms.

Branched-chain Amino Acids

The branched-chain amino acids (BCAAs)—leucine, isoleucine, and valine—are essential. They differ from the other amino acids because they can be used for energy directly in the muscle, without having to go to the liver to be broken down during exercise. It has been suggested that ingesting them before or during long-duration activity may help delay fatigue, but studies have not strongly supported this theory. However, the BCAAs may play a critical role in recovery from exercise by preventing muscle breakdown and also improve immune system function after exercise to exhaustion.[8-10]

Caffeine

Caffeine is one of the most widely used drugs in the world. In some supplements it is listed as guarana or kola nut. It can be found in coffee, tea, chocolate, soft drinks, some pain relievers, some cold medicines, and many weight-loss pills. It has long been known that moderate to high

Table E.5

Caffeine Content of Foods and Beverages

Food/Beverage	Serving Size	Caffeine Content, mg
Coffee		
Brewed	250 mL	100–150
Drip	250 mL	125–175
Instant	250 mL	50–70
Espresso	1 shot	50–110
Tea		
Green (medium)	250 mL	25–40
Black (medium)	250 mL	40–60
Cola drinks	355 mL	35–50
Energy drinks	250 mL	80–150
Chocolate		
Dark	50 mg	20–40
Milk	50 mg	8–16

The values are a range and some products could be outside the range provided as a function of brewing time and other factors. For example, an analysis of 97 espresso shots taken from retail stores in Australia showed a range of 24–214 mg/shot.
Data from Tarnopolsky, M. A. (2010). Caffeine and creatine use in sport. *Annals of Nutrition and Metabolism, 57*(Suppl 2), 1–8. Epub 2011 Feb 22.

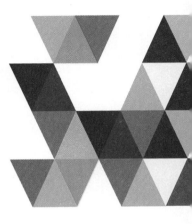

caffeine doses (5–13 grams per kilogram body weight) ingested approximately 1 hour before and during exercise increases endurance exercise performance.[11] Research has also shown caffeine is ergogenic in some short-term, high-intensity exercise and sport situations.[11] Lower caffeine doses (≤ 3 grams per kilogram body weight, or approximately 200 milligrams) taken before exercise also increase athletic performance, and low doses of caffeine taken late in prolonged exercise also show a benefit.[11] The response to caffeine intake can vary from person to person; therefore, it is important to determine whether the ingestion of 200 milligrams of caffeine before or during training and competitions is beneficial on an individual basis.[12] Caffeine has some side effects; individuals who do not regularly consume it can experience gastrointestinal distress, nervousness, rapid heart rate, headaches, and increased blood pressure.[2] **Table E.5** provides the caffeine content of a number of foods and beverages.[11]

Creatine

Creatine is made in the body and can be consumed in the diet, mostly from meat and fish. It is part of creatine phosphate, the key component of the immediate energy system used primarily during sporting events lasting 10 seconds or less (e.g., track sprints). Higher intakes of creatine seem to result in higher levels of creatine phosphate in the muscle cells, thus making more energy available for very high-intensity activity such as strength training and sprinting.[11] Research has also shown creatine supplementation results in small (1–2%) increased gains in strength or speed when combined with appropriate training, while most studies have also reported an acute increase in fat-free mass after 5–7 days of creatine supplementation.[11]

It is important to note that not everyone responds to creatine supplementation the same. Response depends on the frequency and type of training and on the levels produced and present in the body when supplementation begins. Vegetarians and others who do not consume much creatine naturally appear to achieve a greater response from supplementation.[11] Absolutely no result exists without training, and creatine does not benefit aerobic conditioning. Many individuals who have taken it complain of side effects, including headaches, abdominal cramps, and muscle cramps. Long-term creatine use may lead to kidney or liver damage and an increased risk of muscle tears and pulls; however, no research evidence currently supports a connection between creatine and these problems. On the other hand, creatine supplementation in common dosages results in urinary concentrations 90 times greater than normal. This suggests it could damage the kidneys if used long term. As always, follow the dosing outlined with the product and carefully consider taking creatine on an individual basis.[11]

Prohormones and Anabolic Steroids

In 2014, the U.S. government passed the Anabolic Steroid Control Act to expand the list of substances from previous versions of the act to include many prohormones. These substances are now considered Class 3 narcotics, and it is a felony to make, distribute, or possess them. Therefore, any "supplement" claiming to raise hormone levels is either illegal or making false claims.

References

1. Harvard Health. *Making sense of vitamins and minerals: Choosing the foods and nutrients you need to stay healthy.* (2015). Available online at: http://www.health.harvard.edu/heart-health/vitamins-and -minerals-choosing-the-nutrients-you-need-to-stay-healthy; accessed July 20, 2017.
2. Hewlings SH, Medeiros DM. *Nutrition: Real People, Real Choices.* Dubuque, IA: Kendall Hunt; 2011.
3. Atallah R, Fillion KB, Wakil SM, et al. Long-term effects of 4 popular diets on weight loss and cardiovascular risk factors: A systematic review of randomized control trials. *Circ Cardiovasc Qual Outcomes.* 2014;76:815–827.
4. Hall KD, Sacks G, Chandramochan D, et al. Quantification of the effect of the energy imbalance on body weight. *Lancet.* 2011;378:826–837.
5. United States Department of Agriculture (USDA). *How many calories does physical activity use (burn)?* 2015. Available online at: http://www.choosemyplate.gov/physical-activity-calories-burn.
6. Food and Drug Administration (FDA). *Questions and Answers on Dietary Supplements.* 2016. Available online at: http://www.fda.gov/Food/DietarySupplements/UsingDietarySupplements/ucm480069 .htm#what_is; accessed July 20, 2017.
7. Pasiakos SM, McLellan TM, Lieberman HR. The effects of protein supplements on muscle mass, strength, and aerobic and anaerobic power in healthy adults: A systematic review. *Sports Med.* 2015;45(1):111–131.

8. Alvares TS, Meirelles CM, Bhambhani YN, Pascjoalin VM, Gomes PS. L-Arginine as a potential ergogenic aid in healthy subjects. *Sports Med.* 2011;41(3):233–248.

9. Guimaraes-Ferreira L, Cholewa JM, Naimo MA, et al. Synergistic effects of resistance training and protein intake: Practical aspects. *Nutrition.* 2014;30(10):1097–1103.

10. Molfino A, Gioia G, Rossi-Fanelli F, Muscaritoli M. Beta-hydroxy-beta-methylbutyrate supplementation in health and disease: A systematic review of randomized trials. *Amino Acids.* 2013;45(6), 1273–1292.

11. Tarnopolsky MA. Caffeine and creatine use in sport. *Ann Nutr Metab.* 2010;57(Suppl 2):1–8.

12. Spriet LL. Exercise and sports performance with low doses of caffeine. *Sports Med.* 2014;44(Suppl 2): S175–S184.

Glossary

2-beat cueing Counting down from 8 and providing verbal and/or visual cues on counts 2-1, or the last two counts of a phrase.

32-count phrasing A common musical structure used in group fitness where there is an audible build up and closure every 32 counts.

4-beat cueing Counting down from 8 and providing verbal and/or visual cues on counts 4-3-2-1.

A

Abduction Body segment is moving away from the midline of the body.

Abductors Muscles that produce abduction of a limb or joint.

Ability to develop tension The ability to remain the same length, increase length, or decrease length during tension.

Action stage The stage of change in the Transtheoretical Model in which individuals have made specific, overt modifications to their behavior within the past 6 months.

Active stretching Flexibility exercises in which agonists move a limb through a full range of motion, allowing the antagonists to stretch.

Acute variables Components that specify how each exercise is to be performed.

Adaptation phase Second stage of the GAS in which physiological changes take place in order to meet the demands of the newly imposed stress.

Adduction Body segment is moving toward the midline of the body.

Adductors Muscles that produce adduction of a limb or joint.

Adenosine triphosphate (ATP) Energy storage and transfer unit within the cells of the body.

Aerobic metabolism Chemical reactions in the body that require the presence of oxygen to extract energy from carbohydrates, fatty acids, and amino acids.

Aerobic Meaning "with oxygen," the long-term energy production cycle that occurs when sufficient oxygen is present.

Affective influence Influence resulting from emotions.

Afferent neurons Neurons with impulses that move toward the spinal cord and brain from the periphery of the body and are sensory in nature.

Agility Ability to maintain center of gravity over a changing base of support while changing direction at various speeds.

Agonist Muscle that works as the prime mover of a joint exercise.

Alarm phase First stage of the GAS; the initial phase of response to a new stimuli within the Human Movement System.

Altered reciprocal inhibition Process by which an overactive muscle decreases neural drive to its functional antagonist.

Amino acids Building blocks of proteins; composed of a central carbon atom, a hydrogen atom, an amino group, a carboxyl group, and an R-group.

Anaerobic Meaning "without oxygen," the short-term energy production cycle that occurs with insufficient oxygen levels.

Anaerobic metabolism Chemical reactions in the body that do not require the presence of oxygen to create energy through the combustion of carbohydrates.

Anaerobic threshold The point during high-intensity activity when the body can no longer meet its demand for oxygen and anaerobic metabolism predominates; also called the *lactate threshold.*

Anatomic position Standard reference posture where the body stands upright with the arms beside the trunk, and the palms and head both face forward.

Antagonists Muscles that oppose the prime mover.

Anterior oblique subsystem (AOS) Subsystem of the global movement system that creates stability to the trunk, pelvis, and hips and contributes to rotational movements, leg swing (walking), and stabilization. The AOS and POS work together in enabling rotational force production in the transverse plane.

Anterior Toward or on the front side of the body

Appendicular skeleton Portion of the skeleton that includes the bones that support the upper and lower extremities.

Arteries Vessels that transport blood away from the heart.

Ataxia The loss of control of body movements.

Atria Superior chambers of the heart (singular: atrium) that receive blood from outside the heart and deliver it into their corresponding ventricle.

Atrioventricular (AV) node Small mass of specialized cardiac muscle fibers located on the wall of the right atrium of the heart that receives impulses from the sinoatrial (SA) node and directs them to the walls of the ventricles.

Atrioventricular (AV) valves Valves that allow for proper blood flow from the atria to the ventricles.

Autonomy-supportive style Coaching style focused on creating an environment that emphasizes self-improvement, rather than competing against others.

Axial skeleton Portion of the skeletal system consisting of the bones of the skull, rib cage, and vertebral column.

Axon Cylindrical projection from the cell body that transmits nerve impulses to other neurons or effector sites.

B

Background music Using music to set the mood and support the atmosphere.

Balance Ability to maintain the body's center of gravity within its base of support.

Beat The audible, metrical division that occurs within the foundational layer of music.

Beats per minute (BPM) The number of beats in one minute.

Behavior influences Influences that are created as a result of an individual's own behavior.

Biomechanics Study of how forces affect a living body.

Blood glucose Also referred to as "blood sugar"; the sugar that is transported in the body to supply energy to the body's cells, including fueling the brain and other cells in the body that cannot use fat as a fuel.

Body of workout Majority of the fitness class; activities with a singular or integrated focus on cardiorespiratory fitness, muscular strength, muscular endurance, flexibility, or mindfulness.

C

Calorie A scientific unit of energy.

Calorie A scientific unit of heat energy.

Cardiac output ($\dot{Q}$) Heart rate multiplied by stroke volume; a measure of the overall performance of the heart.

Cardiorespiratory system System of the body composed of the cardiovascular and respiratory systems.

Cardiovascular system System of the body composed of the heart, blood, and blood vessels.

Career Instructor Instructor who invests the majority of his or her day teaching, researching, and promoting fitness activities.

Cell body Portion of the neuron that contains the nucleus, lysosomes, mitochondria, and Golgi complex.

Central nervous system (CNS) Division of the nervous system comprising the brain and the spinal cord; primary function is to coordinate activity of all parts of the body.

Class vision A clearly defined intention of a class experience from the participant perspective that drives the outcome and components of a complete class.

Complementary proteins Two or more incomplete proteins that when combined together provide all essential amino acids.

Complete protein Protein that provides all of the essential amino acids in the amount the body needs and is also easy to digest and absorb (e.g., a *high-quality protein*).

Complex carbohydrate A carbohydrate with more than 10 carbon-water units; includes the fiber and starch found in whole grains and vegetables.

Concentric activation Production of tension while shortening in length.

Confidence Feeling or belief of certainty.

Contemplation stage The stage of change in the Transtheoretical Model in which individuals are contemplating making a change within the next 6 months.

Cue-based teaching Use of continuous, reliable, and precise verbal cues that occur simultaneously with movement.

D

Deconditioned A state of lost physical fitness, which may include reduced cardiorespiratory capacity, muscle imbalances, decreased flexibility, and a lack of core and joint stability.

Deep longitudinal subsystem (DLS) Subsystem of the global movement system that creates a contracting tension to absorb and control ground reaction forces during gait.

Dendrite Portion of a neuron responsible for gathering information from other structures.

Dietary Reference Intake (DRI) Framework of dietary standards used to plan and evaluate diets.

Distal Farther from the center of the body or a landmark

Dorsiflexion Anterior flexion of the ankle, where the top of the foot moves up and away from the ground.

Downbeat The first beat of a measure in music.

Dynamic balance Ability to maintain equilibrium through the intended path of motion when external forces are present.

Dynamic posture Positioning of the body during any movement.

Dynamic stretching Multiplanar extensibility with optimal neuromuscular control through a full range of motion.

Dyspnea Difficult or troubled breathing.

E

Eccentric activation Production of tension while increasing in length.

Eccentric function Action of a muscle when generating an eccentric contraction.

Edutainment The balanced combination of education and entertainment used to deliver an instructional experience in the most compelling way possible.

Efferent neurons Neurons with impulses that move out from the brain and spinal cord that send a message for muscles to contract and create movement; commonly called motor neurons.

Elasticity The ability to return to normal or resting length after being stretched.

Electrolytes Minerals in blood and other body fluids that carry an electrical charge.

Essential amino acids Amino acids that cannot be produced by the body and must be acquired by food.

Eversion Bottom of the foot rotates outward (laterally).

Excessive anterior tilt when standing Excessive curve seen in the lower back; tight hip flexors and low back extensors are contributors.

Excessive foot pronation Feet visibly turn out; the sequential combination of dorsiflexion, eversion, and abduction.

Excessive posterior tilt when seated Combine slouching and sitting, and a posterior pelvic tilt will present itself.

Exercise selection Process of choosing exercises that allow for achievement of the desired adaptation.

Exhaustion phase Third stage of the GAS in which stress continues beyond the body's ability to adapt, leading to potential physiological and structural breakdown.

Extensibility The ability to be stretched or lengthened.

Extension Movement at a joint in which the relative angle between two adjoining segments increases.

Extensors Muscles that produce extension of a limb or joint.

External rotation Turning of a limb or body segment away from the midline of the body.

Extrinsic Motivation The performance of an activity to obtain a reward separate from the activity itself.

F

Fatty acid A chain of carbons linked or bonded together; building blocks of fat within the human body.

Fitness community An evolving, growing, and dedicated group of people who follow, trust, and regularly communicate with a Group Fitness Instructor.

Fitness Message A benefit statement or philosophy related to fitness.

Fitness Mission An informative statement about what an instructor does (or wants to do).

Fitness Vision Statement An inspirational statement about what an instructor wants to be in the future.

Five Components of Class Design Five essential pieces that provide a consistent, holistic group exercise experience introduction, movement prep, body of workout, transition, and outro.

Flexion Bending at a joint where the relative angle between two bones decreases.

Flexors Muscles that produce flexion of a limb or joint.

Flow Instructor's ability to create a seamless experience from start to finish.

Force-couple relationship Muscles moving together to produce movement around a joint.

Foreground music Using tempo, lyrics, or song components to drive the movements.

Format-specific movement prep Activities that initiate body-of-the-workout movements at a lower intensity and/or complexity in order to establish neuromuscular connections that protect and support the body in format-specific movements.

Forward head posture Posture that commonly occurs from sitting at a desk and computer for long periods of time.

Freestyle choreography Method of choreography based on the instructor's personal preference, skill set, and knowledge.

Frontal plane Imaginary plane that divides the body into equal front and back halves.

Function Integrated, multiplanar movement that involves acceleration, stabilization, and deceleration.

G

General adaptation syndrome Kinetic chain response and adaptation to imposed demands and stress. (1) How the kinetic chain responds and adapts to imposed demands. (2) How the body responds and adapts to stress.

General movement prep Consists of simple, movements of integrated fitness (such as flexibility, core, and balance) to gradually increase intensity.

Global muscular system System composed of four subsystems that synergistically work together to transfer and stabilize forces through the body to the ground.

Glycogen Complex carbohydrate stored in the liver and muscle cells.

Golgi tendon organs (GTOs) Receptors sensitive to the change in tension of the muscle, and the rate of that change.

H

Hands-on cueing A movement correction technique that requires the instructor to redirect the participant through the use of touch.

Heart palpitations Heart flutters or rapid beating of the heart.

Heart rate (HR) Rate at which the heart pumps; usually measured in beats per minute (bpm).

Hobby Instructor Instructor who balances teaching with other full-time commitments.

Horizontal abduction Lateral-rotational movement *away* from the midline of the body.

Horizontal adduction Medial-rotational movement *toward* the midline of the body.

Hypokalemia Loss of significant amounts of potassium, resulting in weakness, fatigue, constipation, and muscle cramping.

Hyponatremia Loss of significant amounts of sodium, resulting in fluid retention and an increase in the body's water levels.

I

Incomplete protein Food that does not contain all of the essential amino acids in the amount needed by the body.

Inferior toward the bottom part of the body or closer to the feet.

Insertion The relatively mobile attachment site of a muscle's distal end.

Integrated fitness Comprehensive approach combining all exercise components to help a participant achieve higher levels of function.

Integrated performance paradigm A forceful cycle of muscle contraction that involves eccentric loading of the muscle, isometric muscle contraction, and concentric muscle contraction.

Internal rotation Turning of a limb or body segment toward the midline of the body.

Interneurons Receive impulses from afferent (sensory) neurons and conduct signals back out to provide an efferent (motor) response.

Interpersonal influences Influences from those individuals or groups with whom one interacts regularly.

Interval training Training that alternates between intense exertion and periods of rest or lighter exertion.

Intrinsic Motivation The performance of an activity for rewards directly stemming from the activity itself.

Introduction Instructor engagement with participants and explanation of the workout and class expectations.

Inversion Bottom of the foot rotates inwards (medially).

Irritability The ability to respond to internal or external stimuli.

Isolated function A muscle's primary functions, which are the muscle actions produced at a joint when a muscle is being concentrically activated to produce movement of a body segment.

Isometric activation Production of tension while maintaining a constant length.

K

Kilocalorie A unit of energy equal to 1,000 calories.

Kinesiology Study of human movement.

Kinetic Chain The interrelation of the actions of the nervous, muscular, and skeletal systems to create movement.

Kyphosis Abnormal rounding of the thoracic portion of the spine, usually accompanied by rounded shoulders.

L

Lack of ankle dorsiflexion Excessive forward lean; knees do not bend properly during a squat.

Lateral subsystem (LS) Subsystem of the global movement system that provides frontal plane stabilization and pelvo-femoral support during single leg movements such as lunges, leg abduction, and stair climbing.

Lateral Farther from the midline of the body.

Ligament Strong connective tissue that connects bone to bone.

Lipids Group of compounds that includes triglycerides (fats and oils), phospholipids, and sterols.

Load Amount of weight lifted or resistance used during training.

Local muscular system The muscles attaching directly to the spine, whose primary function is to provide trunk stabilization.

Low-density lipoprotein (LDL) The molecule that carries lipids throughout the body and delivers cholesterol that can accumulate on artery walls.

Lower crossed syndrome A postural distortion syndrome characterized by an anterior tilt to the pelvis (arched lower back).

M

Macronutrients Nutrients that provide calories.

Main Movement Cue Explains the intended movement, often as the instructor is simultaneously demonstrating proper form of the movement.

Maintenance stage The stage of change in the Transtheoretical Model that begins 6 months after the criterion has been reached until a time point at which the risk of returning to the old behavior has been terminated.

Mechanoreceptors Sensory receptors responsible for sensing change of position in body tissues.

Medial Toward the midline of the body

Metabolic pathways A series of chemical reactions that either break down or build up compounds in the body.

Metabolism All of the chemical reactions that occur in the body that are required for life. It is the process by which nutrients are acquired, transported, used, and disposed of by the body.

Midline Imaginary vertical line that splits the body into equal halves.

Mirroring Teaching technique in which instructors face their participants and perform movements as if they are the participants' reflection in a mirror.

Mitochondria Organelle found in the cytoplasm of eukaryotic cells that contains genetic material and enzymes necessary for cell metabolism, converting food to energy.

Modality Form or mode of exercise that presents a specific stress to the body.

Modifications Adaptions to movements in order to accommodate specific requests, making moves possible for individuals with specific needs.

Motivational Cue Used to encourage participants during challenging movements or to keep them going when fatigue affects performance.

Motor behavior Motor response to internal and external environmental stimuli.

Motor control How the CNS integrates internal and external sensory information with previous experiences to produce a motor response.

Motor development The change in motor behavior over time throughout the lifespan.

Motor learning The capacity to produce skilled movements through practice and experience.

Motor outputs Response to stimuli that activates movement in organs or muscles.

Movement prep Activities to increase body temperature and prime the body for workout demands.

Multiplanar Occurring in more than one plane of motion.

Muscle imbalance Alteration of muscle length surrounding a joint.

Muscle spindles Receptors sensitive to change in length of the muscle, and the rate of that change.

Musculoskeletal system Combined, interworking system of all muscles and bones in the body.

Musical Style A subset of a genre or claassification of music from certain eras or cultures.

Myofibrils Tubular component of muscle cells containing sarcomeres and protein filaments.

N

Nerve impulses The consecutive linking of neurons by electrochemical signals that travel throughout the nerve fiber.

Nervous system A conglomeration of billions of cells to provide a communication network within the human body.

Neuromuscular control Unconscious trained response of a muscle to a signal regarding dynamic joint stability.

Neuron Functional unit of the nervous system.

Neutral spine The natural position of the spine when the cervical, thoracic, and lumbar curves are in good alignment.

Nonessential amino acids Amino acids produced by the body that do not need to be consumed in dietary sources.

Nonverbal communication Communication other than written or spoken language that creates meaning.

Nonverbal Cue Uses expression, gestures, posture, or other nonverbal forms of communication to keep the class engaged.

Nutrient density Nutrient content of a food relative to its calories.

O

Obesity The condition of being considerably overweight; a person with a BMI of 30 or greater or who is at least 30 pounds over the recommended weight for their height.

Omega-3 fatty acids Fatty acids that have anti-inflammatory effects and help to decrease blood clotting.

Omega-6 fatty acids Fatty acids that promote blood clotting and cell membrane formation.

One-rep maximum (1RM) The maximum force that can be generated in a single repetition.

One-way communication When a communicator (instructor) sends an audio, visual, or kinesthetic signal with no confirmation of receipt from the receiver(s).

Origin The relatively stationary attachment site where a muscle begins.

Outro Final class segment to conclude the workout, praise participants' effort, and invite participants back for the next session.

Overactive traps, rhomboids, and posterior deltoids; overactive anterior delts and pectorals Shoulder-forward posture; "slouching."

Overtraining syndrome (OTS) Excessive frequency, volume, or intensity of training, resulting in fatigue; also caused by a lack of proper rest and recovery.

P

Participant-centered Instruction Movement selection that offers options in intensity and complexity for a variety of skill and fitness levels.

Perceived intensity Perceived exertion is used by participants to guide participants in subjectively defining their training intensity.

Periodization Division of a training program into smaller, progressive stages.

Peripheral nervous system (PNS) All of the nerve fibers that branch off from the spinal cord and extend to the rest of the body.

Perturbation A disturbance of equilibrium; shaking.

Phospholipid Type of lipid in which one fatty acid has been replaced by a phosphate group and one of several nitrogen-containing molecules.

Plantar flexion Posterior extension at the ankle where the top of the foot moves down toward the ground; pointing toes.

Plyometric training Uses quick, powerful movements involving an eccentric contraction, followed immediately by an explosive concentric contraction.

Polyunsaturated fatty acids Fatty acids that have several spots where hydrogen atoms are missing.

Positive reinforcement The practice of offering a reward following a desired behavior to encourage repetition of the behavior.

Positive-based correction (also known as positive correction) Using various forms of verbal and nonverbal feedback to elicit a corrective change in the most encouraging manner possible.

Positive-based Cueing (also known as positive cueing) Choosing words that cue to the solution rather than the problem.

Posterior Toward or on the back side of the body.

Posterior oblique subsystem (POS) Subsystem of the global movement system that provides stabilization of the sacroiliac joint, supports rotational movements in the transverse plane, and assists the DLS during gait.

Postural distortion patterns Common postural malalignments and muscle imbalances that individuals develop based on a variety of factors.

Posture Alignment of all parts of the kinetic chain with the purpose of countering external forces and maintaining structural efficiency.

Power The ability to produce a large amount of force in a short amount of time.

Power Training A form of exercise wherein the focus is on ability of the neuromuscular system to increase the rate of force production (the speed at which the motor units are activated).

Pre-choreographed All components of class are created by a single person, business, or organization with a connecting theme, brand, or experience.

Precontemplation stage Stage of change in the Transtheoretical Model in which individuals do not intend to change their high-risk behaviors in the foreseeable future.

Pre-cue Used to technically set up the movement or movement pattern in a timely, efficient, clearly stated way.

Pre-designed Template that provides overall class direction while allowing instructors to manipulate other variables.

Preparation stage The stage of change in the Transtheoretical Model in which individuals intend to take action in the near future, usually within the next month.

Principle of overload To create physiological changes, an exercise stimulus must be applied at an intensity greater than the body is accustomed to receiving.

Principle of specificity States that the type of exercise stimulus placed on the body will determine the expected physiological outcome.

Progression An option that allows the fitness class participant to increase complexity, impact, or intensity of a movement or movement patterns.

Pronation distortion syndrome A postural distortion syndrome characterized by foot pronation (flat feet) and adducted and internally rotated knees (knock knees).

Pronation Tri-planar movement (eversion, dorsiflexion, abduction).

Pronators Muscles that produce pronation of a limb or body segment.

Prone Body position where one is lying face downward.

Proprioception Cumulative sensory input to the central nervous system from all mechanoreceptors.

Proprioceptively enriched environments Unstable, yet controllable environments.

Protein Long chains of amino acids that serve many essential functional roles in the body.

Proximal Closer to the center of the body.

Q

Quickness Ability to react to a stimulus with an appropriate muscular response without hesitation.

R

Rate of force production Ability of muscles to exert maximal force output in a minimal amount of time.

Rating of perceived exertion (RPE) A technique used to express or validate how hard a participant feels he or she is working during exercise.

Reciprocal inhibition Simultaneous contraction of one muscle and the relaxation of its antagonist to allow movement to take place.

Reflective imaging Teaching technique in which an instructor faces the same direction as the participants and uses a mirror's reflection to teach or cue movements.

Regression An option that allows the fitness class participant to decrease complexity, impact, or intensity of a movement or movement patterns.

Repetition One complete movement of a single exercise.

Repetitive lack of motion Frequent immobility, which holds the potential for repetitive stress injuries.

Respiratory system System of the body composed of the lungs and respiratory passages that collect oxygen from the external environment and transport it to the bloodstream.

Rest period The time taken between sets or exercises to rest or recover.

Resting heart rate (RHR) Number of contractions of the heart occurring in 1 minute while the body is at rest.

Rhythm A pattern of repeated movement or sound.

S

Sagittal plane Imaginary plane that divides the body into equal right and left halves.

Sarcomeres Individual contractile units made up of actin (thin) and myosin (thick) filaments.

Saturated fat Chain of carbons that is saturated with all of the hydrogens that it can hold; there are no double bonds.

Scapular protraction Movement of the shoulder blade forward and away from the spine.

Scapular retraction Movement of the shoulder blades closer to the spine.

Scapular winging Scapula protrudes excessively during prone exercises.

Scoliosis Abnormal lateral twisting or rotating of the spine.

Scope of Practice Knowledge, skills, abilities, processes, and limitations for which an instructor should be held accountable.

Self-efficacy The belief in one's ability to execute a certain behavior.

Self-myofascial release (SMR) Flexibility technique focusing on the neural and fascial systems of the body to decrease receptor excitation and release muscle tension.

Self-talk One's internal dialogue.

Semilunar (SL) valves Valves that allow for proper blood flow away from the heart to the lungs and body.

Sensation influences Physical feelings an individual experiences as they relate to behaviors involved in establishing a healthy lifestyle.

Sensorimotor integration Ability of the nervous system to gather and interpret information to anticipate and execute the proper motor response.

Set A group of consecutive repetitions.

Simple carbohydrate A carbohydrate with fewer than 10 carbon-water units. Includes glucose, sucrose, lactose, galactose, maltose, and fructose.

Sinoatrial (SA) node Specialized area of cardiac tissue located in the right atrium of the heart that initiates the electrical impulses that determine the heart rate; often termed the "pacemaker for the heart."

Special population A group of people who have similar conditions or characteristics that require alterations to the general exercise plan.

Speed The straight-ahead velocity of an individual.

Stabilization Body's ability to remain stable and balanced over the center of gravity in a changing environment.

Static balance Ability to maintain equilibrium in place with no external forces.

Static posture The starting point from which an individual moves; a pose in which the body is standing in its natural, relaxed position.

Static stretching A process of passively taking a muscle to the point of tension and holding the stretch for 30 seconds.

Sterols Subgroup of the steroids and an important class of organic molecules.

Strength Ability of the neuromuscular system to provide internal tension and exert force against external resistance.

Stroke volume (SV) Amount of blood pumped out of the heart with each contraction.

Structural efficiency The structural alignment of the muscular and skeletal systems that allows the body to maintain balance in relation to its center of gravity.

Superior Above a landmark or closer to the head.

Supination Tri-planar movement (plantar flexion, inversion, adduction).

Supinators Muscles that produce supination of a limb or body segment.

Supine Body position where one is lying on the back and facing upward.

Supportive communication Language that creates a climate of trust, caring, and acceptance.

Symmetry Proportion and balance between two items or two sides.

Synergistic dominance When synergists take over function for a weak or inhibited prime mover.

Synergists Muscles that assist the prime mover in a joint action.

Synovial joints Joints that are held together by a fluid-based synovial capsule and ligaments; the type of joint most associated with movement in the body.

T

Talk test A self-evaluation of intensity associated with the ability to talk while exercising.

Tendons Connective tissues that attach muscle to bone and provide an anchor for muscles to produce force.

Tensegrity Term coined by Buckminster Fuller that refers to a structure in which compression and tension are used to give a structure its form, providing stability and efficiency in mass and movement.

Three-dimensional cueing Cueing that incorporates visual, auditory, and kinesthetic learning strategies.

Timed coaching Teaching technique in which an instructor focuses on verbal coaching and motivational phrasing in order to push the participants through timed movement sequences.

Training intensity An individual's level of effort, compared with his or her maximal effort; usually expressed as a percentage.

Training volume The total amount of work performed within a specified time; number of repetitions multiplied by the number of sets in a training session.

Transition Safely takes participants through the gradual physiological change from exertion to rest.

Transtheoretical Model (TTM) States that individuals progress through a series of stages of behavior change, and that movement through these stages is cyclical—not linear.

Transverse plane An imaginary horizontal plane that bisects the body into equal halves, producing a top half and a bottom half.

Triglyceride Chemical or substrate form in which most fat exists in food as well as in the body.

Two-way communication When a communicator (instructor) sends an audio, visual, or kinesthetic signal and the receiver communicates a response back to the sender.

U

Unsaturated fatty acids Fatty acids that are not completely saturated with hydrogen atoms.

Upper crossed syndrome A postural distortion syndrome characterized by a forward head and rounded shoulders.

V

Veins Vessels that transport blood from the extremities back to the heart.

Ventricles Inferior chambers of the heart that receive blood from their corresponding atrium and, in turn, force blood out of the heart into the arteries.

Visual teaching Demonstrating aspirational form and technique while providing a comprehensive view of the movement or pattern from start to finish.

Index

Note: Page numbers followed by *f* and *t* indicate material in figures and tables